CHIMERIC ANTIGEN RECEPTOR (CAR) T CELLS: THE SECOND REVOLUTION IN CELLULAR THERAPY

Kerry Atkinson MBBS MD DTM&H FRACP FRCP

Consultant Physician

Every effort has been made in preparing this book to provide accurate and up-to-date information which is accordance with accepted standards and practice at the time of publication. The author and publisher can make no warranties that the information contained herein is totally free from error, not least because clinical standards are constantly changing through research and regulation. The author and publisher therefore disclaim all liability for direct or consequential damages resulting from the use of material contained in this book. Readers are strongly advised to pay careful attention to information provided by the manufacturer of any drug or equipment that they plan to use. If in any doubt whatsoever, contact the manufacturer and consult the FDA-approval label for the specific medication in question.

Acknowledgements

I would like to acknowledge the help that I received from Jim Severino in designing the covers for this book and for uploading it for me to Kindle Direct Publishing.

Also by Kerry Atkinson

Medical books

1. Graft-versus-Host Disease. Editors, S Burakoff, H J Deeg, J Ferrara, K Atkinson. Marcel Dekker Inc, New York, 1990.
2. Clinical Bone Marrow Transplantation.First edition. Editor, K Atkinson. Cambridge University Press, Cambridge UK, 1994.
3. The BMT Data Book: A Manual for Bone Marrow and Blood Stem Cell Transplantation. K. Atkinson, Cambridge University Press, Cambridge UK, 1998.
4. Clinical Bone Marrow and Blood Stem Cell Transplantation. Second Edition. Editor, K. Atkinson. Cambridge University Press, Cambridge UK, 2000.
5. Clinical Bone Marrow and Blood Stem Cell Transplantation. Third Edition. Eds, K. Atkinson, R Champlin, J Ritz, M Brenner, P Ljungman and W Fibbe. Cambridge University Press, Cambridge UK, 2004.
6. The BMT Data Book. Second edition. R Munker, HM Lazarus and K. Atkinson, Cambridge University Press, Cambridge UK, 2009.
7. The BMT Data Book: Including Cellular Therapy. Third edition. R Munker, C Hildebrandt, HM Lazarus and K. Atkinson, Cambridge University Press, Cambridge UK. 2013.
8. Hematopoietic Cell Transplants: Concepts, Controversies and Future Directions. Eds HM Lazarus, RP Gale, A Keating, A Bacigalupo, R Munker, K Atkinson, A Syed. Cambridge University Press, Cambridge, UK. 2017.
9. The Biology and Therapeutic Application of Mesenchymal Cells. Ed. K Atkinson. Wiley/Blackwell. 2017
10. Revolutionizing Tropical Medicine. Eds. K Atkinson and D Mabey. Wiley/Blackwell Publishers Inc. 2019.
11. Asthma: Targeted Biological Treatments 2020. Kindle Direct Publishing, 2020. e-book and paperback
12. Atopic Dermatitis: Targeted Biological Treatments 2020. Kindle Direct Publishing, 2020. e-book and paperback
13. Psoriasis: Targeted Biological Treatments 2020. Kindle Direct Publishing, 2020. e-book and paperback
14. Crohn's disease and ulcerative colitis: Targeted Biological Treatments 2020. Kindle Direct Publishing, 2020. e-book and paperback

15. Rheumatoid arthritis, Juvenile Idiopathic Arthritis, Ankylosing spondylitis, Psoriatric Arthritis and Gout: Targeted Biological Treatments 2020. Kindle Direct Publishing, 2020. e-book and paperback
16. Small Cell Lung Cancer: Targeted Biological Treatments 2020. Kindle Direct Publishing, 2020. e-book and paperback
17. Chronic Myeloid Leukemia: Targeted Biological Treatments 2020. Kindle Direct Publishing, 2020. e-book and paperback
18. Melanoma: Targeted Biological Treatments 2020, Kindle Direct Publishing 2020. e-book and paperback
19. Dementia - A Caregiver's Guide. Kindle Direct Publishing 2020. e-book
20. Breast Cancer: Targeted Biological Treatments 2021. Kindle Direct Publishing 2021. e-book and paperback
21. Non-melanoma Skin Cancers: Targeted Biological and Specifically Designed Therapeutic agents. 2022. Kindle Direct Publishing 2021. e-book and paperback
22. Hodgkin Lymphoma: Targeted Biological Treatments. 2022. Kindle Direct Publishing 2022. e-book and paperback

Natural history/conservation books

23. Bird facts for everyone. K Atkinson. Outskirts Press Inc., Denver, USA. 2014
24. Birds, Birds, Birds. Kindle Direct Publishing 2020. e-book and paperback
25. A Field Guide to the Wild Habitats of Sydney Australia. Kindle Direct Publishing 2021. e-book and paperback
26. Conserving New Zealand's Endangered Species. Kindle Direct Publishing 2021. e-book and paperback
27. Conserving Australia's Endangered Species. Kindle Direct Publishing 2021. e-book and paperback
28. Nature's Wonders: Britain and Ireland. Kindle Direct Publishing 2021. e-book and paperback.
29. Nature's Wonders: Spain and Bulgaria. Kindle Direct Publishing 2022. e-book and paperback.
30. Nature's Wonders: France's Camargue, the Swiss National Park and Portugal. Kindle Direct Publishing 2022. e-book and paperback.
31. Nature's Wonders: Cuba. Kindle Direct Publishing 2022. e-book and paperback.

32. Natures's Wonders: Japan in Winter Kindle Direct Publishing 2022. e-book and paperback.
33. Nature's Wonders: India Kindle Direct Publishing 2022. e-book and paperback.

Other books

34. Paintings 2019 – 2021. Kindle Direct Publishing 2021. e-book and paperback.
35. Ferrari Road Cars. Kindle Direct Publishing 2022. e-book and paperback.
36. Paintings II. November 2021 – June 2022. e-book and paperback.
37.

Approach

"The only thing I knew how to do
was to keep on keepin' on like a bird that flew
Tangled up in blue"

From the song "Tangled up in blue" by Bob Dylan on his album "Blood on the Tracks" released by Columbia Records in 1975.

Nobel Laureate in Literature, 2016

This photograph of Bob Dylan, reproduced here from Wikimedia Commons, is in the public domain. https://commons.wikimedia.org/wiki/File:Bob-Dylan-arrived-at-Arlanda-surrounded-by-twenty-bodyguards-and-assistants-391770740297_(cropped).jpg. This Swedish photograph is in the public domain in Sweden because it is the work is non-artistic (journalistic, etc.) and has been created before 1 January 1970 (SFS 1960:729, § 49a). (1966). (PD 1970)

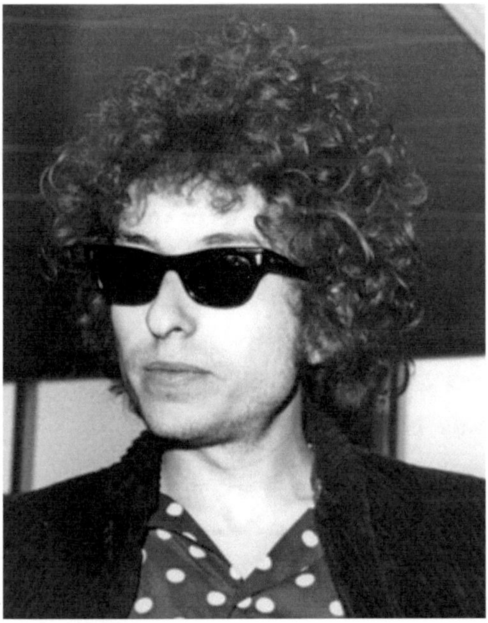

Table of Contents

1. Author's preface

Five major biological revolutions of the second half of the 20th century were

1. The production of monoclonal antibodies
2. The discovery of DNA and how it, RNA and amino acids make proteins
3. Epigenetics and the posttranslational modification of proteins
4. The discovery of cell signalling pathways
5. The cloning of the human genome

Taken together these discoveries in cellular and molecular biology have revealed to scientists appropriate targets for new drugs and the number that have been produced in the last 30 years, and that are still being produced, has hugely enlarged the therapeutic pharmacopeia, producing treatments - even cures - for diseases that were previously untreatable. The majority of these new treatments have been derived because of much more detailed knowledge about how human cells work. They are therefore known as **biological treatments**, often abbreviated to biologics. An example of a biologic is the monoclonal antibody rituximab which reacts specifically with the CD20 antigen present only on B cells, but with no other targets.

In addition, other agents that react specifically with one, or at most, several, targets are **chemically synthesized**: an example is imatinib, which is specific for the tyrosine kinase (TK) domain in abl (the Abelson proto-oncogene), c-kit and PDGF-R (platelet-derived growth factor receptor). Another example is sonedegib, which inhibits activation of the intracellular Hedgehog signalling pathway.

The inclusion of therapeutic agents in this book (and the others in the series) is based on their specificity for a given target. For example, interleukin 2 (IL-2) would not be included since it has a range of biological activities including the proliferation of T cells, the generation of T cell cytotoxic responses and the recall of cytotoxic T cell memory. Likewise interferon-alpha (IFN-α) would not be included since its functions include antiviral activity, antiproliferative activity, NK cell activation, cytokine induction, and interferon-stimulated gene-induction activity. This exclusion applies even though each are made constitutively in the body in response to specific diseases: they are biologic agents, but their targets are broad.

This series of books – one for each disease or disease category - explains what the new treatments are, how they work and how they compare, and interact with, conventional treatment. It is important to state that **no book** in this series makes specific treatment recommendations for any of the diseases covered: such decisions should be initiated and reviewed by an appropriate medical specialist. Much information on each disease is available free of charge from Wikipedia (*wikipedia.org)*, from postgraduate textbooks on each disease and from *UpToDate.com:* the latter website gives information for patients and caregivers free of charge but a subscription is required for more detailed information (uptodate.com). **Rather**, the purpose of this series of books is to give information on newly developed biological and specifically designed treatments and their mechanism of action, enabling hopefully the reader to get a handle on these extensive additions to the medical pharmacopeia.

A distinction is sometimes made between monoclonal antibodies (the mabs) as "immunotherapy", the small specifically designed inhibitory molecules (the nibs) and the receptor blocking agents (the cepts) – the latter sometimes known as decoy receptors. However, since each category of drug has been developed from the comprehensive knowledge of human cell biology discovered over the past seven decades, and as each drug in each category is exquisitely targeted to a specific epitope on a cell surface protein (the mabs), the inhibition of a specific intracellular enzyme process (the nibs), or the blocking of a specific cell surface receptor (the cepts) I prefer to combine the mabs, the nibs and the cepts in the single category of targeted biological treatments. An example from each category are rituximab, imatinib and etanercept.

A fourth type of biological targeted agents has now been FDA-approved for therapeutic use – sonidegib and vismodegib – both of which specifically target the intracellular Hedgehog pathway and are now both FDA-approved for treatment of basal cell carcinoma of the skin

There is now a fifth type of biological targeted therapeutic agents that have been approved by the FDA for therapeutic use: chimeric antigen receptor modified **(CAR) T cells**. The first such agent – tisagenlecleucel – was approved by the USA FDA in 2017 for use in people with acute lymphoblastic leukemia. CAR T cells are an innovative cellular immunotherapeutic approach that involves genetic modification of autologous T cells to express CAR targeting tumor antigen/s as well as a component of the T cell activation pathway – the CD3 zeta chain. T cell surface glycoprotein CD3 zeta chain, also known as T cell receptor T3 zeta chain or CD247, together with T cell receptor alpha/beta and gamma/delta heterodimers and CD3-gamma, -delta, and -epsilon, forms the T cell receptor-CD3 complex. The zeta chain plays an important role in coupling antigen recognition to several intracellular signal-transduction pathways.

CAR T cells represent the second type of cellular therapy to be therapeutically successful and are the subject of this book. The first successful cellular therapy was the use **of hematopoietic stem cells**, introduced in the late 1960s, which offered curative treatment for diseases that were not curable by any other type of thearapy.

These new drug discovery phenomenon is a therapeutic tsunami which shows no sign of slowing. The pharmcopiea has increased enormously and all medical students should consider doing a Master's degree or a PhD in molecular biology. It is only by working in a cellular or molecular biology laboratory (usually combined) that one can really understand how each of these new medications work.

It should be noted that all text on each individual drug is taken directly from the USA FDA's product approval label for that drug, including the drug's generic name, its brand name, the indications for which it is approved, its mechanism of action, boxed warnings and other details on warnings, precautions, adverse events and specific patient populations. These are all in the public domain and can be accessed at https://www.accessdata.fda.gov/scripts/cder/daf/.

Only the prodct label information was take from the FDA. All images and illustrations were taken from a variety of sources. Most of these are in the public domain, but some are licensed by a Creative Commons license. Each image carries the legend written by the creator of the image as well as full attribution details required by the creator. No images were used from the FDA's product approval label for each drug.

A side-effect seen with a number of biologic agents are immune-mediated syndromes. To distinguish them from each other, a brief summary of each is given in

2. Introduction to the new targeted biologic and specifically designed therapeutic agents

Biologics and biosimilars

A **biosimilar** is a biologic medical product highly similar to another already approved biological medicine. Biosimilars are approved according to the same standards of pharmaceutical quality, safety and efficacy that apply to all biological medicines. Biosimilars are officially approved versions of original "innovator" products and can be manufactured when the original product's patent expires. Reference to the innovator product is an integral component of the approval.

It should be noted (as in the text below) that many, if not all, of these new treatments have many, and often serious side-effects, including adverse interactions when combined with other drugs.

Finally, most of these new treatments are extremely expensive ("financial toxicity"), which renders both access to them, and sometimes compliance with them, impossible or suboptimal.

Monoclonal antibodies (mabs)

Background

In 1975, Georges Köhler and César Milstein in the UK succeeded in producing a hybridoma by making fusions of murine myeloma cell lines with murine B cells. This immortalized hybridoma could produce antibodies specific for known antigens. In 1985 the FDA approved the first fully licensed Mab (Muromonab, anti-CD3 for use in preventing kidney transplant rejection. Muromonab was produced using only murine cells and thus the antibodies produced were wholly murine. Subsequently, to decrease immunogenicity of murine antibodies, chimeric antibodies were created in which the constant (Fc) portion of the antibody was human, while the variable (Fab-binding) regions remained of murine origin. After this, humanized mabs were produced in which the framework and constant regions were human, while the hypervariable region remained of murine origin. After this, fully human mabs were produced, lacking any murine component. Finally, it is now possible to produce mabs solely using recombinant DNA technology.

Mabs may be used in many different ways. This is illustrated in Figure 1 for mabs that are developed for the treatment of disease.

Figure 1

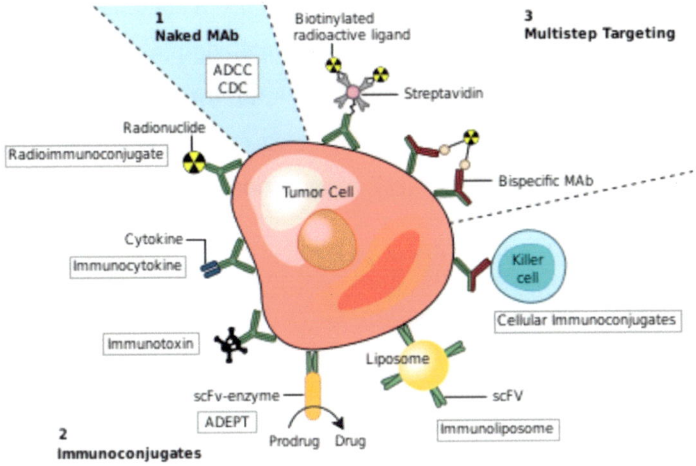

Abbreviations used in Figure 1: antibody directed enzyme prodrug therapy; ADCC: antibody-dependent cell-mediated cytotoxicity; CDC: complement-dependent cytotoxicity; MAb, monoclonal antibody; scFv, single-chain Fv fragment

Nomenclature convention for monoclonal antibodies

Murine mabs have the prefix –o- before mab; eg, abagovomab. (Note: the first murine mab approved by the FDA (Muromonab, anti-CD3) deviated from this nomenclature which was not in place at the time of its approval).

Chimeric mabs have the prefix –xi- before mab; eg, basilixumab

Humanized mabs have the prefix –zu- before mab; eg, trastuzumab

Human mabs have the prefix –u- before mab; eg, atinumab

Examples of these new agents and their mechanism of action in the treatment of non-malignant diseases

Monoclonal antibodies

- Receptor antagonists – eg, dapulimab (anti IL-4 and anti-IL13 signalling) in atopic dermatitis
- Apoptosis (programmed cell death) inducers – eg, rituximab in B cell-mediated autoimmune diseases
- Immune pathway inhibitors – eg, dipilumab for IL-4 and IL-13 signalling in atopic dermatitis, infliximab and adalimumab for TNF inhibition in psoriasis; secukinumab for IL-17 inhibition in psoriasis; ustekinumab for IL-12/Th1 inhibition and IL-23/ILTh17 inhibition in psoriasis; ixekizumab as an anti-IL17A agent in psoriasis; brodalumab as an anti-IL-7 receptor antagonist in psoriasis
- TNF pathway antagonists – eg, adalimumab for psoriasis
- Integrin pathway blockers – eg, natalizumab for Crohn's disease
- Rank ligand inhibitor – eg, denosumab for targeted treatment of postmenopausal women with osteoporosis at high risk for fracture
- Angiogenesis inhibitors – eg, ranibizumab for macular degeneration
- Dabigatran binder – eg, idarucizumab for bleeding due to dabigatran administration
- Proprotein convertase subtilisin kexin type 9 (PCSK9) inhibitor – eg, alirocumab and evolocumab for dyslipidemias
- Bi-specific antibodies – eg, emicizumab-kxwh for hemophilia A
- Monoclonal antibody-delivered toxins or drugs

A list of all monoclonal antibodies and receptor blocking agents that are USA FDA-approved for therapeutic use for either non-malignant disease, malignant disease or both malignant and and non-malignant disease is shown in Table 1 (as of December 2020).

Table 1. A list of all monoclonal antibodies and receptor blocking agents that are USA FDA-approved for therapeutic use

Generic name/brand name/type of mab	Target	FDA-approved indication/s
Abciximab/ ReoPro/ chimeric fab fragment	GPIIb/IIIa	Percutaneous coronary intervention for the prevention of cardiac ischemic complications in patients undergoing percutaneous coronary intervention or in patients with unstable angina not responding to conventional medical therapy when percutaneous coronary intervention is planned within 24 hours
Adalimumab/ Humira/ fully human	TNF	Rheumatoid arthritis (RA), juvenile idiopathic arthritis (JIA), ankylosing spondylitis (AS), psoriatric arthrtitis, Crohn's disease[1], ulcerative colitis, plaque psoriasis, hidradenitis suppura[a], non-infectious uveitis
Adalimumab-abdm/Cyltezo/ fully human, biosimilar	TNF	RA, JIA, AS, psoriatric arthritis, Crohn's disease[1], ulcerative colitis, plaque psoriasis,
Adalimumab-atto/Amjevita/ fully human, biosimilar	TNF	RA, JIA, AS, psoriatric arthritis, Crohn's disease[1], ulcerative colitis, plaque psoriasis
Ado-trastuzumab Emtasine/ Kadcyla/ humanized antibody-microtubule inhibitor conjugate	HER2	HER2-positive, metastatic breast cancer who previously received trastuzumab and a taxane, separately or in combination. Patients should have either: • received prior therapy for metastatic disease, or • developed disease recurrence during or within six months of completing adjuvant therapy. • the adjuvant treatment of patients with HER2-positive early breast cancer who have residual invasive disease after neoadjuvant taxane and trastuzumab-based treatment.
Alemtuzumab/ Campath, Lemtrada/	CD52	Relapsing forms of multiple sclerosis (MS) (previously approved for chronic lymphocytic leukemia but now withdrawn by its manufacturer for this indication in

humanized		order to optimize its launch for treatment of MS)
Alirocumab/ Praluent/fully human	PCSK9 (proprotein convertase subtilisin kexin type 9) inhibitor	Adjunct to diet and maximally tolerated statin therapy for the treatment of adults with heterozygous familial hypercholesterolemia or clinical atherosclerotic cardiovascular disease, who require additional lowering of LDL-cholesterol (LDL-C).
Ansuvimab-zykl / EBANGA™		Treatment of infection caused by Zaire ebolavirus in adult and pediatric patients, including neonates born to a mother who is RT-PCR positive for Zaire ebolavirus infection.
Atezolizumab/ Tecentriq/ humanized	Programmed death ligand 1 (PD-L1)	1. Urothelial carcinoma for the treatment of adult patients with locally advanced or metastatic urothelial carcinoma who are not eligible for cisplatin-containing chemotherapy and whose tumors express PD-L1 or who are not eligible for any platinum-containing chemotherapy regardless of PD-L1 status, or who have disease progression during or following any platinum-containing chemotherapy, or within 12 months of neoadjuvant or adjuvant chemotherapy. This indication is approved under accelerated approval based on tumor response rate and duration of response. Continued approval for this indication may be contingent upon verification and description of clinical benefit in a confirmatory trial(s). 2. Non-small cell lung ancer (NSCLC) in combination with bevacizumab, paclitaxel, and carboplatin for the firstline treatment, of adult patients with metastatic non-squamous NSCLC with no EGFR or ALK genomic tumor aberrations or for the treatment of adult patients with metastatic NSCLC who have disease progression during or following platinum-containing chemotherapy. Patients with EGFR or ALK genomic tumor aberrations should have disease progression on FDA-approved therapy for NSCLC harboring these aberrations prior to receiving TECENTRIQ. 2. Triple-negative breast cancer (TNBC) in combination with paclitaxel for the treatment of adult patients with unresectable locally advanced or metastatic TNBC whose tumors express PD-L1. This indication is approved under accelerated approval based on progression-free survival. Continued approval for this indication may be contingent upon verification and description of clinical benefit in a confirmatory trial(s).
Atoltivimab, maftivimab, and odesivimab-ebgn) injection/ INMAZEB™	INMAZEB is a combination of three recombinant human IgG1κ monoclonal antibodies each targeting the Zaire ebolavirus glycoprotein (GP). Zaire ebolavirus encodes a sole envelope protein, the glycoprotein, which mediates	Zaire ebolavirus in adult and pediatric patients, including neonates born to a mother who is RT-PCR positive for Zaire ebolavirus infection.

	virus attachment and membrane fusion with the host cell membranes. In addition, GP is expressed on the surface of Zaire ebolavirus infected host cells making it a target for antibodies that can mediate killing of these cells by antibody-dependent cellular cytotoxicity and/or other effector functions. The 3 antibodies that make up the combination can bind the GP simultaneously	
Avelumab/ Bavencio/ fully human	PD-L1	1. Adult and pediatric patients 12 years and older with metastatic Merkel cell carcinoma[2a] 2. Patients with locally advanced or metastatic urothelial carcinoma who have disease progression during or following platinum-containing chemotherapy or who have disease progression within 12 months of neoadjuvant or adjuvant treatment with platinum-containing chemotherapy[a]. 3. First-line treatment, in combination with axitinib, of patients with advanced renal cell carcinoma [a]Continued approval for this indication may be contingent upon verification and description of clinical benefit in confirmatory trials
Basiliximab/ Simulect/ chimeric	IL-2 receptor alpha chain (IL-2Rα) blocker	Prophylaxis of acute organ rejection in patients receiving renal transplantation when used as part of an immunosuppressive regimen that includes cyclosporine and corticosteroids
Belimumab/ Benlysta/fully human	B lymphocyte stimulator (BLyS) -specific inhibitor	Active, autoantibody-positive, systemic lupus erythematosus (SLE) in adults who are receiving standard therapy
Benralizumab/ Fasenra/ humanized	Interleukin-5 receptor-α	For the add-on maintenance treatment of patients with severe asthma aged 12 years and older, and with an eosinophilic phenotype
Bevacizumab/ Avastin/ humanized	Vascular endothelial growth factor (VEGF)-specific angiogenesis	1. Metastatic colorectal cancer, with intravenous 5-fluorouracil–based chemotherapy for first- or second-line treatment. 2. Non-squamous non-small cell lung cancer, with carboplatin and paclitaxel for first line treatment of unresectable, locally advanced, recurrent or metastatic

		disease. 3. Metastatic breast cancer, with paclitaxel for treatment of patients who have not received chemotherapy for metastatic HER2-negative breast cancer. 4.Glioblastoma, as a single agent for adult patients with progressive disease following prior therapy 5. Metastatic renal cell carcinoma with interferon-α
Bevacizumab-awwb/Mvasi/ humanized biosimilar	VEGF	1. Metastatic colorectal cancer, in combination with intravenous fluorouracil-based chemotherapy for first- or second-line treatment. 2. Metastatic colorectal cancer, in combination with fluoropyrimidine-irinotecan- or fluoropyrimidine-oxaliplatin-based chemotherapy for second-line treatment in patients who have progressed on a first-line bevacizumab product-containing regimen. 3. Unresectable, locally advanced, recurrent or metastatic non-squamous non-small cell lung cancer, in combination with carboplatin and paclitaxel for first-line treatment. 4. Recurrent glioblastoma in adults. 5. Metastatic renal cell carcinoma in combination with interferon-α. 6. Persistent, recurrent, or metastatic cervical cancer, in combination with paclitaxel and cisplatin, or paclitaxel and topotecan.
Bevlotuxumab/ Zinplava/fully human	Clostridium difficile toxin	Reduction of recurrence of Clostridium difficile infection (CDI) in patients 18 years of age or older who are receiving antibacterial drug treatment of CDI and are at a high risk for CDI recurrence.
Belantamab mafodotin-blmf/ BLENREP Antibody-drug conjugate	Myeloma	Belantamab mafodotin-blmf is an antibody-drug conjugate (ADC). The antibody component is an afucosylated IgG1 directed against BCMA, a protein expressed on normal B lymphocytes and multiple myeloma cells. The small molecule component is MMAF, a microtubule inhibitor. Upon binding to BCMA, belantamab mafodotin-blmf is internalized followed by release of MMAF via proteolytic cleavage. The released MMAF intracellularly disrupts the microtubule network, leading to cell cycle arrest and apoptosis. Belantamab mafodotin-blmf had antitumor activity in multiple myeloma cells and mediated killing of tumor cells through MMAF-induced apoptosis, as well as by tumor cell lysis through antibody-dependent cellular cytotoxicity (ADCC) and antibody-dependent cellular phagocytosis (ADCP).
Blinatumomab/ Blincyto/ murine bispecific CD19-directed CD3 T cell engager	CD19	1. B cell precursor acute lymphoblastic leukemia (ALL) in first or second complete remission with minimal residual disease (MRD) greater than or equal to 0.1%. This indication is approved under accelerated approval based on MRD response rate and hematological relapse-free survival. Continued approval for this indication may be contingent upon verification and description of clinical

		benefit in the confirmatory trials. 2. Relapsed or refractory B cell precursor acute lymphoblastic leukemia
Brentuximab vedotin/ Adcetris/ chimeric, antibody-drug conjugate	CD30	1.Classical Hodgkin lymphoma[3] (cHL) at high risk of relapse or progression as post autologous hematopoietic stem cell transplantation (auto-HSCT) consolidation 2.Classical Hodgkin lymphoma after failure of auto-HSCT or after failure of at least two prior multi-agent chemotherapy regimens in patients who are not auto-HSCT candidates 3. Systemic anaplastic large cell lymphoma (sALCL) after failure of at least one prior multi-agent chemotherapy regimen. Accelerated approval was granted for the sALCL indication based on overall response rate. Continued approval for this indication may be contingent upon verification and description of clinical benefit in confirmatory trials. 4. Primary cutaneous anaplastic large cell lymphoma (pcALCL) or CD30 expressing mycosis fungoides who have received prior systemic therapy
Brodalumab/ Siliq/chimeric	!L-17 receptor	Moderate to severe plaque psoriasis in adult patients who are candidates for systemic therapy or phototherapy and have failed to respond or have lost response to other systemic therapies.
Burosumab-twza/Crysvita/ fully human	Fibroblast growth factor (FGF)23	X-linked hypophosphatemia (XLH) in adult and pediatric patients 6 months of age and older
Canakinuab/ Ilaris/fully human	IL-1β	Cryopyrin-associated periodic syndromes (CAPS), in adults and children 4 years of age and older including familial cold autoinflammatory syndrome (FCAS) and Muckle-Wells Syndrome (MWS)
Capromab pendetide/ Prosta-Scint/ murine radio-labelled (Indium ^{111})	Prostate-specific membrane antigen (PSMA)	1. A diagnostic imaging agent in newly-diagnosed patients with biopsy-proven prostate cancer, thought to be clinically-localized after standard diagnostic evaluation (e.g. chest x-ray, bone scan, CT scan, or MRI), who are at high-risk for pelvic lymph node metastases 2. A diagnostic imaging agent in post-prostatectomy patients with a rising PSA leveland a negative or equivocal standard metastatic evaluation in whom there is a high clinical suspicion of occult metastatic disease.
Certolizumab Pegol/Cimzia/ humanized (pegylated for longer duration of action)	TNF	1.Crohn's disease 2.Rheumatoid arthritis 3.Psoriatic arthritis 4.Ankylosing spondylitis
Cetuximab/ Erbitux/	Epidermal growth factor (EGF)	1.Head and neck cancer

chimeric	receptor	Locally or regionally advanced squamous cell carcinoma of the head and neck in combination with radiation therapy. Recurrent loco-regional disease or metastatic squamous cell carcinoma of the head and neck in combination with platinum-based therapy with 5-FU. Recurrent or metastatic squamous cell carcinoma of the head and neck progressing after platinum-based therapy. 2.Colorectal cancer As a single agent, EGFR-expressing metastatic colorectal cancer after failure of both irinotecan- and oxaliplatin-based regimens or in patients who are intolerant to irinotecan-based regimens. In combination with irinotecan, EGFR-expressing metastatic colorectal carcinoma in patients who are refractory to irinotecan-based chemotherapy.
Cemiplimab/ Libtayo/ humanized	PD-1	Metastatic cutaneous squamous cell carcinoma (CSCC) or locally advanced CSCC who are not candidates for curative surgery or curative radiation.
Daclizumab/ Zenapax/ humanized	IL-2 receptor-α	Prophylaxis of acute organ rejection in patients receiving renal transplants. It is used as part of an immunosuppressive regimen that includes cyclosporine and corticosteroids.
Naxitamab-gqgk/ Danyelza	Naxitamab-gqgk binds to the glycolipid GD2. GD2 is a disialoganglioside that is overexpress-ed on neuroblasto-ma cells and other cells of neuroectod-ermal origin, including the central nervous system and peripheral nerves. In vitro, naxitamab-gqgk was able to bind to cell surface GD2 and induce complement-dependent cytotoxicity (CDC) and antibody dependent- cell-mediated cytotoxicity (ADCC).	DANYELZA is a GD2-binding monoclonal antibody indicated, in combination with granulocyte-macrophage colony-stimulating factor (GMCSF), for the treatment of pediatric patients 1 year of age and older and adult patients with relapsed or refractory high-risk neuroblastoma in the bone or bone marrow who have demonstrated a partial response, minor response, or stable disease to prior therapy
Darzalex/ Zinbryta/	IL-2 receptor	Relapsing forms of multiple sclerosis (MS). Because of its safety profile, the use of ZINBRYTA should generally be reserved for patients who have had an inadequate

humanized		response to two or more drugs indicated for the treatment of MS.
Daratumumab/ Darzalex/fully human	CD38	Multiple myeloma 1.In combination with lenalidomide and dexamethasone in newly diagnosed patients who are ineligible for autologous stem cell transplant and in patients with relapsed or refractory multiple myeloma who have received at least one prior therapy 2.In combination with bortezomib, melphalan and prednisone in newly diagnosed patients who are ineligible for autologous stem cell transplant 3.In combination with bortezomib and dexamethasone in patients who have received at least one prior therapy 4.In combination with pomalidomide and dexamethasone in patients who have received at least two prior therapies including lenalidomide and a proteasome inhibitor 5. As monotherapy, in patients who have received at least three prior lines of therapy including a proteasome inhibitor (PI) and an immunomodulatory agent or who are double-refractory to a PI and an immunomodulatory agent.
Denosumab/ Prolia/fully human	Receptor activator of nuclear factor kappa-B ligand (RANKL)	1.Postmenopausal women with osteoporosis at high risk for fracture 2.Treatment to increase bone mass in men at high risk for fracture receiving androgen deprivation therapy for non-metastatic prostate cancer 3.Treatment to increase bone mass in women at high risk for fracture receiving adjuvant aromatase inhibitor therapy for breast cancer
Denosumab/ Xgeva/fully human	RANKL	1.Prevention of skeletal-related events in patients with multiple myeloma and in patients with bone metastases from solid tumors 2.Treatment of adults and skeletally mature adolescents with giant cell tumor of bone that is unresectable or where surgical resection is likely to result in severe morbidity 3.Treatment of hypercalcemia of malignancy refractory to bisphosphonate therapy
Dinutuximab/ Unituxin/ chimeric	GD2 (a disialo-ganglioside)	In combination with granulocyte-macrophage colony-stimulating factor (GM-CSF), interleukin-2 (IL-2), and 13-cis-retinoic acid (RA), for the treatment of pediatric patients with high-risk neuroblastoma who achieve at least a partial response to prior first-line multiagent, multimodality therapy
Dupilumab/ Dupixent/fully human	IL-4 receptor-α (IL-4RA)	1. For patients aged 12 years and older with moderate-to-severe atopic dermatitis whose disease is not adequately controlled with topical prescription therapies or when those therapies are not advisable. 2. As an add-on maintenance treatment in patients with moderate-to-severe asthma aged 12 years and older with

		an eosinophilic phenotype or with oral corticosteroid-dependent asthma. 3. As an add-on maintenance treatment in adult patients with inadequately controlled chronic rhinosinusitis with nasal polyposis (CRSwNP).
Durvalumab/ Imfinzi/fully human	PD-L1	1.Locally advanced or metastatic urothelial carcinoma who have disease progression during or following platinum-containing chemotherapy or who have disease or progression within 12 months of neoadjuvant or adjuvant treatment with platinum-containing chemotherapy 2. Unresectable, stage III non-small cell lung cancer (NSCLC) whose disease has not progressed following concurrent platinum-based chemotherapy and radiation therapy.
Eculizumab/ Solaris/ humanized	Complement component 5	1.Paroxysmal nocturnal hemoglobinuria (PNH) to reduce hemolysis 2.Atypical hemolytic uremic syndrome (aHUS) to inhibit complement-mediated thrombotic microangiopathy
Elotuzumab/ Empliciti/ humanized	Signalling lymphocytic activation molecule family (SLAMF7, CD319)	In combination with lenalidomide and dexamethasone for the treatment of multiple myeloma who have received one to three prior therapies.
Emicizumab-kxwh/ Hemlibra/ humanized bispecific	Factor IXa, Factor X (bridges activated factor IX and factor X to restore the function of missing activated factor VIII that is needed for effective hemostasis)	Routine prophylaxis to prevent or reduce the frequency of bleeding episodes in adult and pediatric patients ages newborn and older with hemophilia A (congenital factor VIII deficiency) with or without factor VIII inhibitors.
Eptinezumab-jjmr/VYEPTI/ humanized	CGRP	VYEPTI is a calcitonin gene-related peptide antagonist indicated for the preventive treatment of migraine in adults. Eptinezumab-jjmr is a humanized monoclonal antibody that binds to calcitonin gene-related peptide (CGRP) ligand and blocks its binding to the receptor
Erenumab-aooe/Aimovig/ fully human	Calcitonin gene-related peptide receptor (CGRP receptor)	Antagonist indicated for the preventive treatment of migraine in adults
Evolocumab/ Repatha/fully human	Proprotein convertase subtilisin kexin type 9 (PCSK9)	1. To reduce the risk of myocardial infarction, stroke, and coronary revascularization in adults with established cardiovascular disease. 2. As an adjunct to diet, alone or in combination with other

		lipid-lowering therapies (e.g., statins, ezetimibe), for treatment of adults with primary hyperlipidemia (including heterozygous familial hypercholesterolemia) to reduce low-density lipoprotein cholesterol (LDL-C). 3. As an adjunct to diet and other LDL-lowering therapies (e.g., statins, ezetimibe, LDL apheresis) in patients with homozygous familial hypercholesterolemia (HoFH) who require additional lowering of LDL-C.
Gemtuzumab ozogamicin/ Mylotarg/ humanized antibody-drug conjugate (N-acetyl gamma calichea-micin)	CD33	1.Newly-diagnosed CD33-positive acute myeloid leukemia (AML) in adults 2.Relapsed or refractory CD33-positive AML in adults and in pediatric patients 2 years and older
Golimumab/ Simponi/fully human	TNF	1.Moderately to severely active RA in adults, in combination with methotrexate 2.Active psoriatic arthritis in adults, alone or in combination with methotrexate 3.Active AS in adults
Golimumab/ Simponi Aria/ fully human	TNF	1.Moderately to severely RA in combination with methotrexate 2.Active psoriatic arthritis 3.Active AS
Guselkumab/ Tremfya/fully human	IL-23	Adult patients with moderate-to-severe plaque psoriasis who are candidates for systemic therapy or phototherapy
Ibalizumab-uiyk/Trogarzo/ humanized	CD4	In combination with other antiretroviral(s), for the treatment of human immunodeficiency virus type 1 (HIV-1) infection in heavily treatment-experienced adults with multidrug resistant HIV-1 infection failing their current antiretroviral regimen
Ibritumomab tiuxetan/ Zevalin/ murine radio-immunoconjug-ate (the chelate tiuxetan, which tightly binds to $Indium^{111}$ or $Ytrium^{90}$, is covalently linked to ibritumomab. The beta	CD20	1.Relapsed or refractory, low-grade or follicular B cell non-Hodgkin's lymphoma 2. Previously untreated follicular B cell non-Hodgkin lymphoma who achieve a partial or complete response to first-line chemotherapy

emission from Y^{90} induces cellular damage by the formation of free radicals in the target and neighboring cells)		
Idarucizumab/ Praxbind/ humanized fab fragment	Dabigatran (Pradaxa)	Patients treated with Pradaxa® when reversal of the anticoagulant effects of dabigatran is needed: 1. For emergency surgery/urgent procedures 2. In life-threatening or uncontrolled bleeding. This indication is approved under accelerated approval based on a reduction in unbound dabigatran and normalization of coagulation parameters in healthy volunteers. Continued approval for this indication may be contingent upon the results of an ongoing cohort case series study.
Inebilizumab-cdon/ UPLIZNATM	CD19	UPLIZNA is a CD19-directed cytolytic antibody indicated for the treatment of neuromyelitis optica spectrum disorder (NMOSD) in adult patients who are anti-aquaporin-4 (AQP4) antibody positive.
Infliximab/ Remicade/ chimeric	TNF-α	1. Crohn's disease for reducing signs and symptoms and inducing and maintaining clinical remission in adult patients with moderately to severely active disease who have had an inadequate response to conventional therapy. For reducing the number of draining enterocutaneous and rectovaginal fistulas and maintaining fistula closure in adult patients with fistulizing disease. 2. Pediatric Crohn's disease for reducing signs and symptoms and inducing and maintaining clinical remission in pediatric patients with moderately to severely active disease who have had an inadequate response to conventional therapy. 3.Ulcerative colitis for reducing signs and symptoms, inducing and maintaining clinical remission and mucosal healing, and eliminating corticosteroid use in adult patients with moderately to severely active disease who have had an inadequate response to conventional therapy. 4. Pediatric ulcerative colitis for reducing signs and symptoms and inducing and maintaining clinical remission in pediatric patients with moderately to severely active disease who have had an inadequate response to conventional therapy. 5. Rheumatoid arthritis in combination with methotrexate for reducing signs and symptoms, inhibiting the progression of structural damage, and improving physical function in patients with moderately to severely active disease.

		6. Ankylosing spondylitis for reducing signs and symptoms in patients with active disease. 7. Psoriatic arthritis for reducing signs and symptoms of active arthritis, inhibiting the progression of structural damage, and improving physical function. 8. Plaque psoriasis for treatment of adult patients with chronic severe (i.e., extensive and /or disabling) plaque psoriasis who are candidates for systemic therapy and when other systemic therapies are medically less appropriate.
Infliximab-abda/Renflexis /chimeric biosimilar	TNF-α	Similar to Remicade: see https://www.accessdata.fda.gov/drugsatfda_docs/label/2017/761054orig1s000lbl.pdf
Infliximab-dyyb/Inflectra/ chimeric biosimilar	TNF-α	Similar to Remicade. See https://www.accessdata.fda.gov/drugsatfda_docs/label/2016/125544s000lbl.pdf
Infliximab-qbtx/Ixifi chimeric biosimilar	TNF-α	Similar to Remicade. See https://www.accessdata.fda.gov/drugsatfda_docs/label/2017/761072s000lbl.pdf
Inotuzumab ozogamicin/ Besponsa/ humanized; antibody-drug conjugate (N-acetyl gamma calicheamicin)	CD22	Adults with relapsed or refractory B cell precursor acute lymphoblastic leukemia (ALL)
Ipilimomab/ Yervoy/fully human	CTLA-4	Melanoma • Treatment of unresectable or metastatic melanoma in adults and pediatric patients (12 years and older). • Adjuvant treatment of patients with cutaneous melanoma with pathologic involvement of regional lymph nodes of more than 1 mm who have undergone complete resection, including total lymphadenectomy. Renal Cell Carcinoma (RCC) • Treatment of patients with intermediate or poor-risk, previously untreated advanced renal cell carcinoma, in combination with nivolumab. Colorectal Cancer • Treatment of adult and pediatric patients 12 years of age and older with microsatellite instability-high (MSI-H) or mismatch repair deficient (dMMR) metastatic colorectal cancer that has progressed following treatment with a fluoropyrimidine,

		oxaliplatin, and irinotecan, in combination with nivolumab. • This indication is approved under accelerated approval based on overall response rate and duration of response. Continued approval for this indication may be contingent upon verification and description of clinical benefit in confirmatory trials. Hepatocellular Carcinoma • Treatment of patients with hepatocellular carcinoma who have been previously treated with sorafenib, in combination with nivolumab. This indication is approved under accelerated approval based on overall response rate and duration of response. Continued approval for this indication may be contingent upon verification and description of clinical benefit in confirmatory trials. Non-Small Cell Lung Cancer (NSCLC) • Treatment of adult patients with metastatic non-small cell lung cancer expressing PD-L1 (≥1%) as determined by an FDA-approved test, with no EGFR or ALK genomic tumor aberrations, as first-line treatment in combination with nivolumab. • Treatment of adult patients with metastatic or recurrent non-small cell lung cancer with no EGFR or ALK genomic tumor aberrations as first-line treatment, in combination with ipilimumab and 2 cycles of platinum-doublet chemotherapy
Ixekizumab/ Taltz/ humanized	IL-17A antagonist (often referred to as IL-17)	Adults with 1. Moderate-to-severe plaque psoriasis who are candidates for systemic therapy or phototherapy. 2. Active psoriatic arthritis. 3. Active ankylosing spondylitis
Margetuximab-cmkb/ Margenza	Her2/neu	Margenza is a HER2/neu receptor antagonist indicated, in combination with chemotherapy, for the treatment of adult patients with metastatic HER2 positive breast cancer who have received two or more prior anti-HER2 regimens, at least one of which was for metastatic disease
Mepolizumab/ Nucala/ humanized	IL-5	Add-on maintenance treatment of patients with severe asthma aged 12 years and older, and with an eosinophilic phenotype
Mogamuliz-umab/ Poteligeo/ humanized	CCR4 (CC chemo-kines have 2 adjacent cysteine near their amino terminus)	Adult patients with relapsed or refractory mycosis fungoides or Sézary syndrome after at least one prior systemic therapy

Moxetumomab pasudotox Lumoxiti/ murine antibody-drug conjugate. (the toxin called PE38, is a 38kDa fragment of Pseudomonas exotoxin A.	CD22	Adult patients with relapsed or refractory hairy cell leukemia (HCL) who received at least two prior systemic therapies, including treatment with a purine nucleoside analog (PNA)
Natalizumab/ Tysabri/ humanized	α4 integrin	1. Multiple sclerosis (MS): as monotherapy for the treatment of patients with relapsing forms of multiple sclerosis to delay the accumulation of physical disability and reduce the frequency of clinical exacerbations. TYSABRI is generally recommended for patients who have had an inadequate response to, or are unable to tolerate, an alternate MS therapy. 2.Crohn's disease: inducing and maintaining clinical response and remission in adult patients with moderately to severely active Crohn's disease with evidence of inflammation who have had an inadequate response to, or are unable to tolerate, conventional Crohn's disease therapies and inhibitors of TNF-α.
Necitumumab/ Portrazza/ fully human	EGFR	In combination with gemcitabine and cisplatin, for first-line treatment of patients with metastatic squamous non-small cell lung cancer
Nivolumab/ Opdivo/ fully human	PD-1	Melanoma • patients with unresectable or metastatic melanoma, as a single agent or in combination with ipilimumab • patients with melanoma with lymph node involvement or metastatic disease who have undergone complete resection, in the adjuvant setting. Non-Small Cell Lung Cancer (NSCLC) • adult patients with metastatic non-small cell lung cancer expressing PD-L1 (≥1%) as determined by an FDA-approved test, with no EGFR or ALK genomic tumor aberrations, as first-line treatment in combination with ipilimumab. • adult patients with metastatic or recurrent non-small cell lung cancer with no EGFR or ALK genomic tumor aberrations as first-line treatment, in combination with ipilimumab and 2 cycles of platinum-doublet chemotherapy. • patients with metastatic non-small cell lung cancer and progression on or after platinum-based chemotherapy. Patients with EGFR or ALK genomic tumor aberrations should have disease progression on FDA-approved therapy for these aberrations prior to receiving OPDIVO

		. Malignant Pleural Mesothelioma • adult patients with unresectable malignant pleural mesothelioma, as first-line treatment in combination with ipilimumab. Renal Cell Carcinoma (RCC) • patients with intermediate or poor risk advanced renal cell carcinoma, as a first-line treatment in combination with ipilimumab. • patients with advanced renal cell carcinoma, as a first-line treatment in combination with cabozantinib. • patients with advanced renal cell carcinoma who have received prior antiangiogenic therapy. Classical Hodgkin Lymphoma (cHL) • adult patients with classical Hodgkin lymphoma that has relapsed or progressed after • autologous hematopoietic stem cell transplantation (HSCT) and brentuximab vedotin, or • 3 or more lines of systemic therapy that includes autologous HSCT. Squamous Cell Carcinoma of the Head and Neck (SCCHN) • patients with recurrent or metastatic squamous cell carcinoma of the head and neck with disease progression on or after a platinum-based therapy. Urothelial Carcinoma • patients with locally advanced or metastatic urothelial carcinoma • have disease progression during or following platinum-containing chemotherapy • have disease progression within 12 months of neoadjuvant or adjuvant treatment with platinum-containing chemotherapy. Colorectal Cancer • adult and pediatric (12 years and older) patients with microsatellite instability-high (MSI-H) or mismatch repair deficient (dMMR) metastatic colorectal cancer that has progressed following treatment with a fluoropyrimidine, oxaliplatin, and irinotecan, as a single agent or in combination with ipilimumab. Hepatocellular Carcinoma (HCC) • patients with hepatocellular carcinoma who have been previously treated with sorafenib, as a single agent or in combination with ipilimumab.

		Esophageal Squamous Cell Carcinoma (ESCC) • patients with unresectable advanced, recurrent or metastatic esophageal squamous cell carcinoma after prior fluoropyrimidine- and platinum-based chemotherapy. This indication is approved under accelerated approval based on overall response rate and duration of response. Continued approval for this indication may be contingent upon verification and description of clinical benefit in confirmatory trials.
Obiltoxaximab/ Anthim/ chimeric	Protective antigen of the Anthrax toxin	Adult and pediatric patients for treatment of inhalational anthrax due to B. anthracis in combination with appropriate antibacterial drugs and, for prophylaxis of inhalational anthrax when alternative therapies are not available or are not appropriate.
Obinutuzumab /Gazyva/ humanized	CD20	1.In combination with chlorambucil, for the treatment of patients with previously untreated chronic lymphocytic leukemia 2. In combination with bendamustine followed by GAZYVA monotherapy, for the treatment of patients with follicular lymphoma who relapsed after, or are refractory to, a rituximab-containing regimen. 3. In combination with chemotherapy followed by GAZYVA monotherapy in patients achieving at least a partial remission, for the treatment of adult patients with previously untreated stage II bulky, III or IV follicular lymphoma.
Ocrelizumab/ Ocrevus/ humanized	CD20	Relapsing or primary progressive forms of multiple sclerosis
Ofatumumab/ Arzerra/fully human	CD20	Chronic lymphocytic leukemia (CLL) refractory to fludarabine and alemtuzumab.
Olaratumab/ Lartruvo/fully human	PDGFR-α	In combination with doxorubicin, for the treatment of adult patients with soft tissue sarcoma (STS) with a histologic subtype for which an anthracycline-containing regimen is appropriate and which is not amenable to curative treatment with radiotherapy or surgery. This indication is approved under accelerated approval. Continued approval for this indication may be contingent upon verification and description of clinical benefit in the confirmatory trial
Omalizumab/ Xolair/ humanized	IgE	1.Moderate to severe persistent asthma in patients 6 years of age and older with a positive skin test or in vitro reactivity to a perennial aeroallergen and symptoms that are inadequately controlled with inhaled corticosteroids 2.Chronic idiopathic urticaria in adults and adolescents 12 years of age and older who remain symptomatic despite H1 antihistamine treatment
Palivizumab/ Synagis/	F protein of respiratory	Prevention of serious lower respiratory tract disease caused by RSV in children at high risk of RSV disease.

humanized	syncytial virus (RSV)	Notes 1. Safety and efficacy were established in children with bronchopulmonary dysplasia (BPD), infants with a history of premature birth (less than or equal to 35 weeks gestational age), and children with hemodynamically significant congenital heart disease (CHD). 2.The safety and efficacy of Synagis have not been established for treatment of RSV disease
Panitumumab/ Vectibix/ fully human	EGFR	As a single agent for the treatment of metastatic colorectal carcinoma with disease progression on or following fluoropyrimidine, oxaliplatin, and irinotecan chemotherapy regimens. Approval is based on progression-free survival; no data demonstrate an improvement in disease-related symptoms or increased survival with Vectibix. Notes 1. Retrospective subset analyses of metastatic colorectal cancer trials have not shown a treatment benefit for Vectibix in patients whose tumors had KRAS mutations in codon 12 or 13. 2.Use of Vectibix is not recommended for the treatment of colorectal cancer with these mutations
Pembrolizuma b/ Keytruda/ fully human	PD-1	Melanoma • for the treatment of patients with unresectable or metastatic melanoma. • for the adjuvant treatment of patients with melanoma with involvement of lymph node(s) following complete resection. Non-Small Cell Lung Cancer (NSCLC) • in combination with pemetrexed and platinum chemotherapy, as first-line treatment of patients with metastatic nonsquamous NSCLC, with no EGFR or ALK genomic tumor aberrations. • in combination with carboplatin and either paclitaxel or paclitaxel protein-bound, as first-line treatment of patients with metastatic squamous NSCLC. • as a single agent for the first-line treatment of patients with NSCLC expressing PD-L1 [Tumor Proportion Score (TPS) ≥1%] as determined by an FDA-approved test, with no EGFR or ALK genomic tumor aberrations, and is: o stage III where patients are not candidates for surgical resection or definitive chemoradiation, or o metastatic. • as a single agent for the treatment of patients with metastatic NSCLC whose tumors express PD-L1 (TPS ≥1%) as determined by an FDA-approved test, with disease progression on or after platinum-containing chemotherapy. Patients with EGFR or ALK genomic tumor

		aberrations should have disease progression on FDA-approved therapy for these aberrations prior to receiving KEYTRUDA. Small Cell Lung Cancer (SCLC) • for the treatment of patients with metastatic SCLC with disease progression on or after platinum-based chemotherapy and at least one other prior line of therapy. Head and Neck Squamous Cell Cancer (HNSCC) • in combination with platinum and FU for the first-line treatment of patients with metastatic or with unresectable, recurrent HNSCC. • as a single agent for the first-line treatment of patients with metastatic or with unresectable, recurrent HNSCC whose tumors express PD-L1 [Combined Positive Score (CPS) ≥1] as determined by an FDA-approved test. • as a single agent for the treatment of patients with recurrent or metastatic HNSCC with disease progression on or after platinum-containing chemotherapy. Classical Hodgkin Lymphoma (cHL) • for the treatment of adult patients with relapsed or refractory cHL. • for the treatment of pediatric patients with refractory cHL, or cHL that has relapsed after 2 or more lines of therapy. Primary Mediastinal Large B-Cell Lymphoma (PMBCL) • for the treatment of adult and pediatric patients with refractory PMBCL, or who have relapsed after 2 or more prior lines of therapy. • Limitations of Use: KEYTRUDA is not recommended for treatment of patients with PMBCL who require urgent cytoreductive therapy. Urothelial Carcinoma • for the treatment of patients with locally advanced or metastatic urothelial carcinoma who are not eligible for cisplatin-containing chemotherapy and whose tumors express PD-L1 [Combined Positive Score (CPS) ≥10] as determined by an FDA-approved test, or in patients who are not eligible for any platinum-containing chemotherapy regardless of PD-L1 status. • for the treatment of patients with locally advanced or metastatic urothelial carcinoma who have disease progression during or following platinum-containing chemotherapy or within 12 months of neoadjuvant or adjuvant treatment with platinum-containing chemotherapy. • for the treatment of patients with Bacillus Calmette-

		Guerin (BCG)-unresponsive, high-risk, non-muscle invasive bladder cancer (NMIBC) with carcinoma in situ (CIS) with or without papillary tumors who are ineligible for or have elected not to undergo cystectomy. Microsatellite Instability-High or Mismatch Repair Deficient Cancer • for the treatment of adult and pediatric patients with unresectable or metastatic, microsatellite instability-high (MSI-H) or mismatch repair deficient (dMMR) o solid tumors that have progressed following prior treatment and who have no satisfactory alternative treatment options,1 or o colorectal cancer that has progressed following treatment with a fluoropyrimidine, oxaliplatin, and irinotecan. • Limitations of Use: The safety and effectiveness of KEYTRUDA in pediatric patients with MSI-H central nervous system cancers have not been established. Microsatellite Instability-High or Mismatch Repair Deficient Colorectal Cancer (CRC) • for the first-line treatment of patients with unresectable or metastatic MSI-H or dMMR colorectal cancer (CRC). Gastric Cancer • for the treatment of patients with recurrent locally advanced or metastatic gastric or gastroesophageal junction adenocarcinoma whose tumors express PD-L1 [Combined Positive Score (CPS) ≥1] as determined by an FDA-approved test, with disease progression on or after 2 or more prior lines of therapy including fluoropyrimidine- and platinum-containing chemotherapy and if appropriate, HER2/neu-targeted therapy. Esophageal Cancer • for the treatment of patients with locally advanced or metastatic esophageal or gastroesophageal junction (GEJ) (tumors with epicenter 1 to 5 centimeters above the GEJ) carcinoma that is not amenable to surgical resection or definitive chemoradiation either: o in combination with platinum- and fluoropyrimidine-based chemotherapy, or o as a single agent after one or more prior lines of systemic therapy for patients with tumors of squamous cell histology that express PD-L1 (CPS ≥10) as determined by an FDA-approved test. Cervical Cancer • for the treatment of patients with recurrent or metastatic cervical cancer with disease progression on or after chemotherapy whose tumors express PD-L1 [Combined

		Positive Score (CPS) ≥1] as determined by an FDA-approved test. Hepatocellular Carcinoma (HCC) • for the treatment of patients with HCC who have been previously treated with sorafenib. Merkel Cell Carcinoma (MCC) • for the treatment of adult and pediatric patients with recurrent locally advanced or metastatic Merkel cell carcinoma. Renal Cell Carcinoma (RCC) • in combination with axitinib, for the first-line treatment of patients with advanced RCC. Endometrial Carcinoma • in combination with lenvatinib, for the treatment of patients with advanced endometrial carcinoma that is not MSI-H or dMMR, who have disease progression following prior systemic therapy and are not candidates for curative surgery or radiation. Tumor Mutational Burden-High (TMB-H) Cancer • for the treatment of adult and pediatric patients with unresectable or metastatic tumor mutational burden-high (TMB-H) ≥10 mutations/megabase (mut/Mb)] solid tumors, as determined by an FDA-approved test, that have progressed following prior treatment and who have no satisfactory alternative treatment options. • Limitations of Use: The safety and effectiveness of KEYTRUDA in pediatric patients with TMB-H central nervous system cancers have not been established. Cutaneous Squamous Cell Carcinoma (cSCC) • for the treatment of patients with recurrent or metastatic cutaneous squamous cell carcinoma that is not curable by surgery or radiation. Triple-Negative Breast Cancer (TNBC) • in combination with chemotherapy, for the treatment of patients with locally recurrent unresectable or metastatic TNBC whose tumors express PD-L1 [Combined Positive Score (CPS) ≥10] as determined by an FDA approved test. Adult Indications: additional dosing regimen of 400 mg every 6 Weeks • for use at an additional recommended dosage of 400 mg every 6 weeks for all approved adult indications. This indication is approved under accelerated approval based on tumor response rate and durability of response. Continued approval for this indication may be contingent

		upon verification and description of clinical benefit in the confirmatory trials.
Pertuzumab/ Perjeta/ humanized	HER2/neu	In combination with trastuzumab and docetaxel for the treatment of patients with HER2-positive metastatic breast cancer who have not received prior anti-HER2 therapy or chemotherapy for metastatic disease.
Polatuzumab vedotin/Polivy/ Humanized antibody-drug conjugate	CD79	In combination with bendamustine and a rituximab product for the treatment of adult patients with relapsed or refractory diffuse large B cell lymphoma, not otherwise specified, after at least two prior therapies
Ramucirumab/ Cyramza/ fully human	VEGFR2	1. As a single agent or in combination with paclitaxel, for treatment of advanced gastric or gastro-esophageal junction adenocarcinoma, with disease progression on or after prior fluoropyrimidine- or platinum-containing chemotherapy. 2. In combination with docetaxel, for treatment of metastatic non-small cell lung cancer with disease progression on or after platinum-based chemotherapy. Patients with EGFR or ALK genomic tumor aberrations should have disease progression on FDA-approved therapy for these aberrations prior to receiving CYRAMZA
Ranibizumab/ Lucentis/ humanized	VEGFR1, VEGFR2	1. Neovascular (wet) age-related macular degeneration (AMD) 2. Macular edema following retinal vein occlusion (RVO) 3. Diabetic macular edema (DME)
Raxibacumab/ fully human	Protective antigen of Bacillus anthracis[6]	Raxibacumab is indicated for the treatment of adult and pediatric patients with inhalational anthrax due to Bacillus anthracis in combination with appropriate antibacterial drugs, and for prophylaxis of inhalational anthrax when alternative therapies are not available or are not appropriate. Limitations of use: • The effectiveness of raxibacumab is based solely on efficacy studies in animal models of inhalational anthrax. • There have been no studies of raxibacumab in the pediatric population. Dosing in pediatric patients was derived using a population PK approach. • Raxibacumab does not cross the blood-brain barrier and does not prevent or treat meningitis. Raxibacumab should be used in combination with appropriate antibacterial drug
Reslizumab/ Cinqair/ humanized	IL-5	Add-on maintenance treatment of patients with severe asthma aged 18 years and older, and with an eosinophilic phenotype. Limitations of use: CINQAIR is not indicated for • treatment of other eosinophilic conditions

		• relief of acute bronchospasm or status asthmaticus
Rituximab/ Rituxan/ chimeric	CD20	1. Non-Hodgkin's lymphoma o Relapsed or refractory, low grade or follicular, CD20-positive B as a single agent. o Previously untreated follicular, CD20-positive, B cell in combination with first line chemotherapy and, in patients achieving a complete or partial response to RITUXAN in combination with chemotherapy, as single-agent maintenance therapy. o Non-progressing (including stable disease), low-grade, CD20 positive, B cell as a single agent after first-line cyclophosphamide, vincristine, and prednisone (CVP) chemotherapy. o Previously untreated diffuse large B cell, CD20-positive in combination with (cyclophosphamide, doxorubicin, vincristine, and prednisone) (CHOP) or other anthracycline-based chemotherapy regimens. 2. Chronic lymphocytic leukemia (CLL) o Previously untreated and previously treated CD20 positive CLL in combination with fludarabine and cyclophosphamide (FC). 3. Rheumatoid arthritis (RA) in combination with methotrexate in adult patients with moderately-to severely-active RA who have inadequate response to one or more TNF antagonist therapies 4. Granulomatosis with polyangiitis (GPA) (Wegener's granulomatosis) and microscopic polyangiitis (MPA) in adult patients in combination with glucocorticoids 5. Moderate to severe pemphigus vulgaris (PV) in adult patients
Rituximab and hyaluronidase/ chimeric co-formulated with hyaluronidase (a human endoglycos-idase)	CD20	1. Follicular lymphoma (FL) o Relapsed or refractory, follicular lymphoma as a single agent o Previously untreated follicular lymphoma in combination with first line chemotherapy and, in patients achieving a complete or partial response to rituximab in combination with chemotherapy, as single agent maintenance therapy o Non-progressing (including stable disease), follicular lymphoma as a single agent after first-line cyclophosphamide, vincristine, and prednisone (CVP) chemotherapy 2. Diffuse large B cell lymphoma (DLBCL) o Previously untreated diffuse large B cell lymphoma in combination with cyclophosphamide, doxorubicin, vincristine, prednisone (CHOP) or other anthracycline-based chemotherapy regimens

		3. Chronic lymphocytic leukemia (CLL) o Previously untreated and previously treated CLL in combination with fludarabine and cyclophosphamide (FC) Limitations of use: • Initiate treatment with RITUXAN HYCELA only after patients have received at least one full d • RITUXAN HYCELA is not indicated for the treatment of non- conditions.
Sacituzumab govitecan-hziy/ TRODELVY Antibody-drug conjugate	Trop-2 Sacituzumab govitecan-hziy is a Trop-2-directed antibody-drug conjugate. Sacituzumab is a humanized antibody that recognizes Trop-2. The small molecule, SN-38, is a topoisomerase I inhibitor, which is covalently attached to the antibody by a linker. Pharmacology data suggest that sacituzumab govitecan-hziy binds to Trop-2-expressing cancer cells and is internalized with the subsequent release of SN-38 via hydrolysis of the linker. SN-38 interacts with topoisomerase I and prevents re-ligation of topoisomerase I-induced single strand breaks. The resulting DNA damage leads to apoptosis and cell death. Sacituzumab govitecan-hziy decreased tumor growth in mouse xenograft models of triple-negative	TRODELVY is a Trop-2-directed antibody and topoisomerase inhibitor conjugate indicated for the treatment of adult patients with metastatic triple-negative breast cancer (mTNBC) who have received at least two prior therapies for metastatic disease. This indication is approved under accelerated approval based on tumor response rate and duration of response. Continued approval for this indication may be contingent upon verification and description of clinical benefit in confirmatory trials

	breast cancer.	
Sarilumab/ Kevzara/ fully human	IL-6 receptor	Adult patients with moderately to severely active rheumatoid arthritis who have had an inadequate response or intolerance to one or more disease-modifying antirheumatic drugs
Satralizumab-mwge/ Enspryng Humanized	Satralizumab is a humanized monoclonal antibody targeted against human IL-6 receptors. It binds to soluble and membrane-bound IL-6 receptors and prevents the signaling cascade, and subsequent pro-inflammatory effects, associated with its binding to endogenous IL-6.	Treatment of neuromyelitis optica spectrum disorder (NMOSD) in adult patients who are anti-aquaporin-4 (AQP4)
Secukinumab/ Cosentryx/ fully human	IL-17A (also known as IL-17)	Moderate to severe plaque psoriasis in adult patients who are candidates for systemic therapy or phototherapy.
Siltuximab/ Sylvant/ chimeric	IL-6	Multicentric Castleman's disease (MCD) who are human immunodeficiency virus (HIV) negative and human herpesvirus-8 (HHV-8) negative.
Tafasitamab-cxix/ MONJUVI	CD19	MONJUVI is a CD19-directed cytolytic antibody indicated in combination with lenalidomide for the treatment of adult patients with relapsed or refractory diffuse large B cell lymphoma (DLBCL) not otherwise specified, including DLBCL arising from low grade lymphoma, and who are not eligible for autologous stem cell transplant (ASCT). Tafasitamab-cxix is an Fc-modified monoclonal antibody that binds to CD19 antigen expressed on the surface of pre-B and mature B lymphocytes and on several B cell malignancies, including diffuse large B cell lymphoma (DLBCL). Upon binding to CD19, tafasitamab-cxix mediates B cell lysis through apoptosis and immune effector mechanisms, including antibody-dependent cellular cytotoxicity (ADCC) and antibody-dependent cellular phagocytosis (ADCP). This indication is approved under accelerated approval based on overall response rate. Continued approval for this indication may be contingent upon verification and description of clinical benefit in a confirmatory trial(s)
Teprotumumab-trbw/ TEPEZZA	IGFR Teprotumumab-trbw's mechanism	TEPEZZA is an insulin-like growth factor-1 receptor inhibitor indicated for the treatment of Thyroid Eye Disease

	of action in patients with Thyroid Eye Disease has not been fully characterized. Teprotumumab-trbw binds to IGF-1R and blocks its activation and signaling	
Tildrakizumab-asmn/Ilumya/ humanized	IL-23	Adults with moderate-to-severe plaque psoriasis who are candidates for systemic therapy or phototherapy
Tocilizumab/ Actrema/ humanized	IL-6 receptor	1. Rheumatoid arthritis (RA) • Adult patients with moderately to severely active rheumatoid arthritis who have had an inadequate response to one or more disease modifying anti-rheumatic drugs (DMARDs). 2.Giant cell arteritis (GCA) • Adult patients with giant cell arteritis. 3.Polyarticular juvenile idiopathic arthritis (PJIA) • Patients 2 years of age and older with active polyarticular juvenile idiopathic arthritis. 4.Systemic juvenile idiopathic arthritis (SJIA) • Patients 2 years of age and older with active systemic juvenile idiopathic arthritis. 5.Cytokine release syndrome (CRS) • Adults and pediatric patients 2 years of age and older with chimeric antigen receptor (CAR) T cell-induced severe or life-threatening cytokine release syndrome
Tratuzumab/ Herceptin/ humanized	HER2/neu	• HER2 overexpressing breast cancer •HER2-overexpressing metastatic gastric or gastroesophageal junction adenocarcinoma
Trastuzumab-dkst/Ogivri/ humanized biosimilar	HER2/neu	• HER2 overexpressing breast cancer •HER2-overexpressing metastatic gastric or gastroesophageal junction adenocarcinoma
Ustekinumab/ Stelara/ fully human	IL-12, IL-23	1. Adult patients with moderate to severe plaque psoriasis (Ps) who are candidates for phototherapy or systemic therapy. 2. Active psoriatic arthritis (PsA), alone or in combination with methotrexate. 3. Moderately to severely active Crohn's disease (CD) who have failed or were intolerant to treatment with immunomodulators or corticosteroids, but never failed a tumor necrosis factor (TNF) blocker or failed or were

		intolerant to treatment with one or more TNF blockers 4. Adolescent patients (12 years or older) with moderate to severe plaque psoriasis, who are candidates for phototherapy or systemic therapy
Vedolizumab/ Entyvio/ humanized	Binds to the α4β7 integrin and blocks the interaction of α4β7 integrin with mucosal addressin cell adhesion molecule-1 (MAdCAM-1) and inhibits the migration of memory T lymphocytes across the endothelium into inflamed gastro-intestinal parenchymal tissue	1. Adult ulcerative colitis (UC) Adult patients with moderately to severely active UC who have had an inadequate response with, lost response to, or were intolerant to a tumor necrosis factor (TNF) blocker or immunomodulator; or had an inadequate response with, were intolerant to, or demonstrated dependence on corticosteroids • inducing and maintaining clinical response • inducing and maintaining clinical remission • improving endoscopic appearance of the mucosa 2. Achieving corticosteroid-free remission adult Crohn's disease (CD) • Adult patients with moderately to severely active CD who have had an inadequate response with, lost response to, or were intolerant to a TNF blocker or immunomodulator; or had an inadequate response with, were intolerant to, or demonstrated dependence on corticosteroids • achieving clinical response • achieving clinical remission • achieving corticosteroid-free remission

[a]Hidradenitis suppuriva is long term skin disease characterized by the occurrence of inflamed and swollen lumps

One other FDA-approved mab, tositumomab (Bexxar) (anti-CD20), was discontinued in 2014 due to lack of demand

[1]Burrill Bernard Crohn (1884 – 1983) was an American gastroenterologist

[2]Friedrich Sigmund Merkel (1845-1919) was a German anatomist and histopathologist

[3]Thomas Hodgkin (1798 – 1866) was a British physician

[4]Albert Sézary (1880 – 1956) was a French dermatologist and syphilogist

[5] Benjamin Castleman (1906 – 1982) was an American physician and pathologist

Examples of other biological therapeutics approved by the FDA for non-malignant diseases and malignant diseases

- Janus kinase inhibitors – eg, tofacitinib in Crohn's disease, ruxolitinib for steroid-refractory acute graft-versus-host disease
- Bruton's tyrosine kinase inhibitor – eg, ibrutinib for chronic graft-versus-host disease
- Other human tyrosine kinase inhibitors – eg, imatinib for systemic mastocytosis
- Angiogenesis inhibitors – eg, aflibercept for diabetic retinopathy
- Small interfering RNA-based drugs- eg, onasemnogene abeparvovec-xioi (Zolgensma) for familial amyloid polyneuropathy

Enzyme replacement treatments – eg, cerliponase alfa (Brineura) for Batten disease

Enzyme inhibitors – eg, lanadelumab-flyo (Takhzyro) for hereditary angioedema

Anti-sense drugs - eg, fomivirsen for cytomegalovirus retinitis, mipomersen for homozygous familial hypercholesterolemia, eteplirsen for Duchenne muscular dystrophy, nusinersen for spinal muscular atrophy

Cell therapies – Umbilical cord blood stem cells: FDA-approved for over 80 diseases, both non-malignant and malignant.

Gene-modified cell therapies

As of December 2020, the FDA had approved three different chimeric antigen receptor (CAR) T cell therapeutic agents for B cell acute lymphoblastic leukemia and aggressive non-Hodgkin lymphomas.

Gene therapies – eg, onasemnogene abeparvovec-xioi (Zolgensma) to treat spinal muscular atrophy type 1 has been approved for therapeutic use by the FDA. Voretigene neparvovec-rzyl (Luxturna) to treat congenital retinal dystrophy has also been approved by the FDA.

Hedgehog pathway inhibitors – eg sonidegib and vismodegib. These agents are chemically synthesised and FDA-approved for the treatment of advanced cutaneous squamous cell carcinoma or advanced basal cell carcinoma of the skin.

M-TOR inhibitors – eg sirolimus, temsirolimus and everolimus which inhibit the kinase activity of m-TOR, and which are used as immune suppressive agents

A list of small molecule protein kinase inhibitors approved by the USA FDA for therapeutic use (as of December 2020) is shown in Table 2.

Table 2. A list of small molecule protein kinase inhibitors approved by the USA FDA for therapeutic use.

Generic name/ trade name	Target and mechanism of action	FDA-approved indication/s
Abemaciclib/ Verzenio	Cyclin-dependent kinases 4 and 6 (CDK4 and CDK6). CDK4/6 inhibitor activity enforces G1 cell cycle arrest, and thus inhibits cellular proliferation	• In combination with an aromatase inhibitor as initial endocrine-based therapy for the treatment of postmenopausal women with hormone receptor (HR)-positive, human epidermal growth factor receptor 2 (HER2)-negative advanced or metastatic breast cancer. • in combination with fulvestrant for the treatment of women with hormone receptor (HR)-positive, human epidermal growth factor receptor 2 (HER2)-negative advanced or metastatic breast cancer with disease progression following endocrine therapy. • as monotherapy for the treatment of adult patients with HR positive, HER2-negative advanced or metastatic breast cancer with disease progression following endocrine therapy and prior chemotherapy in the metastatic setting.
Acalabrutinib/ Calquence	Bruton's tyrosine kinase[1]. (BTK). BTK is a signalling molecule of the B cell antigen receptor (BCR) and cytokine receptor pathways	1. Mantle cell lymphoma (MCL) who have received at least one prior therapy. This indication is approved under accelerated approval based on overall response rate. Continued approval for this indication may be contingent upon verification and description of clinical benefit in

		confirmatory trials 2. Chronic lymphocytic leukemia (CLL) or small lymphocytic lymphoma (SLL)
Afatinib/ Golotrif	ErbB (derived avian erythroblastosis oncogeneB). Signalling through the ErbB1/2/4 family of receptors promotes cell proliferation and opposes apoptosis. (ErbB is also known as, HER-2, HER-2/neu, HER2, NEU, CD340). Afatinib covalently binds to the kinase domains of EGFR (ErbB1), HER2 (ErbB2), and HER4 (ErbB4) and irreversibly inhibits tyrosine kinase autophosphorylation, resulting in downregulation of ErbB signalling.	1. First-line treatment of patients with metastatic non-small cell lung cancer (NSCLC) whose tumors have non-resistant epidermal growth factor receptor (EGFR) mutations 2. Treatment of patients with metastatic, squamous NSCLC progressing after platinum-based chemotherapy
Alectinib/ Alecensa	ALK, RET. Alectinib is a tyrosine kinase inhibitor that targets ALK and RET. In non-clinical studies, alectinib inhibited ALK phosphorylation and ALK-mediated activation of the downstream signalling proteins STAT3 and AKT, and decreased tumor cell viability in multiple cell lines harboring ALK fusions, amplifications, or activating mutations.	Anaplastic lymphoma kinase (ALK)-positive metastatic non-small cell lung cancer (NSCLC)
Avapritinib/AYVAKIT	PDGFRA and PDGFRA D842 mutants Avapritinib is a tyrosine kinase inhibitor that targets PDGFRA and PDGFRA D842 mutants as well as multiple KIT exon 11, 11/17 and 17 mutants with half maximal inhibitory concentrations (IC50s) less than 25 nM. Certain mutations in PDGFRA and KIT can result in the autophosphorylation and constitutive activation of these receptors which can contribute to tumor cell proliferation. Other potential targets for avapritinib include wild type KIT, PDGFRB, and CSFR1. In in vitro cellular assays, avapritinib inhibited the autophosphorylation of KIT D816V and PDGFRA D842V, mutants associated with resistance to approved kinase inhibitors, with IC50 of 4 nM and 30 nM, respectively.	AYVAKIT is a kinase inhibitor indicated for the treatment of adults with unresectable or metastatic gastrointestinal stromal tumor (GIST) harboring a platelet-derived growth factor receptor alpha (PDGFRA) exon 18 mutation, including PDGFRA D842V mutations.

	Avapritinib also had anti-tumor activity in mice implanted with an imatinib-resistant patientderived xenograft model of human GIST with activating KIT exon 11/17 mutations.	
Axitinib/Inlyta	Vascular endothelial growth factor receptors (VEGFR) 1/2/3. Axitinib has been shown to inhibit receptor tyrosine kinases including vascular endothelial growth factor receptors VEGFR-1, VEGFR-2, and VEGFR-3	Advanced renal cell carcinoma after failure of one prior systemic therapy
Baricitinib/ Olumiant	JAK1/2. Janus kinases phosphorylate activated cytokine receptors. These phosphorylated receptors in turn recruit STAT transcrip-tion factors which modulate gene transcription	Adult patients with moderately to severely active rheumatoid arthritis who have had an inadequate response to one or more TNF antagonist therapies
Binimetinib/ Mektovi	MEK1/2. MEK inhibitors inhibit the mitogen-activated protein kinase kinase enzymes MEK1and/or MEK2. They can be used to affect the MAPK/ERK pathway which is often overactive in some cancers	In combination with encorafenib, for the treatment of patients with unresectable or metastatic melanoma with a BRAF V600E or V600K mutation, as detected by an FDA-approved test.
Bosutinib/ Bosulif	BCR-ABL Bosutinib inhibits the BCR-ABL kinase that promotes CML	Treatment of adult patients with chronic, accelerated, or blast phase Ph+ chronic myelogenous leukemia (CML) with resistance or intolerance to prior therapy
Brigatinib/ Alunbrig	ALK. Brigatinib is a tyrosine kinase inhibitor with in vitro activity at clinically achievable concentrations against multiple kinases including ALK, ROS1, insulin-like growth factor-1 receptor (IGF-1R), and FLT-3 as well as EGFR deletion and point mutations. Brigatinib inhibited autophosphorylation of ALK and ALK-mediated phosphorylation of the downstream signalling proteins STAT3, AKT, ERK1/2, and S6 in in vitro and in vivo assays.	Patients with anaplastic lymphoma kinase (ALK)-positive metastatic non-small cell lung cancer (NSCLC) who have progressed on or are intolerant to crizotinib. This indication is approved under accelerated approval based on tumor response rate and duration of response. Continued approval for this indication may be contingent upon verification and description of clinical benefit in a confirmatory trial
Cabozantinib/ Cabometyx	RET, VEGFR2. Cabozantinib inhibits the tyrosine kinase activity of RET, MET, VEGFR-1, -2 and -3, KIT, TRKB, FLT-3, AXL, ROS1, TYRO3, MER, and TIE-2. These receptor tyrosine kinases are	1.Patients with advanced renal cell carcinoma (RCC) 2. Patients with hepatocellular carcinoma (HCC) who have been previously treated with sorafenib

	involved in both normal cellular function and pathologic processes such as oncogenesis, metastasis, tumor angiogenesis, drug resistance, and maintenance of the tumor microenvironment.	
Cabozantinib/ Cometriq	RET, VEGFR2	Patients with progressive, metastatic medullary thyroid cancer (MTC)
Capmatinib/ TABRECTATM	MET Capmatinib is a kinase inhibitor that targets MET, including the mutant variant produced by exon 14 skipping. MET exon 14 skipping results in a protein with a missing regulatory domain that reduces its negative regulation leading to increased downstream MET signaling. Capmatinib inhibited cancer cell growth driven by a mutant MET variant lacking exon 14 at clinically achievable concentrations and demonstrated anti-tumor activity in murine tumor xenograft models derived from human lung tumors with either a mutation leading to MET exon 14 skipping or MET amplification. Capmatinib inhibited the phosphorylation of MET triggered by binding of hepatocyte growth factor or by MET amplification, as well as METmediated phosphorylation of downstream signaling proteins and proliferation and survival of MET-dependent cancer cells.	TABRECTA is a kinase inhibitor indicated for the treatment of adult patients with metastatic non-small cell lung cancer (NSCLC) whose tumors have a mutation that leads to mesenchymal-epithelial transition (MET) exon 14 skipping as detected by an FDA-approved test. This indication is approved under accelerated approval based on overall response rate and duration of response. Continued approval for this indication may be contingent upon verification and description of clinical benefit in confirmatory trial(s).
Ceritinib/ Zykadia	ALK. Targets of ceritinib inhibition identified in either biochemical or cellular assays at clinically relevant concentrations include ALK, insulin-like growth factor 1 receptor (IGF-1R), insulin receptor (InsR), and ROS1. Among these, ceritinib is most active against ALK. Ceritinib inhibited autophosphorylation of ALK, ALK-mediated phosphorylation of the downstream signalling protein STAT3, and proliferation of ALK-dependent cancer cells in in vitro and in vivo assays.	Patients with metastatic non-small cell lung cancer (NSCLC) whose tumors are anaplastic lymphoma kinase (ALK)-positive
Cobimetinib/ Cotellic	MEK1/2. Cobimetinib is a reversible inhibitor of mitogen-activated protein kinase (MAPK)/extracellular signal regulated	Unresectable or metastatic melanoma with a BRAF V600E or V600K mutation, in combination with vemurafenib

	kinase 1 (MEK1) and MEK2. MEK proteins are upstream regulators of the extracellular signal related kinase (ERK) pathway, which promotes cellular proliferation. BRAF V600E and K mutations result in constitutive activation of the BRAF pathway which includes MEK1 and MEK2.	
Crizotinib/ Xalkori	ALK, ROS1. Crizotinib is an inhibitor of receptor tyrosine kinases including ALK, Hepatocyte growth factor receptor (HGFR, c-Met), ROS1 (c-ros), and Recepteur d'Origine Nantais (RON). Translocations can affect the ALK gene resulting in the expression of oncogenic fusion proteins. The formation of ALK fusion proteins results in activation and dysregulation of the gene's expression and signalling which can contribute to increased cell proliferation and survival in tumors expressing these proteins.	Patients with metastatic non-small cell lung cancer (NSCLC) whose tumors are anaplastic lymphoma kinase (ALK) or ROS1-positive
Dabrafenib/ Tafinlar	B-RAF. Dabrafenib is an inhibitor of some mutated forms of BRAF kinases with in vitro IC50 values of 0.65, 0.5, and 1.84 nM for BRAF V600E, BRAF V600K, and BRAF V600D enzymes, respectively. Dabrafenib also inhibits wild-type BRAF and CRAF kinases with IC50 values of 3.2 and 5.0 nM, respectively, and other kinases such as SIK1, NEK11, and LIMK1 at higher concentrations. Some mutations in the BRAF gene, including those that result in BRAF V600E, can result in constitutively activated BRAF kinases that may stimulate tumor cell growth.	TAFINLAR is a kinase inhibitor indicated as a single agent for the treatment of patients with unresectable or metastatic melanoma with BRAF V600E mutation as detected by an FDA-approved test. • TAFINLAR in combination with trametinib is indicated for the treatment of patients with unresectable or metastatic melanoma with BRAF V600E or V600K mutations as detected by an FDA-approved test. The use in combination is based on the demonstration of durable response rate. Improvement in disease-related symptoms or overall survival has not been demonstrated for TAFINLAR in combination with trametinib. Limitation of Use: TAFINLAR is not indicated for treatment of patients with wild-type BRAF melanoma.
Dacomitinib/ Vizimpro	EGFR. Dacomitinib is an irreversible inhibitor of the kinase activity of the human epidermal growth factor receptor (EGFR) family (EGFR/HER1, HER2, and HER4) and certain EGFR	First-line treatment of patients with metastatic non-small cell lung cancer (NSCLC) with epidermal growth factor receptor (EGFR) exon 19 deletion or exon 21 L858R substitution mutations

	activating mutations (exon 19 deletion or the exon 21 L858R substitution mutation).	
Dasatinib/ Sprycell	BCR-ABL. Dasatinib, at nanomolar concentrations, inhibits the following kinases: BCR-ABL, SRC family (SRC, LCK, YES, FYN), c-KIT, EPHA2, and PDGFR-β. Based on modeling studies, dasatinib is predicted to bind to multiple conformations of the ABL kinase.	1. Newly diagnosed adults with Philadelphia chromosome-positive (Ph+) chronic myeloid leukemia (CML) in chronic phase. The trial is ongoing and further data will be required to determine long-term outcome. 2. Adults with chronic, accelerated, or myeloid or lymphoid blast phase Ph+ CML with resistance or intolerance to prior therapy including imatinib. 3. Adults with Philadelphia chromosome-positive acute lymphoblastic leukemia (Ph+ ALL) with resistance or intolerance to prior therapy
Encorafenib/Braftovi	B-RAF. Encorafenib is a kinase inhibitor that targets BRAF V600E, as well as wild-type BRAF and CRAF in in vitro cell-free assays with IC50 values of 0.35, 0.47, and 0.3 nM, respectively. Mutations in the BRAF gene, such as BRAF V600E, can result in constitutively activated BRAF kinases that may stimulate tumor cell growth. Encorafenib was also able to bind to other kinases in vitro including JNK1, JNK2, JNK3, LIMK1, LIMK2, MEK4, and STK36 and substantially reduce ligand binding to these kinases at clinically achievable concentrations (≤ 0.9 μM).	BRAFTOVI is a kinase inhibitor indicated: • in combination with binimetinib, for the treatment of patients with unresectable or metastatic melanoma with a BRAF V600E or V600K mutation, as detected by an FDA-approved test. • in combination with cetuximab, for the treatment of adult patients with metastatic colorectal cancer (CRC) with a BRAF V600E mutation, as detected by an FDA-approved test, after prior therapy. Limitations of Use: BRAFTOVI is not indicated for treatment of patients with wild-type BRAF melanoma or wild-type BRAF CRC.
Entrectinib/ Rozlytrek	TRKA/B/C, ROS1, ALK. Entrectinib is an inhibitor of the tropomyosin receptor tyrosine kinases (TRK) TRKA, TRKB, and TRKC (encoded by the neurotrophic tyrosine receptor kinase [NTRK] genes NTRK1, NTRK2, and NTRK3, respectively), proto-oncogene tyrosine-protein kinase ROS1 (ROS1), and anaplastic lymphoma kinase (ALK). Fusion proteins that include TRK, ROS1, or ALK kinase domains can drive tumorigenic potential through hyperactivation of	• Adult patients with metastatic non-small cell lung cancer (NSCLC) whose tumors are ROS1-positive • Adult and pediatric patients 12 years of age and older with solid tumors that: o have a neurotrophic tyrosine receptor kinase (NTRK) gene fusion without a known acquired resistance mutation o are metastatic or where

	downstream signalling pathways leading to unconstrained cell proliferation.	surgical resection is likely to result in severe morbidity o have progressed following treatment or have no satisfactory alternative therapy. This indication is approved under accelerated approval based on tumor response rate and durability of response. Continued approval for this indication may be contingent upon verification and description of clinical benefit in the confirmatory trials.
Erdafitinib/ Balversa	FGFR1/2/3/4. Erdafitinib is a kinase inhibitor that binds to and inhibits enzymatic activity of FGFR1, FGFR2, FGFR3 and FGFR4 based on in vitro data. Erdafitinib also binds to RET, CSF1R, PDGFRA, PDGFRB, FLT4, KIT, and VEGFR2. Erdafitinib inhibited FGFR phosphorylation and signalling and decreased cell viability in cell lines expressing FGFR genetic alterations, including point mutations, amplifications, and fusions. Erdafitinib demonstrated antitumor activity in FGFR-expressing cell lines and xenograft models derived from tumor types, including bladder cancer.	Treatment of adult patients with locally advanced or metastatic urothelial carcinoma that has • susceptible FGFR3 or FGFR2 genetic alterations and • progressed during or following at least one line of prior platinum-containing chemotherapy including within 12 months of neoadjuvant or adjuvant platinum-containing chemotherapy. This indication is approved under accelerated approval based on tumor response rate. Continued approval for this indication may be contingent upon verification and description of clinical benefit in confirmatory trials
Erlotinib/ Tarceva	EGFR. The mechanism of the clinical antitumor action of erlotinib is not fully characterized. Erlotinib inhibits the intracellular phosphorylation of tyrosine kinase associated with the epidermal growth factor receptor (EGFR). Specificity of inhibition with regard to other tyrosine kinase receptors has not been fully characterized. EGFR is expressed on the cell surface of normal cells and cancer cells.	1. Maintenance treatment of patients with locally advanced or metastatic non-small cell lung cancer (NSCLC) whose disease has not progressed after four cycles of platinum-based first-line chemotherapy. 2.Treatment of locally advanced or metastatic non-small cell lung cancer after failure of at least one prior chemotherapy regimen. 3.First-line treatment of patients with locally advanced, unresectable or metastatic pancreatic cancer, in combination with gemcitabine
Fedratinib/ Inrebic	JAK2, FLT3. Fedratinib is an oral kinase inhibitor with activity against wild type and mutationally activated Janus Associated Kinase 2 (JAK2) and	Treatment of adult patients with intermediate-2 or high-risk primary or secondary (post-polycythemia vera or post-essential thrombocythemia)

	FMS-like tyrosine kinase 3 (FLT3). Fedratinib is a JAK2-selective inhibitor with higher inhibitory activity for JAK2 over family members JAK1, JAK3 and TYK2. Abnormal activation of JAK2 is associated with myeloproliferative neoplasms (MPNs), including myelofibrosis and polycythemia vera	myelofibrosis (MF)
Fostamatinib/ Tavalisse	SYK. Fostamatinib is a tyrosine kinase inhibitor with demonstrated activity against spleen tyrosine kinase (SYK). The major metabolite of fostamatinib, R406, inhibits signal transduction of Fc-activating receptors and B cell receptor. The fostamatinib metabolite R406 reduces antibody-mediated destruction of platelets.	Treatment of thrombocytopenia in adult patients with chronic immune thrombocytopenia (ITP) who have had an insufficient response to a previous treatment.
Gefitinib/ Iressa	EGFR. The epidermal growth factor receptor (EGFR) is expressed on the cell surface of both normal and cancer cells and plays a role in the processes of cell growth and proliferation. Some EGFR activating mutations (exon 19 deletion or exon 21 point mutation L858R) within NSCLC cells have been identified as contributing to the promotion of tumor cell growth, blocking of apoptosis, increasing the production of angiogenic factors and facilitating the processes of metastasis. Gefitinib reversibly inhibits the kinase activity of wild-type and certain activating mutations of EGFR, preventing autophosphorylation of tyrosine residues associated with the receptor, thereby inhibiting further downstream signalling and blocking EGFR-dependent proliferation. Gefitinib binding affinity for EGFR exon 19 deletion or exon 21 point mutation L858R mutations is higher than its affinity for the wild-type EGFR. Gefitinib also inhibits IGF and PDGF-mediated signalling at clinically relevant concentrations; inhibition of other tyrosine kinase receptors has not been fully characterized.	First-line treatment of patients with metastatic non-small cell lung cancer (NSCLC) whose tumors have epidermal growth factor receptor (EGFR) exon 19 deletions or exon 21 (L858R) substitution mutations. Limitation of use: the safety and efficacy of IRESSA have not been established in patients whose tumors have EGFR mutations other than exon 19 deletions or exon 21 (L858R) substitution mutations
Gilteritinib/ Xospata	Flt3. Gilteritinib is a small molecule that inhibits multiple receptor tyrosine kinases, including FMS-like tyrosine	Treatment of adult patients who have relapsed or refractory acute myeloid leukemia (AML) with a FLT3 mutation

	kinase 3 (FLT3). Gilteritinib demonstrated the ability to inhibit FLT3 receptor signalling and proliferation in cells exogenously expressing FLT3 including FLT3-ITD, tyrosine kinase domain mutations (TKD) FLT3-D835Y and FLT3-ITD-D835, and it induced apoptosis in leukemic cells expressing FLT3-ITD.	
Ibrutinib/ Imbruvica	BTK. Ibrutinib is a small-molecule inhibitor of BTK. Ibrutinib forms a covalent bond with a cysteine residue in the BTK active site, leading to inhibition of BTK enzymatic activity. BTK is a signalling molecule of the B cell antigen receptor (BCR) and cytokine receptor pathways. BTK's role in signalling through the B cell surface receptors results in activation of pathways necessary for B cell trafficking, chemotaxis, and adhesion. Non-clinical studies show that ibrutinib inhibits B cell proliferation and survival in vivo as well as cell migration and substrate adhesion in vitro.	Treatment of adult patients with: 1. Mantle cell lymphoma (MCL) who have received at least one prior therapy. Accelerated approval was granted for this indication based on overall response rate. Continued approval for this indication may be contingent upon verification and description of clinical benefit in a confirmatory trial. 2. Chronic lymphocytic leukemia (CLL)/Small lymphocytic lymphoma (SLL) Chronic lymphocytic leukemia (CLL)/Small lymphocytic lymphoma (SLL) with 17p deletion 3. Waldenström's macroglobulinemia (WM) 4. Marginal zone lymphoma (MZL) who require systemic therapy and have received at least one prior anti-CD20-based therapy. Accelerated approval was granted for this indication based on overall response rate. Continued approval for this indication may be contingent upon verification and description of clinical benefit in a confirmatory trial. 5. Chronic graft-versus-host disease (cGVHD) after failure of one or more lines of systemic therapy
Imatinib/ Gleevec	Imatinib is tyrosine kinase specific for the TK domain in abl (the Abelson proto-oncogene), c-kit and PDGF-R (platelet-derived growth factor receptor.	1. Newly diagnosed adult and pediatric patients with Philadelphia chromosome positive chronic myeloid leukemia (Ph+ CML) in chronic phase 2. Patients with Philadelphia chromosome positive chronic myeloid leukemia (Ph+ CML) in blast crisis (BC), accelerated phase (AP), or in chronic phase

		(CP) after failure of interferon-alpha therapy 3. Adult patients with relapsed or refractory Philadelphia chromosome positive acute lymphoblastic leukemia (Ph+ ALL) 4. Pediatric patients with newly diagnosed Philadelphia chromosome positive acute lymphoblastic leukemia (Ph+ ALL) in combination with chemotherapy 5. Adult patients with myelodysplastic/myeloproliferative diseases (MDS/MPD) associated with platelet-derived growth factor receptor (PDGFR) gene re-arrangements 6. Adult patients with aggressive systemic mastocytosis (ASM) without the D816V c-Kit mutation or with c-Kit mutational status unknown 7. Adult patients with hypereosinophilic syndrome (HES) and/or chronic eosinophilic leukemia (CEL) who have the FIP1L1-PDGFR-α fusion kinase and for patients with HES and/or CEL who are FIP1L1 PDGFR-α fusion kinase negative or unknown 8. Adult patients with unresectable, recurrent and/or metastatic dermatofibrosarcoma protuberans (DFSP) 9. Patients with kit (CD117) positive unresectable and/or metastatic gastrointestinal stromal tumors (GIST) 10. Adjuvant treatment of adult patients following resection of kit (CD117) positive GIST
Lapatinib/ Tykerb	EGFR, ErbB2/HER2. Lapatinib is a 4-anilinoquinazoline kinase inhibitor of the intracellular tyrosine kinase domains of both Epidermal Growth Factor Receptor (EGFR [ErbB1]) and of Human Epidermal Receptor Type 2 (HER2 [ErbB2]). Lapatinib inhibits ErbB-driven tumor cell growth in vitro and in various animal models.	TYKERB, a kinase inhibitor, is indicated in combination with: • capecitabine, for the treatment of patients with advanced or metastatic breast cancer whose tumors overexpress HER2 and who have received prior therapy including an anthracycline, a taxane, and trastuzumab. • letrozole for the treatment of

		postmenopausal women with hormone receptor positive metastatic breast cancer that overexpresses the HER2 receptor for whom hormonal therapy is indicated. TYKERB in combination with an aromatase inhibitor has not been compared to a trastuzumab-containing chemotherapy regimen for the treatment of metastatic breast cancer
Larotrectinib/ Vitrakvi	TRKA/B/C. Larotrectinib is an inhibitor of the tropomyosin receptor kinases (TRK), TRKA, TRKB, and TRKC. In a broad panel of purified enzyme assays, larotrectinib inhibited TRKA, TRKB, and TRKC. TRKA, B, and C are encoded by the genes NTRK1, NTRK2, and NTRK3. Chromosomal rearrangements involving in-frame fusions of these genes with various partners can result in constitutively-activated chimeric TRK fusion proteins that can act as an oncogenic driver, promoting cell proliferation and survival in tumor cell lines.	Treatment of adult and pediatric patients with solid tumors that • have a neurotrophic receptor tyrosine kinase (NTRK) gene fusion without a known acquired resistance mutation • are metastatic or where surgical resection is likely to result in severe morbidity, and • have no satisfactory alternative treatments or that have progressed following treatment. This indication is approved under accelerated approval based on overall response rate and duration of response. Continued approval for this indication may be contingent upon verification and description of clinical benefit in confirmatory trials.
Lenvatinib/ Lenvima	VEGFR, FGFR, RET, PDGFR, KIT. Lenvatinib is a kinase inhibitor that inhibits the kinase activities of vascular endothelial growth factor (VEGF) receptors VEGFR1 (FLT1), VEGFR2 (KDR), and VEGFR3 (FLT4). Lenvatinib inhibits other kinases that have been implicated in pathogenic angiogenesis, tumor growth, and cancer progression in addition to their normal cellular functions, including fibroblast growth factor (FGF) receptors FGFR1, 2, 3, and 4; platelet derived growth factor receptor alpha (PDGFRα), KIT, and RET. Lenvatinib also exhibited antiproliferative activity in hepatocellular carcinoma cell lines dependent on activated FGFR signalling with a concurrent inhibition of FGF-receptor substrate 2α (FRS2α) phosphorylation. The combination of lenvatinib and	Treatment of patients with 1. Locally recurrent or metastatic, progressive, radioactive iodine-refractory differentiated thyroid cancer (DTC). 2. In combination with everolimus, for the treatment of patients with advanced renal cell carcinoma (RCC) following one prior antiangiogenic therapy. 3. For the first-line treatment of patients with unresectable hepatocellular carcinoma (HCC)

	everolimus showed increased antiangiogenic and antitumor activity as demonstrated by decreases in human endothelial cell proliferation, tube formation, and VEGF signalling in vitro, and by decreases in tumor volume in mouse xenograft models of human renal cell cancer that were greater than those with either drug alone.	
Lonafarnib	Lonafarnib inhibits farnesyltransferase to prevent farnesylation and subsequent accumulation of progerin and progerin-like proteins in the inner nuclear membrane.	ZOKINVY is a farnesyltransferase inhibitor indicated in patients 12 months of age and older with a body surface area of 0.39 m^2 and above • To reduce risk of mortality in Hutchinson-Gilford Progeria Syndrome • For treatment of processing-deficient Progeroid Laminopathies with either: o Heterozygous LMNA mutation with progerin-like protein accumulation o Homozygous or compound heterozygous ZMPSTE24 mutations
Lorlatinib/ Lorbrena	ALK, ROS1 and others. Lorlatinib is a kinase inhibitor with in vitro activity against ALK and ROS1 as well as TYK1, FER, FPS, TRKA, TRKB, TRKC, FAK, FAK2, and ACK. Lorlatinib demonstrated in vitro activity against multiple mutant forms of the ALK enzyme, including some mutations detected in tumors at the time of disease progression on crizotinib and other ALK inhibitors.	Treatment of patients with anaplastic lymphoma kinase (ALK)-positive metastatic non-small cell lung cancer (NSCLC) whose disease has progressed on • crizotinib and at least one other ALK inhibitor for metastatic disease • or on alectinib as the first ALK inhibitor therapy for metastatic disease • or on ceritinib as the first ALK inhibitor therapy for metastatic disease. This indication is approved under accelerated approval based on tumor response rate and duration of response. Continued approval for this indication may be contingent upon verification and description of clinical benefit in a confirmatory trial.
Midostaurin/ Rydapt	Flt3. Midostaurin is a small molecule that	Treatment of adult patients with: newly diagnosed acute myeloid

	inhibits multiple receptor tyrosine kinases. In vitro biochemical or cellular assays have shown that midostaurin or its major human active metabolites CGP62221 and CGP52421 inhibit the activity of wild type FLT3, FLT3 mutant kinases (ITD and TKD), KIT (wild type and D816V mutant), PDGFRα/β, VEGFR2, as well as members of the serine/threonine kinase PKC (protein kinase C) family.	leukemia (AML) that is FLT3 mutation-positive in combination with standard cytarabine and daunorubicin induction and cytarabine consolidation. Limitations of use: RYDAPT is not indicated as a single-agent induction therapy for the treatment of patients with AML, aggressive systemic mastocytosis (ASM), systemic mastocytosis with associated hematological neoplasm (SM-AHN), or mast cell leukemia (MCL).
Neratinib/ Nerlynx	ErbB2/HER2. A kinase inhibitor that irreversibly binds to Epidermal Growth Factor Receptor (EGFR), Human Epidermal Growth Factor Receptor 2 (HER2), and HER4. In vitro, neratinib reduces EGFR and HER2 autophosphorylation, downstream MAPK and AKT signalling pathways, and showed antitumor activity in EGFR and/or HER2 expressing carcinoma cell lines. Neratinib human metabolites M3, M6, M7 and M11 inhibited the activity of EGFR, HER2 and HER4 in vitro. In vivo, oral administration of neratinib inhibited tumor growth in mouse xenograft models with tumor cell lines expressing HER2 and EGFR.	NERLYNX is a kinase inhibitor indicated: • As a single agent, for the extended adjuvant treatment of adult patients with early stage HER2-positive breast cancer, to follow adjuvant trastuzumabbased therapy. • In combination with capecitabine, for the treatment of adult patients with advanced or metastatic HER2-positive breast cancer who have received two or more prior anti-HER2 based regimens in the metastatic setting.
Netarsudil/ Rhopressa	ROCK1/2 (Rho associated coiled-coil containing protein kinase 1) Netarsudil is a rho kinase inhibitor, which is believed to reduce intra-ocular pressure (IOP) by increasing the outflow of aqueous humor through the trabecular meshwork route. The exact mechanism is unknown.	RHOPRESSA® (netarsudil ophthalmic solution) 0.02% is a Rho kinase inhibitor indicated for the reduction of elevated intraocular pressure in patients with open-angle glaucoma or ocular hypertension
Nilotinib/ Tasigna	BCR-ABL. Nilotinib is an inhibitor of the BCR-ABL kinase.	1. Treatment of newly diagnosed adult patients with Philadelphia chromosome positive chronic myeloid leukemia (Ph+ CML) in chronic phase. 2. Treatment of chronic phase (CP) and accelerated phase (AP) Ph+ CML in adult patients resistant to or intolerant to prior therapy that included imatinib.
Nintedanib/ Vargatef	Multiple kinases. Nintedanib is a small molecule that	The treatment of idiopathic pulmonary fibrosis (IPF).

	inhibits multiple receptor tyrosine kinases (RTKs) and non-receptor tyrosine kinases (nRTKs). Nintedanib inhibits the following RTKs: platelet-derived growth factor receptor (PDGFR) α and β, fibroblast growth factor receptor (FGFR) 1-3, vascular endothelial growth factor receptor (VEGFR) 1-3, and Fms-like tyrosine kinase-3 (FLT3). Among them, FGFR, PDGFR, and VEGFR have been implicated in IPF pathogenesis. Nintedanib binds competitively to the adenosine triphosphate (ATP) binding pocket of these receptors and blocks the intracellular signalling which is crucial for the proliferation, migration, and transformation of fibroblasts representing essential mechanisms of the IPF pathology.	
Osimertinib/ Tagrisso	EGFR Osimertinib is a kinase inhibitor of the epidermal growth factor receptor (EGFR), which binds irreversibly to certain mutant forms of EGFR (T790M, L858R, and exon 19 deletion) at approximately 9- fold lower concentrations than wild-type. In vitro, osimertinib also inhibited the activity of HER2, HER3, HER4, ACK1, and BLK at clinically relevant concentrations. In cultured cells and animal tumor implantation models, osimertinib exhibited anti-tumor activity against NSCLC lines harboring EGFR-mutations (T790M/L858R, L858R, T790M/exon 19 deletion, and exon 19 deletion) and, to a lesser extent, wild-type EGFR amplifications	1. The first-line treatment of patients with metastatic NSCLC whose tumors have epidermal growth factor receptor (EGFR) exon 19 deletions or exon 21 L858R mutations 2. The treatment of patients with metastatic EGFR T790M mutation-positive NSCLC whose disease has progressed on or after EGFR TKI therapy
Palbociclib/ Ibrance	CDK4/6	IBRANCE is a kinase inhibitor indicated for the treatment of adult patients with hormone receptor (HR)-positive, human epidermal growth factor receptor 2 (HER2)-negative advanced or metastatic breast cancer in combination with: • an aromatase inhibitor as initial endocrine-based therapy in postmenopausal women or in men; or • fulvestrant in patients with disease progression following endocrine therapy.

Pazopanib/ Votrient	VEGFR1/2/3 Pazopanib is a multi-tyrosine kinase inhibitor of vascular endothelial growth factor receptor (VEGFR)-1, VEGFR-2, VEGFR-3, platelet-derived growth factor receptor (PDGFR)-α and -β, fibroblast growth factor receptor (FGFR) -1 and -3, cytokine receptor (Kit), interleukin-2, receptor inducible T cell kinase (Itk), leukocyte-specific protein tyrosine kinase (Lck), and transmembrane glycoprotein receptor tyrosine kinase (c-fms). In vitro, pazopanib inhibited ligand-induced autophosphorylation of VEGFR-2, Kit and PDGFR-β receptors. In vivo, pazopanib inhibited VEGF-induced VEGFR-2 phosphorylation in mouse lungs, angiogenesis in a mouse model, and the growth of some human tumor xenografts in mice.	The treatment of patients with: 1. Advanced renal cell carcinoma 2. Advanced soft tissue sarcoma who have received prior chemotherapy. Limitations of use: the efficacy of VOTRIENT for the treatment of patients with adipocytic soft tissue sarcoma or gastrointestinal stromal tumors has not been demonstrated.
Pemigatinib/ PEMAZYRE™	FGFR2 Pemigatinib is a small molecule kinase inhibitor that targets FGFR1, 2 and 3 with IC50 values of less than 2 nM. Pemigatinib also inhibited FGFR4 in vitro at a concentration approximately 100 times higher than those that inhibit FGFR1, 2, and 3. Pemigatinib inhibited FGFR1-3 phosphorylation and signaling and decreased cell viability in cancer cell lines with activating FGFR amplifications and fusions that resulted in constitutive activation of FGFR signaling. Constitutive FGFR signaling can support the proliferation and survival of malignant cells. Pemigatinib exhibited anti-tumor activity in mouse xenograft models of human tumors with FGFR1, FGFR2, or FGFR3 alterations resulting in constitutive FGFR activation including a patient-derived xenograft model of cholangiocarcinoma that expressed an oncogenic FGFR2 Transformer-2 beta homolog (TRA2b) fusion protein.	PEMAZYRE is a kinase inhibitor indicated for the treatment of adults with previously treated, unresectable locally advanced or metastatic cholangiocarcinoma with a fibroblast growth factor receptor 2 (FGFR2) fusion or other rearrangement as detected by an FDA-approved test. This indication is approved under accelerated approval based on overall response rate and duration of response. Continued approval for this indication may be contingent upon verification and description of clinical benefit in a confirmatory trial(s).
Pexidartinib/ Turalio	Multiple kinases. Pexidartinib is a small molecule tyrosine kinase inhibitor that targets colony stimulating factor 1 receptor (CSF1R), KIT proto-oncogene receptor tyrosine kinase (KIT), and FMS-like tyrosine kinase 3 (FLT3)	The treatment of adult patients with symptomatic tenosynovial giant cell tumor (TGCT) associated with severe morbidity or functional limitations and not amenable to improvement with surgery.

	harboring an internal tandem duplication (ITD) mutation. Overexpression of the CSF1R ligand promotes cell proliferation and accumulation in the synovium. In vitro, pexidartinib inhibited proliferation of cell lines dependent on CSF1R and ligand-induced autophosphorylation of CSF1R. Pexidartinib also inhibited the proliferation of a CSF1R dependent cell line in vivo.	
Ponatinib/ Iclusig	ABL Ponatinib inhibited the in vitro tyrosine kinase activity of ABL and T315I mutant ABL with IC50 concentrations of 0.4 and 2.0 nM, respectively. Ponatinib inhibited the in vitro activity of additional kinases with IC50 concentrations between 0.1 and 20 nM, including members of the VEGFR, PDGFR, FGFR, EPH receptors and SRC families of kinases, and KIT, RET, TIE2, and FLT3. Ponatinib inhibited the in vitro viability of cells expressing native or mutant BCR-ABL, including T315I. In mice, treatment with ponatinib reduced the size of tumors expressing native or T315I mutant BCR-ABL when compared to controls.	Iclusig is a kinase inhibitor indicated for the: 1. Treatment of adult patients with chronic phase, accelerated phase, or blast phase chronic myeloid leukemia (CML) or Ph+ ALL for whom no other tyrosine kinase inhibitor (TKI) therapy is indicated. 2. Treatment of adult patients with T315I-positive CML (chronic phase, accelerated phase, or blast phase) or T315I-positive Philadelphia chromosome positive acute lymphoblastic leukemia (Ph+ ALL)
Pralsetinib/Gavreto	Kinase inhibitor of wild-type RET and oncogenic RET fusions and mutations.	For the treatment of adult patients with metastatic RET fusion-positive non-small cell lung cancer (NSCLC) as detected by an FDA approved test
Regorafenib/ Tafinlar	VEGFR1/2/3 Regorafenib is a small molecule inhibitor of multiple membrane-bound and intracellular kinases involved in normal cellular functions and in pathologic processes such as oncogenesis, tumor angiogenesis, and maintenance of the tumor microenvironment. In in vitro biochemical or cellular assays, regorafenib or its major human active metabolites M-2 and M-5 inhibited the activity of RET, VEGFR1, VEGFR2, VEGFR3, KIT, PDGFR-alpha, PDGFR-beta, FGFR1, FGFR2, TIE2, DDR2, Trk2A, Eph2A, RAF-1, BRAF, BRAFV600E , SAPK2, PTK5, and Abl at concentrations of regorafenib that	Metastatic colorectal cancer (CRC) who have been previously treated with fluoropyrimidine-, oxaliplatin- and irinotecan-based chemotherapy, an anti-VEGF therapy, and, if KRAS wild type, an anti-EGFR therapy

	have been achieved clinically. In in vivo models, regorafenib demonstrated anti-angiogenic activity in a rat tumor model, and inhibition of tumor growth as well as anti-metastatic activity in several mouse xenograft models including some for human colorectal carcinoma.	
Ribociclib/ Kisqali	CDK4/6 Ribociclib is an inhibitor of cyclin-dependent kinase (CDK) 4 and 6. These kinases are activated upon binding to Dcyclins and play a crucial role in signalling pathways which lead to cell cycle progression and cellular proliferation. The cyclin D-CDK4/6 complex regulates cell cycle progression through phosphorylation of the retinoblastoma protein (pRb). In vitro, ribociclib decreased pRb phosphorylation leading to arrest in the G1 phase of the cell cycle and reduced cell proliferation in non-Hodgkin's lymphoma cell lines. In vivo, treatment with single agent ribociclib in a rat xenograft model with human tumor cells led to decreased tumor volumes, which correlated with inhibition of pRb phosphorylation.	IBRANCE is a kinase inhibitor indicated for the treatment of adult patients with hormone receptor (HR)-positive, human epidermal growth factor receptor 2 (HER2)-negative advanced or metastatic breast cancer in combination with: • an aromatase inhibitor as initial endocrine-based therapy in postmenopausal women or in men; or • fulvestrant in patients with disease progression following endocrine therapy
Ripretinib/ QINLOCK™	KIT, PDGFRA	QINLOCK is a kinase inhibitor indicated for the treatment of adult patients with advanced gastrointestinal stromal tumor (GIST) who have received prior treatment with 3 or more kinase inhibitors, including imatinib. Ripretinib is a tyrosine kinase inhibitor that inhibits KIT proto-oncogene receptor tyrosine kinase (KIT) and platelet derived growth factor receptor A (PDGFRA) kinase, including wild type, primary, and secondary mutations. Ripretinib also inhibits other kinases in vitro, such as PDGFRB, TIE2, VEGFR2, and BRAF.
Ruxolitinib/ Jakafi	JAK1/2/3,Tyk Ruxolitinib, a kinase inhibitor, inhibits Janus Associated Kinases (JAKs) JAK1 and JAK2 which mediate the signalling of a number of cytokines and growth factors that are important for hematopoiesis and immune	Jakafi is a kinase inhibitor indicated for treatment of patients with intermediate or high-risk myelofibrosis, including primary myelofibrosis, post-polycythemia vera myelofibrosis and post-essential thrombocythemia

	function. JAK signalling involves recruitment of STATs (signal transducers and activators of transcription) to cytokine receptors, activation and subsequent localization of STATs to the nucleus leading to modulation of gene expression. Myelofibrosis (MF) is a myeloproliferative neoplasm (MPN) known to be associated with dysregulated JAK1 and JAK2 signalling. In a mouse model of JAK2V617F-positive MPN, oral administration of ruxolitinib prevented splenomegaly, preferentially decreased JAK2V617F mutant cells in the spleen and decreased circulating inflammatory cytokines (eg, TNF-α, IL-6).	myelofibrosis
Selpercatinib/ RETEVMO	RET Selpercatinib is a kinase inhibitor. Selpercatinib inhibited wild-type RET and multiple mutated RET isoforms as well as VEGFR1 and VEGFR3 with IC50 values ranging from 0.92 nM to 67.8 nM. In other enzyme assays, selpercatinib also inhibited FGFR 1, 2, and 3 at higher concentrations that were still clinically achievable. In cellular assays, selpercatinib inhibited RET at approximately 60-fold lower concentrations than FGFR1 and 2 and approximately 8-fold lower concentration than VEGFR3. Certain point mutations in RET or chromosomal rearrangements involving in-frame fusions of RET with various partners can result in constitutively activated chimeric RET fusion proteins that can act as oncogenic drivers by promoting cell proliferation of tumor cell lines. In in vitro and in vivo tumor models, selpercatinib demonstrated anti-tumor activity in cells harboring constitutive activation of RET protein resulting from gene fusions and mutations, including CCDC6-RET, KIF5B-RET, RET V804M, and RET M918T. In addition, selpercatinib showed anti-tumor activity in mice intracranially implanted with a patient-derived RET fusion positive tumor.	RETEVMO is a kinase inhibitor indicated for the treatment of: • Adult patients with metastatic RET fusion-positive non-small cell lung cancer (NSCLC)1 • Adult and pediatric patients 12 years of age and older with advanced or metastatic RET-mutant medullary thyroid cancer (MTC) who require systemic therapy • Adult and pediatric patients 12 years of age and older with advanced or metastatic RET fusion-positive thyroid cancer who require systemic therapy and who are radioactive iodine-refractory (if radioactive iodine is appropriate). 1 This indication is approved under accelerated approval based on overall response rate and duration of response. Continued approval for this indication may be contingent upon verification and description of clinical benefit in confirmatory Selpercatinib is a kinase inhibitor. Selpercatinib inhibited wild-type RET and multiple mutated RET isoforms as well as VEGFR1 and VEGFR3 with IC50 values ranging from 0.92 nM to 67.8 nM. In other enzyme assays, selpercatinib also inhibited FGFR 1, 2, and 3 at higher concentrations that were still clinically achievable. In cellular assays, selpercatinib inhibited RET at approximately

		60-fold lower concentrations than FGFR1 and 2 and approximately 8-fold lower concentration than VEGFR3. Certain point mutations in RET or chromosomal rearrangements involving in-frame fusions of RET with various partners can result in constitutively activated chimeric RET fusion proteins that can act as oncogenic drivers by promoting cell proliferation of tumor cell lines. In in vitro and in vivo tumor models, selpercatinib demonstrated anti-tumor activity in cells harboring constitutive activation of RET protein resulting from gene fusions and mutations, including CCDC6-RET, KIF5B-RET, RET V804M, and RET M918T. In addition, selpercatinib showed Reference ID: 4605720 anti-tumor activity in mice intracranially implanted with a patient-derived RET fusion positive tumor trial(s).
Selumetinib/ KOSELUGO	MEK1/2 Selumetinib is an inhibitor of mitogen-activated protein kinase kinases 1 and 2 (MEK1/2). MEK1/2 proteins are upstream regulators of the extracellular signal-related kinase (ERK) pathway. Both MEK and ERK are critical components of the RAS-regulated RAF-MEK-ERK pathway, which is often activated in different types of cancers. In genetically modified mouse models of NF1 that generate neurofibromas that recapitulate the genotype and phenotype of human NF1, oral dosing of selumetinib inhibited ERK phosphorylation, and reduced neurofibroma numbers, volume, and proliferation.	KOSELUGO is a kinase inhibitor indicated for the treatment of pediatric patients 2 years of age and older with neurofibromatosis type 1 (NF1) who have symptomatic, inoperable plexiform neurofibromas (PN).
Sorafenib/ Nexavar	VEGFR1/2/3 Sorafenib has been shown to inhibit multiple intracellular (c-CRAF, BRAF and mutant BRAF) and cell surface kinases (KIT, FLT- 3, RET, RET/PTC, VEGFR-1, VEGFR- 2, VEGFR- 3, and PDGFR-ß). Several of these kinases are thought to be involved in tumor cell signalling, angiogenesis and apoptosis. Sorafenib inhibited tumor growth of HCC, RCC, and DTC human tumor	Treatment of 1.Unresectable hepatocellular carcinoma (HCC) 2. Advanced renal cell carcinoma (RCC) 3. Locally recurrent or metastatic, progressive, differentiated thyroid carcinoma (DTC) refractory to radioactive iodine treatment

	xenografts in immunocompromised mice. Reductions in tumor angiogenesis were seen in models of HCC and RCC upon sorafenib treatment, and increases in tumor apoptosis were observed in models of HCC, RCC, and DTC.	
Sunitinib/ Sutent	Multiple kinases. Sunitinib is a small molecule that inhibits multiple receptor tyrosine kinases (RTKs), some of which are implicated in tumor growth, pathologic angiogenesis, and metastatic progression of cancer. Sunitinib was evaluated for its inhibitory activity against a variety of kinases (>80 kinases) and was identified as an inhibitor of platelet-derived growth factor receptors (PDGFRα and PDGFRβ), vascular endothelial growth factor receptors (VEGFR1, VEGFR2 and VEGFR3), stem cell factor receptor (KIT), Fms-like tyrosine kinase-3 (FLT3), colony stimulating factor receptor Type 1 (CSF-1R), and the glial cell-line derived neurotrophic factor receptor (RET). Sunitinib inhibited the phosphorylation of multiple RTKs (PDGFRβ, VEGFR2, KIT) in tumor xenografts expressing RTK targets in vivo and demonstrated inhibition of tumor growth or tumor regression and/or inhibited metastases in some experimental models of cancer. Sunitinib demonstrated the ability to inhibit growth of tumor cells expressing dysregulated target RTKs (PDGFR, RET, or KIT) in vitro and to inhibit PDGFRβ- and VEGFR2-dependent tumor angiogenesis in vivo.	The treatment of: 1. Gastrointestinal stromal tumor (GIST) after disease progression on or intolerance to imatinib mesylate. 2. Advanced renal cell carcinoma (RCC). 3. Progressive, well-differentiated pancreatic neuroendocrine tumors (pNET) in patients with unresectable locally advanced or metastatic disease
Tofacitinib/ Xeljanz/ Xeljanz XR	JAK Tofacitinib is a Janus kinase (JAK) inhibitor. JAKs are intracellular enzymes which transmit signals arising from cytokine or growth factor-receptor interactions on the cellular membrane to influence cellular processes of hematopoiesis and immune cell function. Within the signalling pathway, JAKs phosphorylate and activate Signal Transducers and Activators of Transcription (STATs) which modulate intracellular activity including gene expression.	1. Rheumatoid arthritis: XELJANZ/XELJANZ XR is indicated for the treatment of adult patients with moderately to severely active rheumatoid arthritis who have had an inadequate response or intolerance to methotrexate. It may be used as monotherapy or in combination with methotrexate or other non-biologic disease-modifying antrheumatic drugs (DMARDs). ○ Limitations of use: use of XELJANZ/XELJANZ XR in

	Tofacitinib modulates the signalling pathway at the point of JAKs, preventing the phosphorylation and activation of 26 Reference ID: 4467787 STATs. JAK enzymes transmit cytokine signalling through pairing of JAKs (e.g., JAK1/JAK3, JAK1/JAK2, JAK1/TyK2, JAK2 /JAK2). Tofacitinib inhibited the in vitro activities of JAK1/JAK2, JAK1/JAK3, and JAK2/JAK2 combinations with IC50 of 406, 56, and 1377 nM, respectively. However, the relevance of specific JAK combinations to therapeutic effectiveness is not known.	combination with biologic DMARDs or potent immunosuppressants such as azathioprine and cyclosporine is not recommended. 2. Psoriatic arthritis: XELJANZ/XELJANZ XR is indicated for the treatment of adult patients with active psoriatic arthritis who have had an inadequate response or intolerance to methotrexate or other disease-modifying anti-rheumatic drugs (DMARDs). ○ Limitations of use: use of XELJANZ/XELJANZ XR in combination with biologic DMARDs or potent immunosuppressants such as azathioprine and cyclosporine is not recommended. 3. Ulcerative colitis: XELJANZ is indicated for the treatment of adult patients with moderately to severely active ulcerative colitis (UC), who have had an inadequate response or who are intolerant to TNF blockers. ○ Limitations of use: use of XELJANZ in combination with biological therapies for UC or with potent immunosuppressants such as azathioprine and cyclosporine is not recommended.
Trametinib/ Mekinist	MEK1/2 Trametinib is a reversible inhibitor of mitogen-activated extracellular signal-regulated kinase 1 (MEK1) and MEK2 activation and of MEK1 and MEK2 kinase activity. MEK proteins are upstream regulators of the extracellular signal-related kinase (ERK) pathway, which promotes cellular proliferation. BRAF V600E mutations result in constitutive activation of the BRAF pathway which includes MEK1 and MEK2. Trametinib inhibits cell growth of various BRAF V600 mutation-positive tumors in vitro and in vivo. Trametinib and dabrafenib target two different kinases in the RAS/RAF/MEK/ERK pathway. Use of trametinib and dabrafenib in combination resulted in greater growth inhibition of BRAF V600 mutation-positive tumor cell	MEKINIST is a kinase inhibitor indicated as a single agent for the treatment of patients with unresectable or metastatic melanoma with BRAF V600E or V600K mutations as detected by an FDA-approved test. MEKINIST is indicated, in combination with dabrafenib, for: • the treatment of patients with unresectable or metastatic melanoma with BRAF V600E or V600K mutations as detected by an FDA-approved test. • the adjuvant treatment of patients with melanoma with BRAF V600E or V600K mutations, as detected by an FDA-approved test, and involvement of lymph node(s),

	lines in vitro and prolonged inhibition of tumor growth in BRAF V600 mutation positive tumor xenografts compared with either drug alone.	following complete resection. • the treatment of patients with metastatic non-small cell lung cancer (NSCLC) with BRAF V600E mutation as detected by an FDA-approved test. Limitation of Use: MEKINIST is not indicated for treatment of patients with melanoma who have progressed on prior BRAF-inhibitor therapy
Tucatinib/TUKYSA	HER2 Tucatinib is a tyrosine kinase inhibitor of HER2. In vitro, tucatinib inhibits phosphorylation of HER2 and HER3, resulting in inhibition of downstream MAPK and AKT signaling and cell proliferation, and showed antitumor activity in HER2 expressing tumor cells. In vivo, tucatinib inhibited the growth of HER2 expressing tumors. The combination of tucatinib and trastuzumab showed increased anti-tumor activity in vitro and in vivo compared to either drug alone.	TUKYSA is a kinase inhibitor indicated in combination with trastuzumab and capecitabine for treatment of adult patients with advanced unresectable or metastatic HER2-positive breast cancer, including patients with brain metastases, who have received one or more prior anti-HER2-based regimens in the metastatic setting
Vemurafenib/ Zalora	B-Raf Vemurafenib is a low molecular weight, orally available inhibitor of some mutated forms of BRAF serine-threonine kinase, including BRAF V600E. Vemurafenib also inhibits other kinases in vitro such as CRAF, ARAF, wild-type BRAF, SRMS, ACK1, MAP4K5, and FGR at similar concentrations. Some mutations in the BRAF gene including V600E result in constitutively activated BRAF proteins, which can cause cell proliferation in the absence of growth factors that would normally be required for proliferation. Vemurafenib has anti-tumor effects in cellular and animal models of melanoma with mutated BRAF V600E.	ZELBORAF® is a kinase inhibitor indicated for the treatment of patients with unresectable or metastatic melanoma with BRAF V600E mutation as detected by an FDA-approved test. Limitation of Use: ZELBORAF is not indicated for treatment of patients with wild-type BRAF melanoma.
Upadacitinib/Rinvaq	Janus kinase inhibitor	The treatment of adults with moderately to severely active rheumatoid arthritis who have had an inadequate response or intolerance to methotrexate. Limitation of use: use of RINVOQ in combination with other JAK inhibitors, biologic DMARDs, or with potent immunosuppressants

		such as azathioprine and cyclosporine is not recommended

To this list can now be added the CAR T cell therapies approved by the USA FDA for therapeutic use (Table 3).

Table 3. FDA-approved CAR T cell therapies.

Generic name	**Brand name**	**Target antigen**	**Targeted disease**	**Patient population**
Tisagenlecleucel	Kymriah	CD19	B cell acute lymphoblastic leukemia (ALL); B cell non-Hodgkin lymphoma (NHL)	Children and young adults with refractory or relapsed (r/r) B cell ALL Adults with r/y B cell NHL
Axicabtagene ciloleucel	Yescarta	CD19	B cell NHL Follicular lymphoma	Adults with r/r B cell NHL Adults with r/r follicular NHL
Brexucabtagene	Tecartus	CD19	Mantle cell lymphoma	Adults with

autoleucel			(MCL) B cell ALL	r/r MCL Adults with r/r B cell ALL
Lisocabtagene maraleucel	Breyanzi	CD19	B cell NHL	Adults with r/ry B cell NHL
Idecabtagene vicleucel	Abecma	B cell maturation antigen (BCMA)	Multiple myeloma (MM)	Adults with r/r MM
Ciltacabtagene autoleucel	Carvikti	BCMA	MM	Adults with r/r MM

[1]Ogden Carr Bruton (1908 - 2003) was an American pediatrician

Summary of treatments derived from of the biological discoveries in the last 70 years

94 monoclonal antibodies (including biosimilars) and 59 small molecule protein kinase inhibitors are now FDA-approved for therapeutic purposes. Additional classes of therapeutics include new cellular therapies including gene-modified cellular therapies and gene therapies.

All these agents will be described in detail in each book on diseases for which they have been approved.

This book deals only with the use of **CAR T cell therapies.** It is one in a series of books on the impact of targeted biological and specifically designed therapeutic agents across the whole field of medicine in a series called Medicine 2020.

3. The biology of normal human cells

To fully understand how these new therapeutic agents work it is useful to understand how cells work – in particular what signalling pathways they use. Normal cells and cells in tissues affected by non- diseases use signalling pathways often different from those used by cells.

All human cells are derived from a single totipotent stem cell which is produced by the fusion of a single sperm with a single ovum. This totipotent stem cell has all the genes on its chromosomes responsible for the future growth and development of the fetus, including reproductive capacity. Cell biology is concerned with the physiological properties, metabolic processes, signalling pathways, life cycle, chemical composition and interactions of cells with their environment. Cell biology involves genetics, biochemistry, molecular biology, immunology and cytochemistry. Human cells are eukaryotes - they contain organelles. The generalized structure of a eukaryotic cell is shown in Figure 2.

Figure 2. A diagram of a mammalian cell

This image has been released into the public domain by its author, LadyofHats (Mariana Ruiz). Source: own work using Adobe Illustrator. Image renamed from Image:Animal cell structure.svg. https://commons.wikimedia.org/wiki/File:Animal_cell_structure_en.svg. No changes have been made to this image.

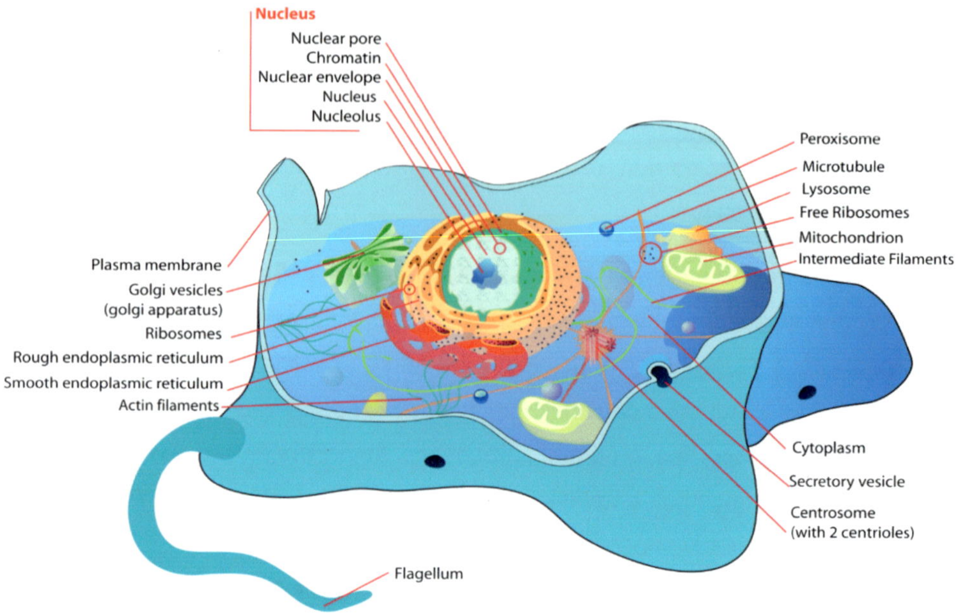

Most of the processes of eukaryotic cells are performed by a mixture of small organic molecules, inorganic ions, hormones and water. Approximately 75-85% of the cell's volume is due to water making it an indispensable solvent as a result of its polarity and structure. The shape of cells are generally round and spherical or oval.

The main constituents of the cell include proteins and lipids which are either free-flowing or membrane-bound, along with different internal compartments known as organelles. The cytoplasm is all of the material within a cell, enclosed by the cell membrane, except for the cell nucleus. The material inside the nucleus and contained within the nuclear membrane is termed the nucleoplasm. A cell's DNA, contained on the cell's chromosomes, is located within the cell's nucleus. The main components of the cytoplasm are cytosol – a gel-like substance, the organelles – the cell's internal sub-structures - and various cytoplasmic inclusions. Cell are composed of hydrophilic and hydrophobic regions. The hydrophilic regions of the cell are on both the inside and outside of the cell, while the hydrophobic regions are within the phospholipid bilayer of the cell membrane. A diagram of a mammalian cell membrane is shown in Figure 3. This shows the detailed diagram of lipid bilayer cell membrane. The cell membrane, also called the plasma membrane or plasmalemma, biological molecules, primarily proteins and lipids, which are involved in a vast array of cellular processes. It also serves as the attachment point for both the intracellular cytoskeleton and, if present, the cell wall.

Figure 3.

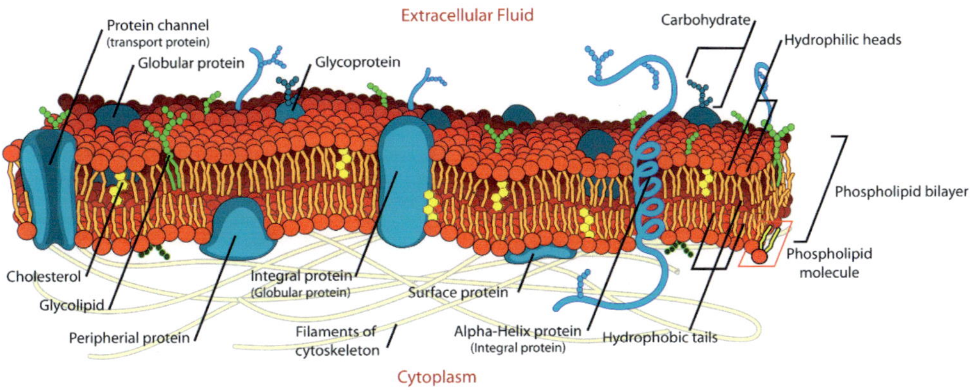

This image, reproduced here from Wikimedia Commons, has been released into the public domain by its author, LadyofHats (Mariana Ruiz). Source: Own work. Image renamed from File:Cell membrane detailed diagram.svg. https://commons.wikimedia.org/wiki/File:Cell_membrane_detailed_diagram_en.svg. No changes have been made to this image.

In order for molecules to participate in reactions within the cell, they need to be able to cross this membrane layer to get into the cell. They accomplish this process of gaining access to the cell via osmotic pressure, diffusion, concentration gradients, and membrane channels. Inside the cell are extensive internal suB cellular membrane-bounded compartments called organelles.

Figure 4. Some of the cell surface proteins and internal signalling pathways of a normal human cell.

This image, reproduced here from Wikimedia Commons is in the public domain in the United States because it is a work prepared by an officer or employee of the United States Government as part of that person's official duties under the terms of Title 17, Chapter 1, Section 105 of the US Code. Source: http://dir.niehs.nih.gov/dirlst/imagemap/cell.jpg. https://commons.wikimedia.org/wiki/File:NIEHScell.jpg. No changes have been made to this image.

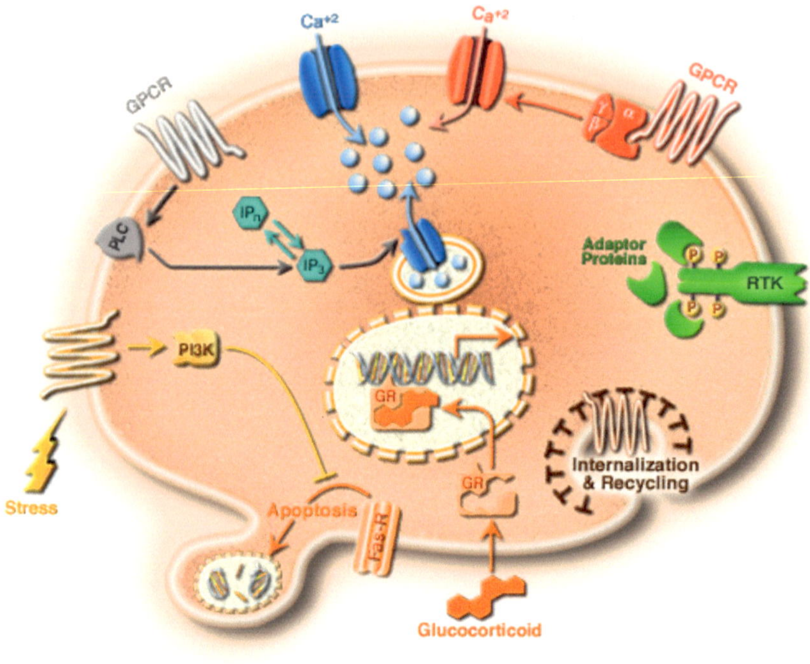

Cell growth pertains to the increase in the number of cells present in an organism as it grows and develops; in order for the organism to grow the number of cells present must increase. To enable cell growth and development the cell goes through the steps of the cell cycle: DNA replication, cell division, regeneration, specialization, and cell death. The cell cycle is divided into four distinct phases, G1, S, G2, and M. The G phases (cell growth) make up approximately 95% of the cycle. After proliferation cells then differentiate to become specialized in order to form specialized tissues, then organs and ultimately systems. The G phases along with the S phase – DNA replication, damage and repair - are considered to be the interphase portion of the cycle. While the M phase (mitosis and cytokinesis) is the cell division portion of the cycle. The cell cycle is regulated by a series of signalling factors and complexes such as cyclin-dependent kinases and p53. When the cell has completed its growth process, and if it is found to be damaged or altered, it undergoes cell death, either by apoptosis or necrosis, in order to eliminate the threat it can cause to the organism's survival. Some of the main cell surface proteins and internal signalling processes are shown in Figure 3.

Essential cell processes include

- Active transport and passive transport – the movement of molecules into and out of cells
- Adhesion - holding cells and tissues together
- Cell movement - chemotaxis, contraction and cilia
- Cell signalling - regulation of cell behaviour by signals from outside and inside the cell
- Division – the process by which cells reproduce either by mitosis (to produce clones of the parent cell) or meiosis (to produce haploid gametes either male [sperm)] or female [ova]) dependent on the gender of the organism
- DNA repair - cell death and cell senescence
- Metabolism - glycolysis, respiration, photosynthesis, and chemosynthesis
- Signal transduction - the process by which the activities in the cell are regulated
- Transcription and mRNA splicing - gene expression

Three of the most important processes – signal transduction, gene expression and apoptosis (also known as programmed cell death) - are described furtherl below. Some of the most important pathways for understanding the basis of targeted therapies, such as the pathways for angiogenesis, interkeukin (IL) 4, IL-12 and IL-23 and the TNF pathways are described in chapters dealing with the therapeutic use of molecules involved in these pathways.

Signal transduction and cell signalling pathways

Signal transduction is the process by which a chemical or physical signal is transmitted through a cell as a series of molecular events, most commonly protein phosphorylation catalyzed by protein kinases, which ultimately results in a cellular response. Proteins responsible for detecting stimuli such as ligands are termed receptors The changes elicited by ligand binding to a receptor give rise to a biochemical cascade otherwise known as a signalling path. A simplified representation of major signal transduction pathways in mammals is shown in Figure 5.

Figure 5

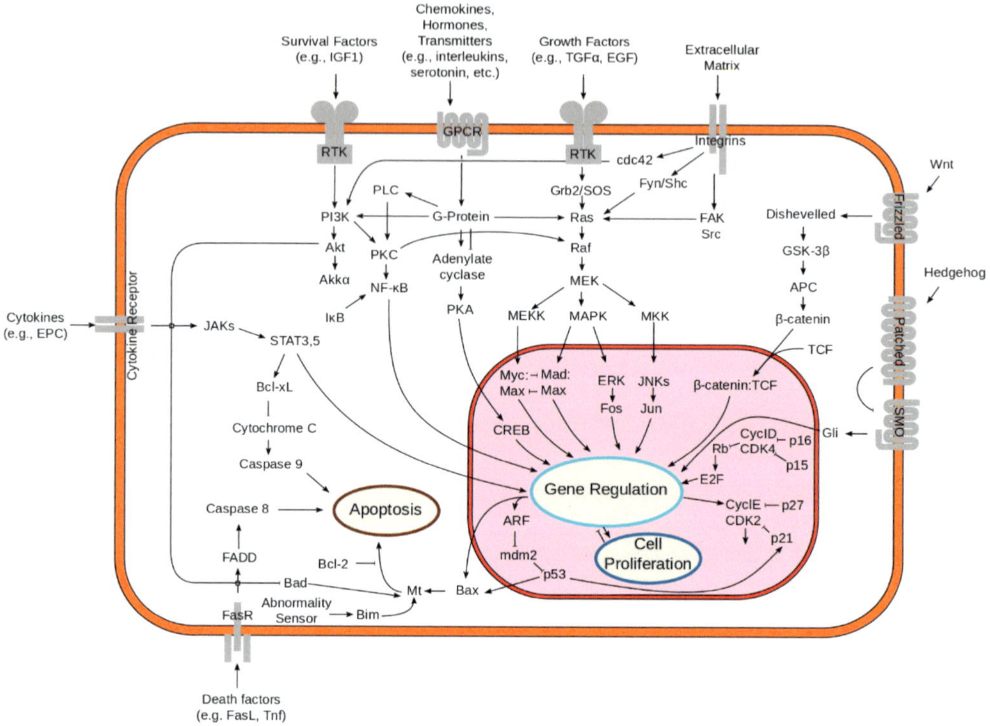

Figure 5. A simplified representation of major signal transduction pathways in mammals. This image is reproduced here from Wikimedia Commons since permission has been granted by its creator, Cybertory, to copy, distribute and/or modify this document under the terms of the GNU Free Documentation License, Version 1.2 or any later version published by the Free Software Foundation. Author: By Cybertory - This file was derived from: Signal transduction v1.png, CC BY-SA 3.0, https://commons.wikimedia.org/w/index.php?curid=12081090; https://en.wikipedia.org/wiki/Creative_Commons_license. No changes have been made to the image

When signalling pathways interact with one another they form networks, which allow cellular responses to be coordinated, often by combinatorial signalling events. At the molecular level, such responses include changes in the transcription or translation of genes, and post-translational and conformational changes in proteins, as well as changes in their location. These molecular events are the basic mechanisms controlling cell growth, proliferation, metabolism and many other processes. In multicellular organisms, signal transduction pathways have evolved to regulate cell communication in a wide variety of ways.

Each component (or node) of a signalling pathway is classified according to the role it plays with respect to the initial stimulus. Ligands are termed first messengers, while receptors are the signal transducers, which then activate primary effectors. Such effectors are often linked to second messengers, which can activate secondary effectors, and so on. Depending on the efficiency of the nodes, a signal can be amplified (a concept known as signal gain), so that one signalling molecule can generate a response involving hundreds to millions of molecules With the advent of computational biology, the analysis of signalling pathways and networks has become an essential tool to understand cellular functions and disease, including signalling rewiring mechanisms underlying responses to acquired drug resistance.

Ligands

The majority of signal transduction pathways involve the binding of signalling molecules, known as ligands, to receptors that trigger events inside the cell. The binding of a signalling molecule with a receptor causes a change in the conformation of the receptor, known as receptor activation. Most ligands are soluble molecules from the extracellular medium which bind to cell surface receptors. These include growth factors, cytokines and neurotransmitters. Components of the extracellular matrix such as fibronectin and hyaluronan can also bind to such receptors (integrins and CD44, respectively). In addition, some molecules such as steroid hormones are lipid-soluble and thus cross the plasma membrane to reach nuclear receptors.

Some receptors such as HER2/neu are capable of ligand-independent activation when overexpressed or mutated. This leads to constitutive activation of the pathway, which may or may not be overturned by compensation mechanisms. In the case of HER2, which acts as a dimerization partner of other EGFRs, constitutive activation leads to hyperproliferation and cancer – primarily some cases of breast cancer and gastric cancer (HER2/neu is also known as receptor tyrosine-protein kinase erbB-2, CD340, proto-oncogene Neu and ERBB2). A ribbon diagram of the Fab fragment of trastuzumab, a monoclonal antibody, bound to the extracellulardomain of HER2 is shown in Figure 6.

Figure 6.

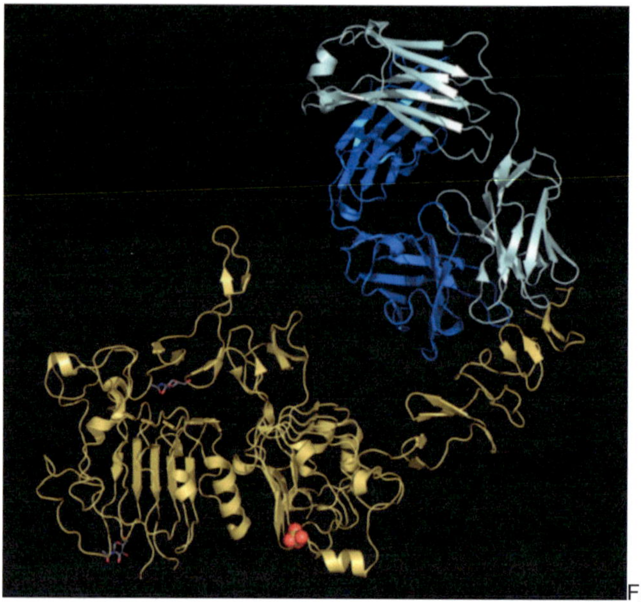

Figure 6

Figure 6. Ribbon diagram of the Fab fragment of trastuzumab, a monoclonal antibody, bound to the extracellular domain of HER2. Legend: Trastuzumab Fab fragment, heavy chain ; Trastuzumab Fab fragment, light chain ; HER2, extracellular domain This image, reproduced here from Wikimedia Commons, is in the public domain because its creator, Fvasconcellos, has placed it there. https://commons.wikimedia.org/wiki/File:Trastuzumab_Fab-HER2_complex_1N8Z.png#/media/File:Trastuzumab_Fab-HER2_complex_1N8Z.png; https://commons.wikimedia.org/wiki/User:Fvasconcellos. Created using Accelrys DS Visualizer Pro 1.6 and GIMP. More information: Cho HS, Mason K, Ramyar KX, et al. (2003). "Structure of the extracellular region of HER2 alone and in complex with the Herceptin Fab". Nature 421 (6924): 756–60. PMID 12610629. doi:10.1038/nature01392. No changes have been made to this image.

Extracellular receptors, ligand binding, messengers and adaptor proteins

Extracellular receptors are integral transmembrane proteins that span the plasma membrane (Figure 2) of the cell, with one part of the receptor on the outside of the cell and the other on the inside. Signal transduction occurs as a result of a ligand binding to the outside region of the receptor (the ligand does not pass through the membrane). Ligand-receptor binding induces a change in the conformation of the inside part of the receptor, a process sometimes called "receptor activation". This results in either the activation of an enzyme domain of the receptor or the exposure of a binding site for other intracellular signalling proteins within the cell, eventually propagating the signal through the cytoplasm (Figure 5).

In mammalian cells most intracellular proteins activated by a ligand/receptor interaction possess an enzymatic activity; examples include tyrosine kinases and phosphatases. Often such enzymes are covalently linked to the receptor. Some of them create second messengers such as cyclic AMP and IP3, the latter controlling the release of intracellular calcium stores into the cytoplasm. Other activated proteins interact with adaptor proteins (an example is shown Figure 4) that facilitate signalling protein interactions and coordination of signalling complexes necessary to respond to a particular stimulus. Enzymes and adaptor proteins are both responsive to various second messenger molecules.

Many adaptor proteins and enzymes activated as part of signal transduction possess specialized protein domains that bind to specific secondary messenger molecules. For example, calcium ions bind to the EF hand domains of calmodulin, allowing it to bind and activate calmodulin-dependent kinase.

The following major extracellular receptor/ligand binding pathways will be discussed in more detail below:

- G protein-coupled receptors
- Tyrosine, seronine/threonine- and histidine-specific protein kinases
- Integrins
- Toll-like receptors
- Ligand-gated ion binding channels

G proteins, also known as guanine nucleotide-binding proteins, are a family of proteins that act as molecular switches inside cells, and are involved in transmitting signals from a variety of stimuli outside a cell to its interior. Their activity is regulated by factors that control their ability to bind to and hydrolyze guanosine triphosphate (GTP) to guanosine diphosphate (GDP). When they are bound to GTP, they are 'on', and, when they are bound to GDP, they are 'off'.

They possess seven transmembrane domains and are linked to a heterotrimeric G protein. A ribbon diagram of a G protein is shown in Figure 7. Beta and gamma subunits of G-protein are shown by blue and red, respectively, in the phosducin-transducin beta-gamma complex. (Phosducin binds tightly to the beta gamma subunits (Gt beta gamma) of the heterotrimeric G protein transducin, preventing Gt beta gamma reassociation with Gt alpha-GDP and thereby inhibiting the G-protein cycle).

Figure 7. Ribbon diagram of a G protein

This image, reproduced here from Wikimedia Commons, has been released into the public domain by its creator, Andrei Lomize, has placed it there. By Andrei Lomize - Own work, Public Domain,

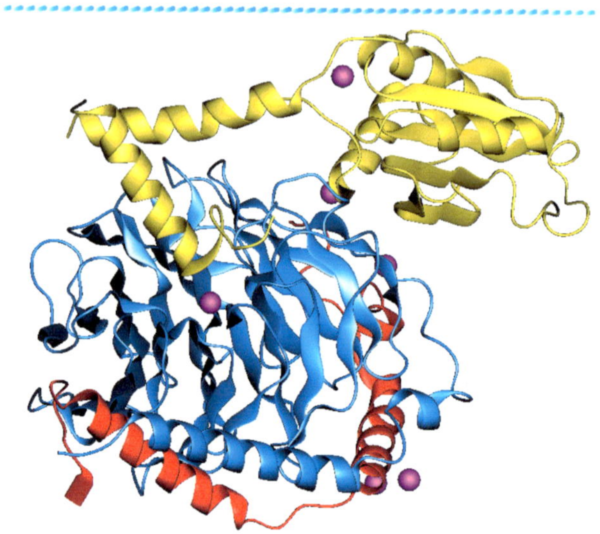

Tyrosine and seronine/threonine-specific protein kinases

Receptor tyrosine kinases (RTKs) are transmembrane proteins with an intracellular kinase domain and an extracellular domain that binds ligands (Figure 4); examples include growth factor receptors such as the insulin receptor. To perform signal transduction, RTKs need to form dimers in the plasma membrane. The dimer is stabilized by ligands binding to the receptor. The interaction between the cytoplasmic domains stimulates the autophosphorylation of tyrosine residues within the intracellular kinase domains of the RTKs, causing conformational changes. Subsequent to this, the receptors' kinase domains are activated, initiating phosphorylation signalling cascades of downstream cytoplasmic molecules that facilitate various cellular processes such as cell differentiation and metabolism. Many serine/threonine and dual-specificity protein kinases are important for signal transduction, either acting downstream of receptor tyrosine kinases, or as membrane-embedded or cell-soluble versions in their own right. The process of signal transduction involves around 560 known protein kinases and pseudokinanases, encoded by the human kinome. The kinome of an organism is the complete set of protein kinases encoded in its genome.

As is the case with GPCRs, proteins that bind GTP play a major role in signal transduction from the activated RTK into the cell. In this case, the G proteins are members of the Ras, Rho (see Figure 4 above), and Raf families, referred to collectively as small G proteins. They act as molecular switches usually tethered to membranes by isoprenyl groups linked to their carboxyl ends. Upon activation, they assign proteins to specific membrane subdomains where they participate in signalling. Activated RTKs in turn activate small G proteins that activate guanine nucleotide exchange factors such as SOS1. Once activated, these exchange factors can activate more small G proteins, thus amplifying the receptor's initial signal. The mutation of certain RTK genes, as with that of GPCRs, can result in the expression of receptors that exist in a constitutively activated state. Such mutated genes may act as oncogenes. An example is the BCR-ABL gene, which is translated to the BCR-ABL protein, a growth factor responsible for the development of chronic myeloid leukemia (CML). The first tyrosine kinase inhibitor developed that was therapeutically successful is imatinib, now routinely used as first-line treatment of CML, obviating the need in many cases of the only curative treatment for CML – allogeneic hematopoietic stem cell transplantaion, a procedure that had a treatment-related mortality of 20-30%.

Integrins

Integrins are produced by a wide variety of cells. They play a role in cell attachment to other cells and the extracellular matrix and in the transduction of signals from extracellular matrix components such as fibronectin and collagen (Figure 8).

Figure 8. An overview of integrin-mediated signal transduction, adapted from Hehlgens et al. (2007).

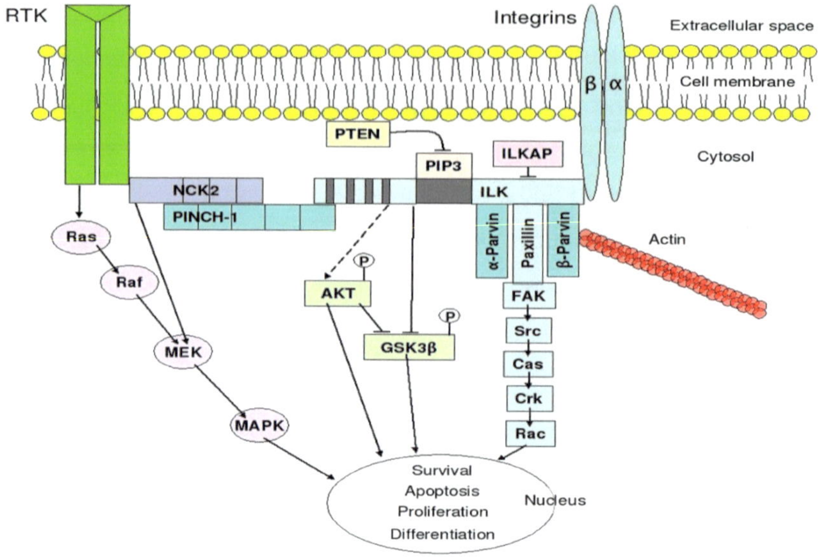

This image, reproduced here from Wikimedia Commons, has been released into the public domain by its author, K.murphy at English Wikipedia. https://commons.wikimedia.org/wiki/File:Integrin_sig_trans_overview.jpeg. Original source: Hehlgans S, Haase M, Cordes N (Jan 2007). "Signalling via integrins: implications for cell survival and anticancer strategies". Biochimica et Biophysica Acta. 1775 (1): 163–80. doi:10.1016/j.bbcan.2006.09.001. PMID 17084981.

Ligand binding to the extracellular domain of integrins changes the protein's conformation, clustering it at the cell membrane to initiate signal transduction. Integrins lack kinase activity; hence, integrin-mediated signal transduction is achieved through a variety of intracellular protein kinases and adaptor molecules, the main coordinator being integrin-linked kinase. As shown in Figure 7, cooperative integrin-RTK signalling determines the timing of cellular survival, apoptosis, proliferation and differentiation.

Toll-like receptors

When activated, toll-like receptors (TLRs) take adapter molecules within the cytoplasm of cells in order to propagate a signal.

Figure 9. Cellular signalling pathways activated by Toll-like receptors. Dashed grey lines represent unknown associations.

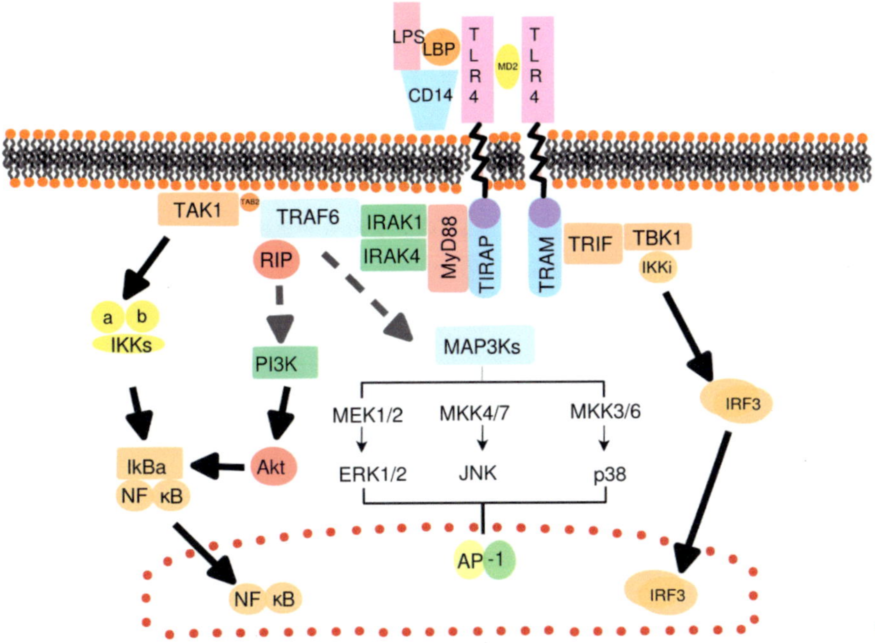

Four adaptor molecules are known to be involved in signalling. These are Myd88, TIRAP, TRIF, and TRAM. These adapter molecules activate other intracellular molecules such as IRAK1, IRAK4, TBK1, and IKKi that amplify the signal, eventually leading to the induction or suppression of genes that cause certain responses. Thousands of genes are activated by TLR signalling, implying that this method constitutes an important gateway for gene modulation.

Messenger systems

First messengers are the signalling molecules (hormones, neurotransmitters and paracrine/autocrine agents) that reach the cell from the extracellular fluid and bind to their specific receptors.

Second messengers are the substances that enter the cytoplasm and act within the cell to trigger a response. Second messengers serve as chemical relays from the plasma membrane to the cytoplasm, thus carrying out intracellular signal transduction.

Calcium

The release of calcium ions from the endoplasmic reticulum (Figure 1) into the cytosol results in its binding to signalling proteins that are then activated. It is then sequestered in the smooth endoplasmic reticulum and the mitochondria (Figure 1). Calcium is used in many processes including muscle contraction, neurotransmitter release from nerve endings, and cell migration. The three main pathways that lead to its activation are GPCR pathways, RTK pathways, and gated ion channels. It regulates proteins either directly or by binding to an enzyme.

Cellular responses

Gene activations and metabolism alterations are examples of cellular responses to extracellular stimulation that require signal transduction. Gene activation leads to further cellular effects, since the products of responding genes include instigators of activation. Transcription factors produced as a result of a signal transduction cascade can activate even more genes. Hence, an initial stimulus can trigger the expression of a large number of genes, leading to physiological events. Examples are the increased uptake of glucose from the blood stream and the migration of neutrophils to sites of infection.

Mammalian cells require stimulation for cell division and survival. In the absence of growth factor, apoptosis (programmed cell death – see below) ensues. Such requirements for extracellular stimulation are necessary for controlling cell behavior. Signal transduction pathways are perceived to be so central to biological processes that a large number of diseases are attributed to their dysregulation. Three basic types of signals determine cellular growth:

1. **Stimulatory signals (growth factors)**

Transcription-dependent response

Steroids are an example of this. They bind DNA, which needs to be transcribed. The produced mRNA needs to be translated, and the produced protein/peptide can undergo posttranslational modification (PMT).

Transcription-independent response

Epidermal growth factor (EGF) is an example. It binds to the epidermal growth factor receptor (EGFR), which causes dimerization and autophosphorylation of the EGFR, which in turn activates the intracellular signalling pathway.

2. **Inhibitory signals (cell-cell contact)**

3. **Permissive signals (cell-matrix interactions)**

The combination of these signals are integrated in an altered cytoplasmic machinery which leads to altered cell behaviour.

Major cell signalling pathways

The following are some of the major cell signalling pathways, demonstrating how ligands binding to their receptors can affect second messengers and eventually result in altered cellular responses.

- MAPK/ERK pathway: a pathway that couples intracellular responses to the binding of growth factors to cell surface receptors. This pathway is very complex and includes many protein components. In many cell types, activation of this pathway promotes cell division, and many forms of cancer are associated with aberrations in it.

- cAMP-dependent pathway: cAMP works by activating protein kinase A (PKA, cAMP-dependent protein kinase (Figure 11). Further effects depend mainly on cAMP-dependent protein kinase, which vary based on the type of cell involved.

- IP3/DAG pathway: PLC cleaves the phospholipid phosphatidylinositol 4,5-bisphosphate (PIP2), yielding diacyl glycerol (DAG) and inositol 1,4,5-triphosphate (IP3). DAG remains bound to the membrane, and IP3 is released as a soluble structure into the cytosol. IP3 then diffuses through the cytosol to bind to IP3 receptors, particular calcium channels in the endoplasmic reticulum (ER). These channels are specific to calcium and allow the passage of only calcium to move through. This causes the cytosolic concentration of calcium to increase, in turn precipitating a cascade of intracellular changes and activity. In addition, calcium and DAG together work to activate PKC, which then phosphorylates other molecules, leading to altered cellular activity.

DNA, RNA and genes

DNA is a molecule composed of two chains that coil around each other to form a double helix carrying the genetic instructions used in the growth, development, functioning, and reproduction of all known organisms and many viruses. DNA and ribonucleic acid (RNA) are nucleic acids. Nucleic acids, together with proteins, lipids and complex carbohydrates (polysaccharides), are one of the four major types of macromolecules that are essential for all known forms of life.

The two DNA strands are also known as polynucleotides as they are composed of simpler monomeric units called nucleotides. Each nucleotide is composed of one of four nitrogen-containing nucleobases (cytosine [C], guanine [G], adenine [A] or thymine [T]), a sugar called deoxyribose, and a phosphate group.

Figure 10 is a graphic of DNA replication. The nitrogenous bases of the two separate polynucleotide strands are bound together, according to base pairing rules (A with T and C with G), with hydrogen bonds to make double-stranded DNA in a helical form.

Figure 10. A graphic of DNA replication.

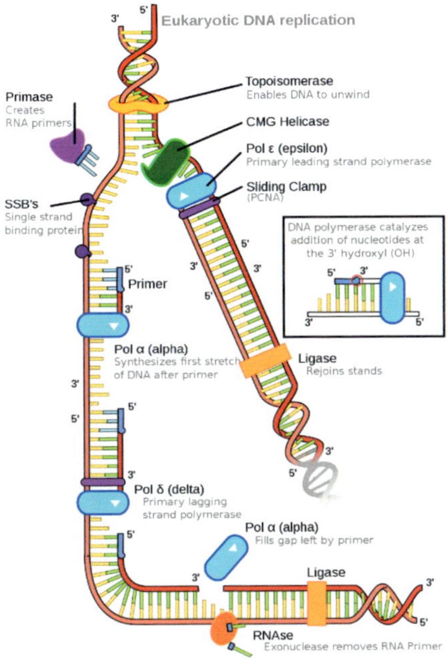

Genes

A gene is a sequence of nucleotides in DNA or RNA that codes for a molecule that has a function. Genes are contained on the chromosomes in the cell nucleus. During gene expression, the DNA is first copied into RNA. The RNA can be directly functional or be the intermediate template for a protein that performs a function. A chromosome consists of a long strand of DNA containing many genes. A human chromosome can have up to 500 million base pairs of DNA with thousands of genes. Gene expression is the process by which information from a gene is used in the synthesis of a functional gene product. These products are often proteins, When the end-product is a protein, genes are first transcribed into RNA, and this transcript is then translated into protein. Several steps in the gene expression process may be modulated, including transcription, RNA splicing, translation and post-translational modification of the protein. Gene regulation gives the cell control over structure and function, and is the basis for cellular differentiation, morphogenesis and the versatility and adaptability of any organism.

Genes are expressed by being transcribed into RNA, and this transcript may then be translated into protein.

Figure 11. Diagram showing how translation of messenger RNA and protein synthesis takes place in ribosomes.

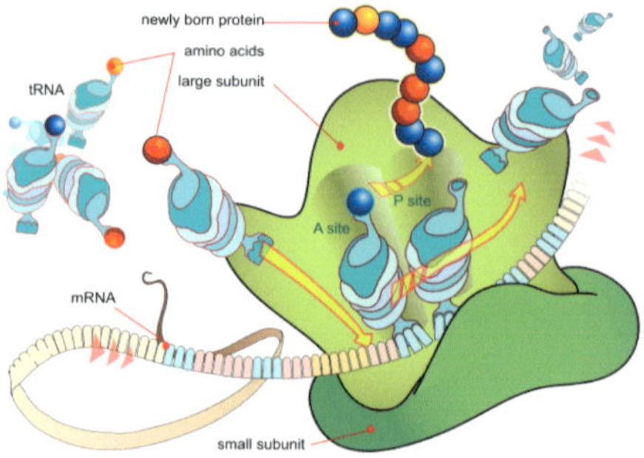

Figure 11. This work has been released into the public domain by its author, LadyofHats. By LadyofHats - Own work based on:[1], [2], [3], [4], [5], [6], [7], and [8]., Public Domain, https://commons.wikimedia.org/w/index.php?curid=4889777; https://en.wikipedia.org/wiki/Translation_(biology)#/media/File:Ribosome_mRNA_translation_en.svg. No changes have been made to this image.

Protein folding

A polypeptide (protein) folds into its characteristic and functional three-dimensional structure from a random coil. Each protein exists as an unfolded polypeptide or random coil when translated from a sequence of messenger (m) RNA into a linear chain of amino acids (Figure 12, left hand image). Amino acids interact with each other to produce a well-defined three-dimensional structure.

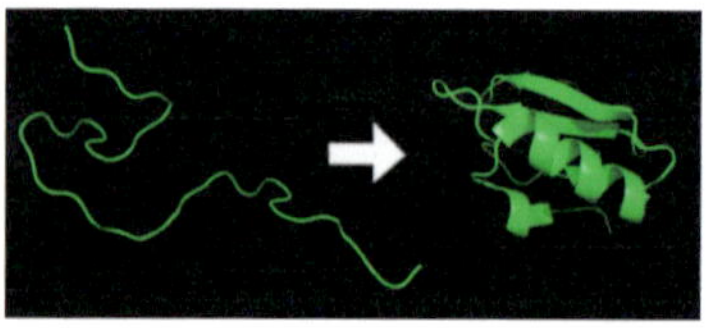

Figure 12 shows a protein before (left) and after (right) folding

.

This image, reproduced here from Wikimedia Commons, is in the public domain because its creator has placed it there. By No machine-readable author provided. Dr Kjaergaard assumed (based on copyright claims). - No machine-readable source provided. Own work assumed (based on copyright claims). Public Domain, https://commons.wikimedia.org/w/index.php?curid=1967109. https://en.wikipedia.org/wiki/Protein_folding#/media/File:Protein_folding.png. No changes have been made to this image.

4. The biology of malignant human cells.

Defects in genes (DNA), epigenetic factors and mismatch repair systems can all cause human cells to become malignant.

Genes

With the exception of congenital disorders, malignant human cells have an abnormality of their genetic systems, and differ in this regard to abnormal, but non-malignant, as well as to normal human cells. Carcinogenesis is the formation of a cancer, whereby normal cells are transformed into cancer cells. The process is characterized by changes at the cellular, genetic, and epigenetic levels and abnormal cell division. Cell division is a physiological process that occurs in almost all tissues and under a variety of circumstances. Normally the balance between proliferation and programmed cell death, in the form of apoptosis, is maintained to ensure the integrity of tissues and organs. According to the prevailing accepted theory of carcinogenesis, the somatic mutation theory, mutations in DNA and epimutations that lead to cancer disrupt these orderly processes by disrupting the programming regulating the processes, upsetting the normal balance between proliferation and cell death. This results in uncontrolled cell division and the evolution of those cells by natural selection in the body. Only certain mutations lead to cancer whereas the majority of mutations do not.

A series of several mutations to certain classes of genes is usually required before a normal cell will transform into a malignant cell.

In order for a normal cell to transform into a malignant cell, the genes that regulate cell growth and differentiation must be altered.

The affected genes are divided into two broad categories. Oncogenes are genes that promote cell growth and reproduction. Tumor suppressor genes are genes that inhibit cell division and survival. Malignant transformation can occur through the formation of novel oncogenes, the inappropriate over-expression of normal oncogenes, or by the under-expression or disabling of tumor suppressor genes. Typically, changes in multiple genes are required to transform a normal cell into a cancer cell (Figure 13)

Figure 13 illustrates that cancers are caused by a series of mutations. Each mutation alters the behavior of the cell to some extent.

Figure 13.

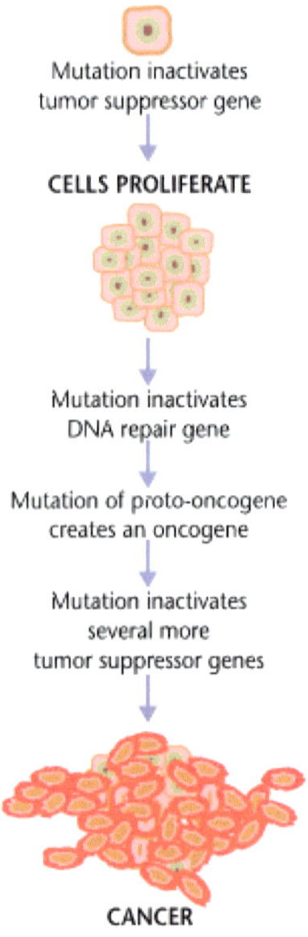

The abnormal biological properties of human malignant cells can be summarized as follows:

- Acquisition of self-sufficiency in growth signals, leading to unchecked growth.
- Loss of sensitivity to anti-growth signals, also leading to unchecked growth.
- Loss of capacity for apoptosis, allowing growth despite genetic errors and external anti-growth signals.
- Loss of capacity for senescence, leading to limitless replicative potential (immortality).
- Acquisition of sustained angiogenesis, allowing the tumor to grow beyond the limitations of passive nutrient diffusion.
- Acquisition of ability to invade neighbouring tissues, the defining property of invasive carcinoma.
- Acquisition of ability to seed metastases at distant sites, a late-appearing property of some malignant tumors (carcinomas or others).

Involved in these steps is

- Loss of capacity to repair genetic errors, leading to an increased mutation rate (genomic instability), thus accelerating all the above changes.

Often, the multiple genetic changes that result in cancer may take many years to accumulate. During this time, the biological behavior of the pre-malignant cells slowly changes from the properties of normal cells to those with cancer-like properties (Figure 14).

Figure 14. Figure 14 shows that tissue can be organized in a continuous spectrum from normal to malignant.

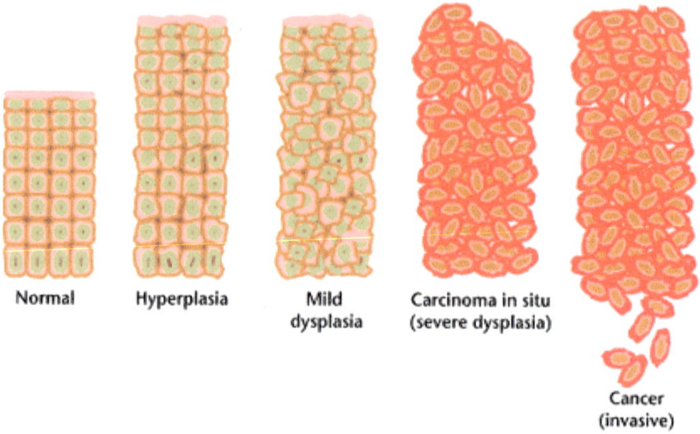

Epigenetic factors also plays a major role in the development of human cancers.

Epigenetic modifications to the DNA of cancer cells do not involve a change in the nucleotide sequence, but instead involve a change in the way the genetic code is expressed. Epigenetic alterations may be just as important, or even more important, than genetic mutations in a cell's transformation to malignancy. In malignant cells loss of expression of genes occurs about 10 times more frequently by transcription silencing (caused by epigenetic promoter hypermethylation of CpG islands) than by mutations. In different types of cancer, a variety of epigenetic mechanisms can be perturbed, such as silencing of tumor suppressor genes and activation of oncogenes by altered CpG island methylation patterns, histone modifications, and dysregulation of DNA-binding proteins (Figure 15)

Figure 15. This figure shows epigenetic patterns in a normal and cancer cells.

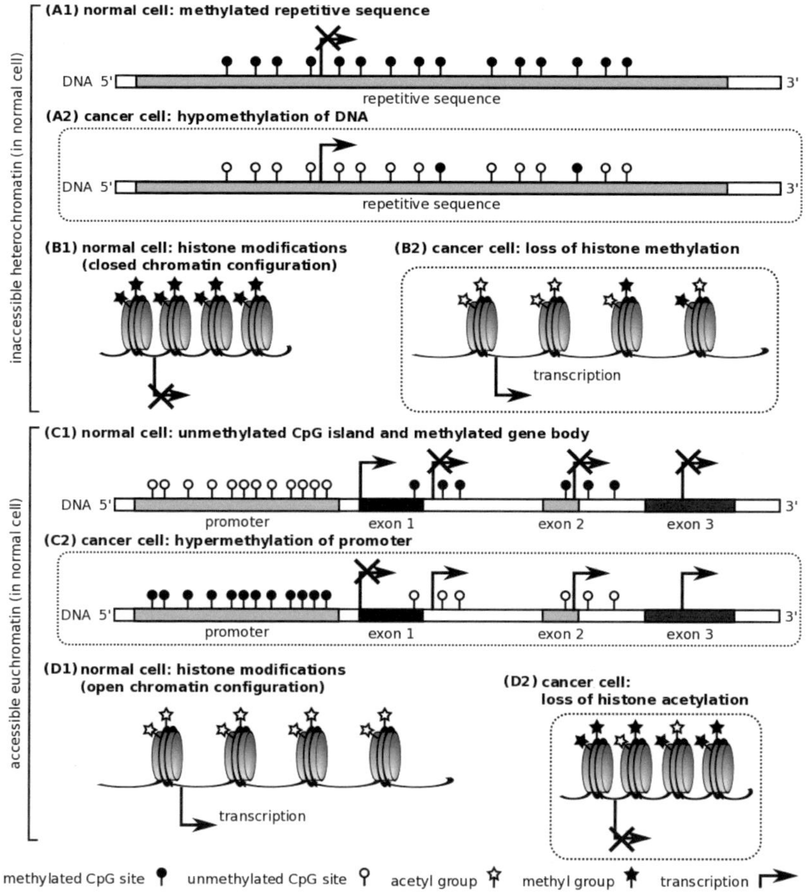

Figure 16 shows a DNA molecule that is methylated on both strands on the center cytosine. DNA methylation plays an important role for epigenetic gene regulation in development and cancer. The image shows the crystal structure of a short DNA helix with sequence "accgcCGgcgcc", which is methylated on both strands at the center cytosine.

Figure 16. A DNA molecule that is methylated on both strands on the center cytosine.

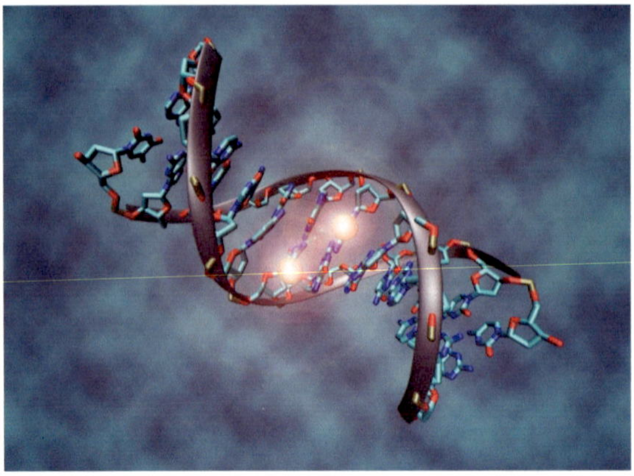

DNA mismatch repair systems

If DNA repair is deficient, DNA damage tends to accumulate. Such excess DNA damage can increase mutational errors during DNA replication. Excess DNA damage can also increase epigenetic alterations due to errors during DNA repair. Such mutations and epigenetic alterations can give rise to malignancy. Germ line mutations in DNA repair genes cause only 2–5% of colon cancer cases. However, altered expression of microRNAs, causing DNA repair deficiencies, are frequently associated with cancers and may be an important causal factor for such cancers.

In non-hereditary cancers, a deficiency in DNA repair is occasionally found to be due to a mutation in a DNA repair gene, but reduced or absent expression of DNA repair genes is much more frequently due to epigenetic alterations that reduce or silence gene expression.

Cancer therapy procedures such as chemotherapy and radiotherapy work by overwhelming the capacity of the malignant cells to repair DNA damage, resulting in their death. Cells that are most rapidly dividing – most typically cancer cells – are preferentially affected. An important side-effect is that other non-cancerous but rapidly dividing cells such as progenitor cells in the gut, skin, and hematopoietic system are also affected. Modern cancer treatments attempt to localize the DNA damage to cells and tissues only associated with cancer, either by physical means (concentrating the therapeutic agent in the region of the tumor) or by biochemical means (exploiting a feature unique to cancer cells in the body).

5. Overview of B cell acute lymphoblastic leukemia

B cell acute lymphoblastic leukemia (ALL) is a cancer of B lymphocytes in the bone marrow characterized by the development of large numbers of lymphoblasts (Figure 17). Symptoms may include feeling tired, pale skin color, fever, easy bleeding or bruising, enlarged lymph nodes, or bone pain. ALL progresses rapidly, metastasizes widely including into the central nervoussystem and is typically fatal within weeks or months if left untreated. In most cases, the cause is unknown.

Figure 17. A Wright's stained bone marrow aspirate smear of patient with precursor B cell acute lymphoblastic leukemia.

The large cells with purple nuclei are malignant lymphoblasts typical of B cell ALL.

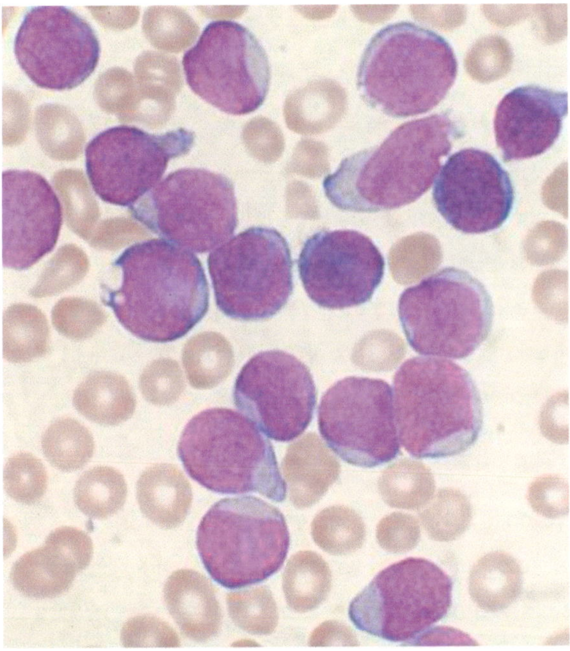

Over the past several decades, there have been strides to increase the efficacy of treatment regimens, resulting in increased survival rates. The aim of treatment is to induce a lasting remission, defined as the absence of detectable leukemia cells in the body (usually less than 5% blast cells in the bone marrow). ALL is typically treated initially with chemotherapy aimed at inducing remission. This is then followed by further chemotherapy typically over a number of years. Treatment usually also includes intrathecal chemotherapy since systemic chemotherapy has limited penetration into the central nervous system and the central nervous system is a common site for relapse of acute lymphoblastic leukemia. Treatment can also include radiation therapy if spread to the brain has occurred. Allogeneic hematopoietic stem cell transplantation may be used if the disease recurs following standard treatment. Additional treatments such as **chimeric antigen receptor (CAR) T cell immunotherapy** (the topic of this book) are now being used and 2 such medications have been approved by the USA FDA for relapsed or refractory B cell ALL.

ALL affected about 876,000 people globally in 2015 and resulted in about 111,000 deaths. It occurs most commonly in children, particularly those between the ages of two and five. In the United States it is the most common cause of cancer and death from cancer among children. ALL is notable for being the first disseminated cancer to be cured. Survival for children increased from under 10% in the 1960s to 90% in 2015. Survival rates remain lower for babies (50%) and adults (35%).

6. Overview of diffuse large B cell non-Hodgkin lymphoma.

B cell non-Hodgkin lymphomas are typically divided into low and high grade lymphomas, corresponding to indolent (slow-growing) lymphomas and aggressive (rapidly growing) lymphomas, respectively. Indolent lymphomas are also known as follicular lymphomas corresponding to the description of their architecture within an involved lymph node, while aggressive lymphomas usually invade tissues in a diffuse pattern (Figure 18). As a generalisation, indolent lymphomas respond to treatment and are kept in remission with long-term survival of many years, but are not cured. Aggressive lymphomas usually require intensive treatments, with some having a good prospect for a cure.

Prognosis and treatment depends on the specific type of lymphoma as well as the stage and grade of the lymphoma. Treatment includes radiation and chemotherapy. Early-stage indolent B-cell lymphomas can often be treated with radiation alone, with long-term non-recurrence. Early-stage aggressive disease is treated with chemotherapy and often radiation, with a 70–90% cure rate. Late-stage aggressive disease is treated with chemotherapy, with cure rates of over 70%.

If chemotherapy or radiotherapy fail, hematopoietic stem cell transplantation is a possible option.

New treatments for lymphomas include **CAR T cell therapies**. As of June 24th 2022, the USA FDA had approved 3 CAR T cell therapies for relapsed or refractory B cell non-Hodgkin lymphomas, 1 for relapsed or refractory mantle cell lymphoma, and 1 for relapsed or refractory follicular lymphoma (Table 3).

Figure 18. Micrograph of a large B cell lymphoma. Lymph node fine needle aspirate specimen. (Field stain).

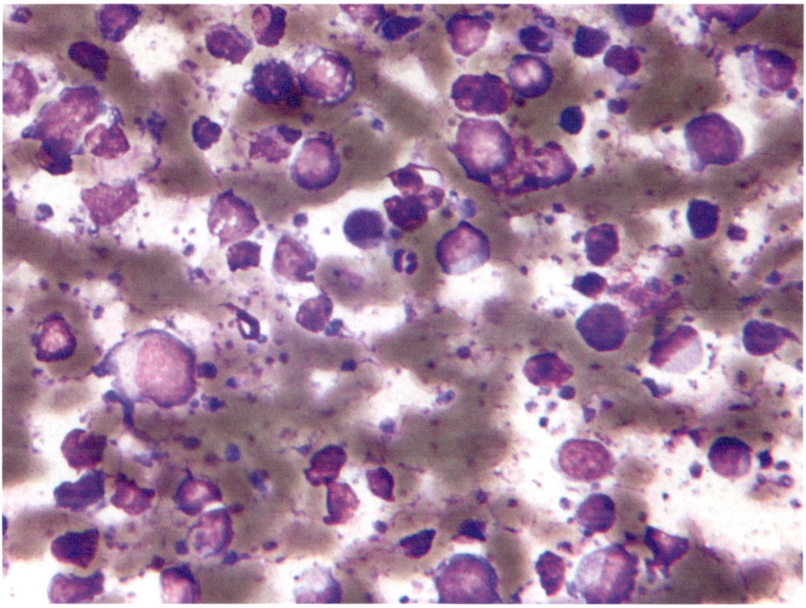

7. Overview of multiple myeloma

Multiple myeloma (MM) is a cancer of plasma cells, that normally produce antibodies. Often, no symptoms are noticed initially. As it progresses, bone pain, anemia, kidney dysfunction, and infections may occur. Complications may include amyloidosis.

Multiple myeloma is diagnosed based on blood or urine tests finding abnormal antibodies, bone marrow biopsy finding malignant plasma cells, and medical imaging finding bone lesions. Another common finding is high blood calcium levels.

Multiple myeloma is treatable, but generally incurable. Remissions may be brought about with corticosteroids, chemotherapy, targeted therapy, and hematopoietic stem cell transplantation. Bisphosphonates and radiation therapy are sometimes used to reduce pain from bone lesions.

It usually occurs around the age of 60 and is uncommon before the age of 40. Without treatment, the median survival in the prechemotherapy era was about 7 months. After the introduction of chemotherapy, prognosis improved significantly with a median survival of 24 to 30 months and a 10-year survival rate of 3%. Further improvements in prognosis have occurred because of the introduction of newer biologic therapies and better salvage options, with median survivals now exceeding 60 to 90 months.

Bone pain affects almost 70% of people with multiple myeloma and is one of the most common symptoms. Myeloma bone pain usually involves the spine and ribs, and worsens with activity. Persistent, localized pain may indicate a pathological bone fracture. Involvement of the vertebrae may lead to spinal cord compression or kyphosis. Myeloma bone disease is due to the overexpression of receptor activator for nuclear factor κ B ligand (RANKL) by bone marrow stromal cells. RANKL activates osteoclasts, which resorb bone. The resultant bone lesions are usually osteolytic in nature, but occasionally they can be denser than the surrounding normal bone (osteoblastic lesions). The breakdown of bone leads to the release of calcium ions into the blood, leading to hypercalcemia and its associated symptoms.

The anemia found in myeloma is usually normocytic and normochromic. It results from the replacement of normal bone marrow by infiltrating tumor cells and inhibition of normal hematopoiesis by cytokines.

Impaired kidney function may develop, either acutely or chronically, and with any degree of severity. The most common cause of kidney failure in multiple myeloma is due to proteins secreted by the malignant cells. Myeloma cells produce **monoclonal proteins** of varying types, most commonly immunoglobulins and free light chains, resulting in abnormally high levels of these proteins in the blood. Depending on the size of these proteins, they may be excreted through the kidneys. Kidneys can be damaged by the effects of the abnormal immunoglobulins or light chains. Increased bone resorption leads to hypercalcemia and causes nephrocalcinosis, thus contributing to kidney failure. Amyloidosis is a distant third in the causation. People with amyloidosis have high levels of amyloid protein that can be excreted through the kidneys and cause damage to the kidneys and other organs. Light chains produce myriad effects that can manifest as the Fanconi syndrome (type II kidney tubular acidosis).

The most common infections are pneumonias and pyelonephritis. Common pneumonia pathogens include S. pneumoniae, S. aureus, and K. pneumoniae, while common pathogens causing pyelonephritis include E. coli and other Gram-negative organisms. The greatest risk period for the occurrence of infection is in the initial few months after the start of chemotherapy. The increased risk of infection is due to immune deficiency. Although the total immunoglobulin level is typically elevated in multiple myeloma, the majority of the antibodies are ineffective monoclonal antibodies (paraproteins) from the clonal plasma cells. A selected group of people with documented hypogammaglobulinemia due tomyeloma may benefit from replacement immunoglobulin therapy to reduce the risk of infection.

Some symptoms (e.g., weakness, confusion, and fatigue) may be due to anemia or hypercalcemia. Headache, visual changes, and retinopathy may be the result of hyperviscosity of the blood depending on the properties of the paraprotein. Rasicular pain, loss of bowel or bladder control (due to involvement of spinal cord leading to cord compression) or carpal tunnel syndrome, and other neuropathies (due to infiltration of peripheral nerves by amyloid) may occur. It may give rise to paraplegia in late-presenting cases.

When the disease is well-controlled, neurological symptoms may result from current treatments, some of which may cause peripheral neuropathy, manifesting as numbness or pain in the hands, feet, and lower legs.

Initial symptoms may involve pain, numbness, swelling, expansion of the jaw, tooth mobility, and radiolucency. Multiple myeloma in the mouth can mimic common dental problems such as periapical abscess or periodontal abscess, gingivitis, periodontitis, or other gingival enlargement or masses.

Monoclonal gammopathy of undetermined significance (MGUS) increases the risk of developing multiple myeloma. MGUS transforms to multiple myeloma at the rate of 1% to 2% per year, and almost all cases of multiple myeloma are preceded by MGUS.

Smoldering multiple myeloma increases the risk of developing multiple myeloma. Individuals diagnosed with this premalignant disorder develop multiple myeloma at a rate of 10% per year for the first 5 years, 3% per year for the next 5 years, and then 1% per year.

Rarely, Epstein–Barr virus (EBV) is associated with multiple myeloma, particularly in individuals who have an immunodeficiency due to, for example, HIV/AIDS, organ transplantation, or a chronic inflammatory condition such as rheumatoid arthritis. EBV-positive multiple myeloma is classified by the World Health Organization (2016) as one form of the Epstein–Barr virus-associated lymphoproliferative diseases and termed Epstein–Barr virus-associated plasma cell myeloma. EBV-positive disease is more common in people with plasmacytoma rather than the multiple myeloma form of plasma cell cancer.

B lymphocytes develop in the bone marrow and thenmigrate to the lymph nodes. As they progress, they mature and display different proteins on their cell surfaces. When they are activated to secrete antibodies, they are known as plasma cells.

Multiple myeloma develops in B lymphocytes after they have left the part of the lymph node known as the germinal center. The normal cell type most closely associated with MM cells is generally taken to be either an activated memory B cell or the precursor to plasma cells, the plasmablast.

The immune system tightly controls the proliferation of B cells and the secretion of antibodies under tight control. When chromosomes and genes are damaged, often through rearrangement, this control is lost. Often, a promoter gene moves translocates to a chromosome, where it stimulates an antibody gene to overproduction.

A chromosomal translocation between the immunoglobulin heavy chain gene (on chromosome 14, locus q32) and an oncogene (often 11q13, 4p16.3, 6p21, 16q23 and 20q11 is frequently observed in people with multiple myeloma. This mutation results in dysregulation of the oncogene which is thought to be an important initiating event in the pathogenesis of myeloma. The result is a proliferation of a plasma cell clone and genomic instability that leads to further mutations and translocations. The chromosome 14 abnormality is observed in about 50% of all cases of myeloma. Deletion of parts of chromosome 13 is also observed in about 50% of cases.

Production of cytokines (especially IL-6) by the malignant plasma cells causes much of their localised damage, such as osteoporosis, and creates a microenvironment in which the malignant cells thrive. Angiogenesis is increased.

The abnormal antibodies are deposited in various organs, leading to kidney failure, polyneuropathy, and other myeloma-associated symptoms.

In a study that investigated the DNA methylation profile of multiple myeloma cells and normal plasma cells, a gradual demethylation from stem cells to plasma cells was observed. The observed methylation pattern of CpG within intronic regions with enhancer-related chromatin marks in multiple myeloma is similar to that of undifferentiated precursor and stem cells. These results may represent a de novo epigenetic reprogramming in multiple myeloma, leading to the acquisition of a methylation pattern related to stemness. Other studies have identified a multiple myeloma specific gene silencing pattern associated with the polycomb repressive complex 2 (PRC2). Increased expression of the PRC2 subunit, EZH2 have been described to be a common feature in multiple myeloma, resulting in an accumulation and redistribution of histone H3 lysine 27 trimethylation which increases with disease severity.

Chromosomal abnormalities commonly found in this disease, like trisomy of multiple odd-numbered chromosomes, t(11;14), and del(13q), are not associated with a worse prognosis. However, about 25% of patients with newly diagnosed disease have abnormalities associated with a worse prognosis, such as t(4;14), t(14;16), and del(17p). Other less common abnormalities associated with a worse prognosis include t(14;20) and ≥4 copies of 1q. Associated genetic mutations include ATM, BRAF, CCND1, DIS3, FAM46C, KRAS, NRAS and TP53.

The genetic and epigenetic changes occur progressively. The initial change, often involving one chromosome 14 translocation, establishes a clone of bone marrow plasma cells that causes the asymptomatic disorder MGUS. Further genetic or epigenic changes produce a new clone of bone marrow plasma cells, usually descendant from the original clone, that causes the more serious, but still asymptomatic premalignant disorder smoldering multiple myeloma. This myeloma is characterized by a rise in the number of bone marrow plasma cells or levels of the circulating myeloma protein above that seen in MGUS. Subsequent genetic and epigenetic changes lead to a new, more aggressive clone of plasma cells, which cause further rises in the level of the circulating myeloma protein, further rises in the number of bone marrow plasma cells, or the development of one or more of a specific set of "CRAB" symptoms, which are the basis for diagnosing malignant multiple myeloma and treating the disease.

In a small percentage of multiple myeloma cases, further genetic and epigenetic changes lead to the development of a plasma cell clone that moves from the bone marrow into the circulatory system, invades distant tissues, and thereby causes the most malignant of all plasma cell dyscrasias, plasma cell leukemia.

Blood tests

Figure 19. Serum protein electropheretogram showing a paraprotein (peak in the gamma zone) in a person with multiple myeloma

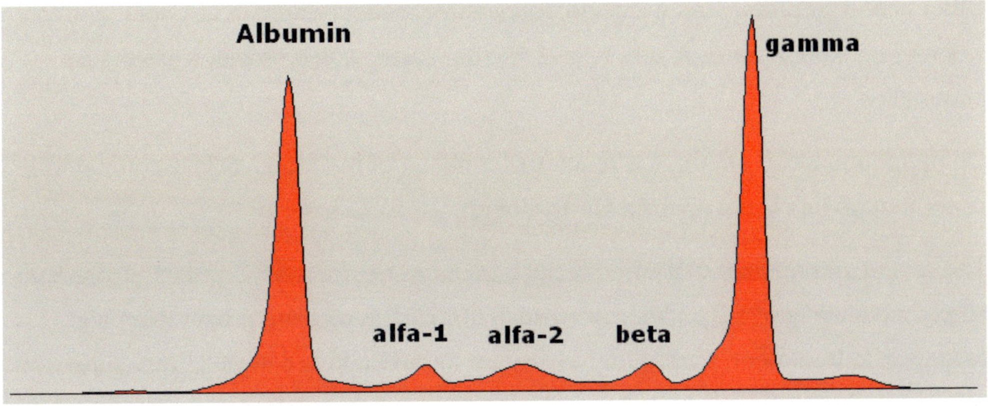

The globulin level may be normal in established disease. However, protein electrophoresis of the blood and urine, may show the presence of a paraprotein, with or without reduction of normal immunoglobulins. One type of paraprotein is the Bence Jones protein, which is a urinary paraprotein composed of free light chains. Quantitative measurements of the paraprotein are necessary to establish a diagnosis and to monitor the disease.

In multiple myeloma IgG paraproteins are most common, followed by IgA and IgM. IgD and IgE myeloma are very rare. In addition, light and or heavy chains of immunoglobulins may be secreted in isolation: κ- or λ-light chains or any of the five types of heavy chains (α-, γ-, δ-, ε- or μ-heavy chains). People without evidence of a monoclonal protein may have "nonsecretory" myeloma (not producing immunoglobulins); this represents about 3% of all people with multiple myeloma.

Additional findings may include a raised calcium level since osteoclasts are breaking down bone, releasing it into the bloodstream, raised serum creatinine level due to reduced kidney function, which is mainly due to casts of paraprotein deposition in the kidney, although the cast may also contain complete immunoglobulins, Tamm-Horsfall protein and albumin.

Other useful laboratory tests include quantitative measurement of IgA, IgG, and IgM to look for immune paresis, and beta-2 microglobulin, which provides prognostic information.

On peripheral blood smear, the rouleaux formation of red blood cells is commonly seen, though this is not specific for myeloma..

The recent introduction of a commercial immunoassay for measurement of free light chains potentially offers an improvement in monitoring disease progression and response to treatment, particularly where the paraprotein is difficult to measure accurately by electrophoresis (for example in light chain myeloma, or where the paraprotein level is very low). Initial research also suggests that measurement of free light chains may also be used, in conjunction with other markers, for assessment of the risk of progression from MGUS to multiple myeloma.

This assay, the serum free light chain assay, has recently been recommended by the International Myeloma Working Group for the screening, diagnosis, prognosis, and monitoring of plasma cell dyscrasias.

Figure 20. Bone marrow aspirate showing a microphotograph of bone marrow in which the normal cellular elements have been replaced by a population of malignant plasma cells, recognizable by their characteristic eccentric nuclei. H&E stain.

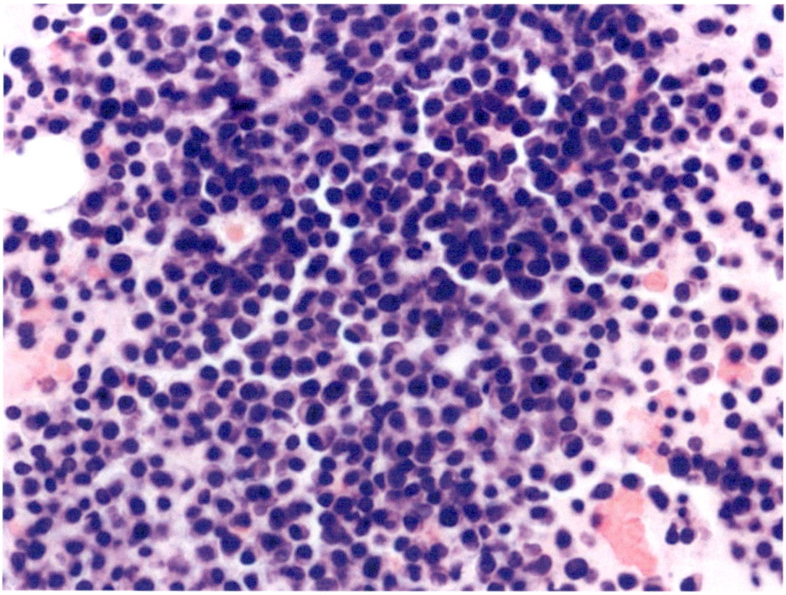

Figure 21. Plasmacytoma, H&E stain. This micrograph shows abundant malignant plasma cells with the occasional Mott cell, a plasma cell with an intracytoplasmic Russell bodies (an eosinophilic uniformly staining membrane bound body which contains immunoglobulin).

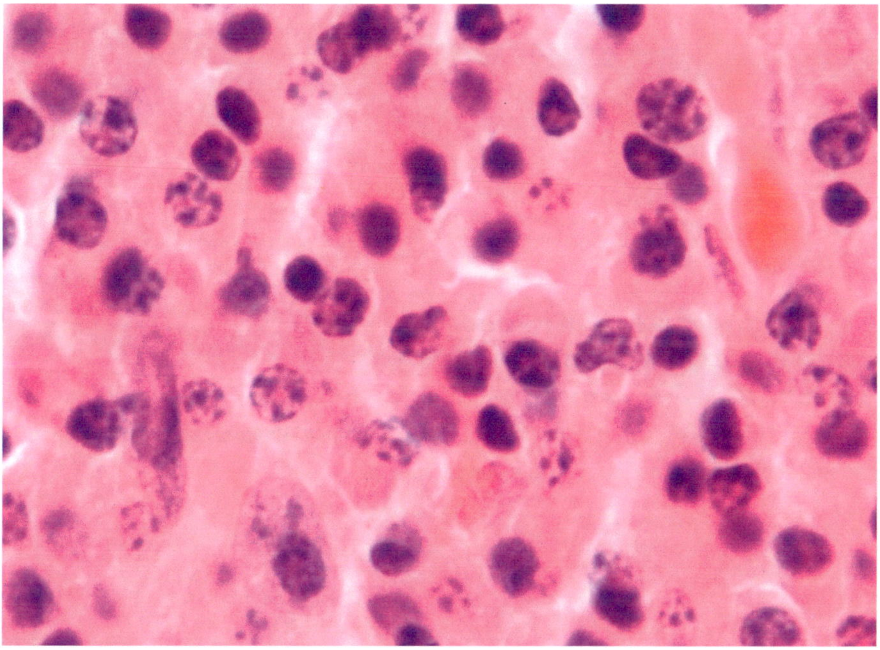

This image is by Nephron - Own work, CC BY-SA 3.0, https://commons.wikimedia.org/w/index.php?curid=7350559; https://en.wikipedia.org/wiki/Multiple_myeloma#/media/File:Plasmacytoma1.jpg. This file is licensed under the Creative Commons Attribution-Share Alike 3.0 Unported license. No changes were made to this image.

Figure 22. Micrograph showing myeloma cast nephropathy in a kidney biopsy: Hyaline casts are PAS positive (dark pink/red – right of image). Myelomatous casts are PAS negative (pale pink – left of image), PAS stain.

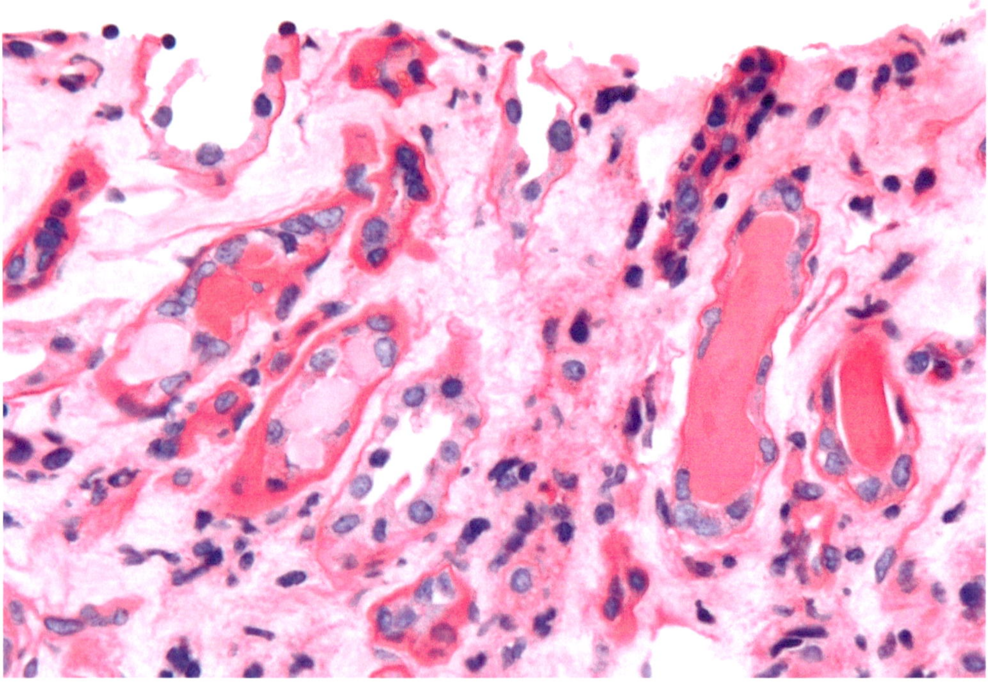

This image is by Nephron - Own work, CC BY-SA 3.0, https://commons.wikimedia.org/w/index.php?curid=17547364; https://en.wikipedia.org/wiki/Multiple_myeloma#/media/File:Cast_nephropathy_-_2_cropped_-_very_high_mag.jpg. This file is licensed under the Creative Commons Attribution-Share Alike 3.0 Unported license. No changes were made to this image.

A bone marrow biopsy is usually performed to estimate the percentage of bone marrow occupied by plasma cells. This percentage is used in the diagnostic criteria for myeloma. Immunohistochemistry can detect plasma cells that express immunoglobulin in the cytoplasm and occasionally on the cell surface; myeloma cells are often CD56, CD38, CD138, and CD319 positive and CD19, CD20, and CD45 negative. Flow cytometry is often used to establish the clonal nature of the plasma cells, which will generally express only kappa or lambda light chain. Cytogenetics may also be performed in myeloma for prognostic purposes, including a myeloma-specific fluorescent in situ hybridization and virtual karyotype.

Historically, CD138 has been used to isolate myeloma cells for diagnostic purposes. However, this antigen disappears rapidly ex vivo. Recently, however, the surface antigen CD319 (SLAMF7) was discovered to be considerably more stable and allows robust isolation of malignant plasma cells from delayed or even cryopreserved samples.

The prognosis varies widely depending upon various risk factors. The Mayo Clinic has developed a risk-stratification model termed Mayo Stratification for Myeloma and Risk-adapted Therapy (mSMART), which divides people into high-risk and standard-risk categories. People with deletion of chromosome 13 or hypodiploidy by conventional cytogenetics, t(4;14), t(14;16), t(14;20) or 17p- by molecular genetic studies, or with a high plasma cell labeling index (3% or more) are considered to have high-risk myeloma.

The diagnostic examination of a person with suspected multiple myeloma typically includes a skeletal survey. Myeloma activity sometimes appears as "lytic lesions" (with local disappearance of normal bone due to resorption) and on the skull X-ray as "punched-out lesions" (raindrop skull). Lesions may also be sclerotic, which are seen as radiodense. Magnetic resonance imaging is more sensitive than simple X-rays in the detection of lytic lesions, and may supersede a skeletal survey, especially when vertebral disease is suspected. Occasionally, a CT scan is performed to measure the size of soft-tissue plasmacytomas.

Figure 23. X-ray of the forearm with multiple lytic lesions.

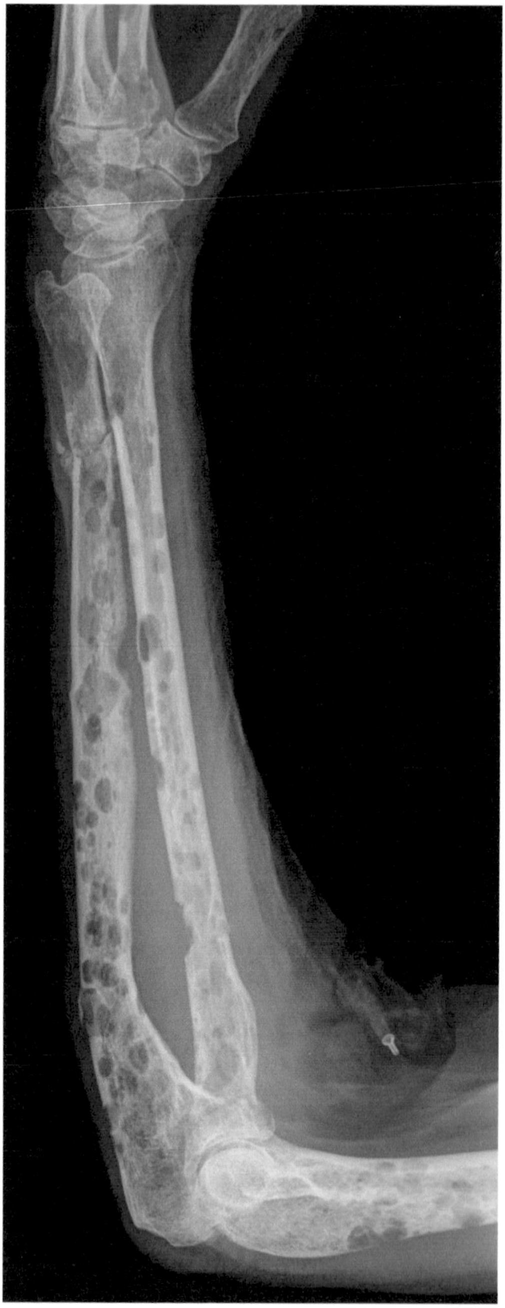

arm.png. This file is licensed under the Creative Commons Attribution-Share Alike 3.0 Unported license. No changes were made to this image.

Figure 24. Pathological fracture of the lumbar spine due to multiple myeloma.

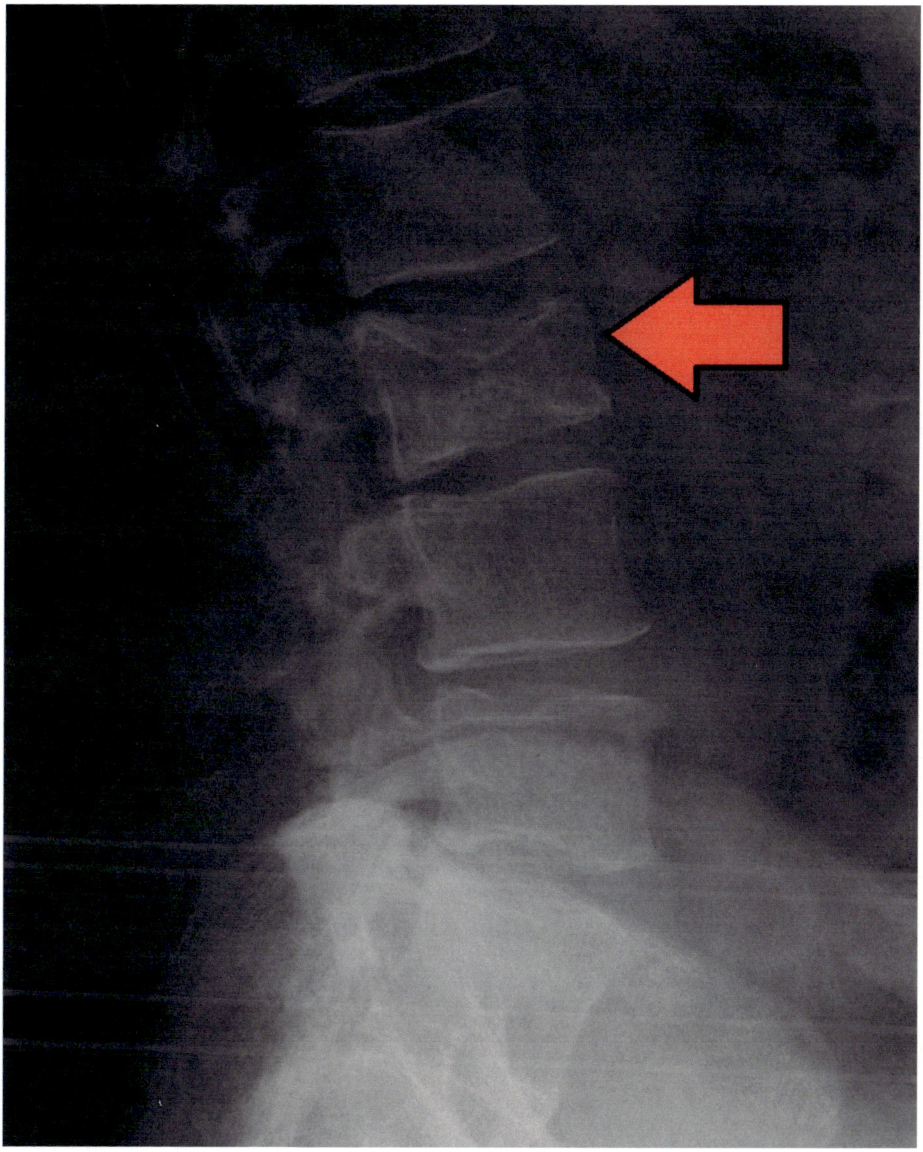

This image is by James Heilman, MD - Own work, CC BY-SA 4.0, https://commons.wikimedia.org/w/index.php?curid=49320717; https://en.wikipedia.org/wiki/Multiple_myeloma#/media/File:PathFracMMPlainMark.png. This file is licensed under the Creative Commons Attribution-Share Alike 4.0 International license. No changes were made to this image.

Figure 25. CT scan of the lower vertebral column in a man with multiple myeloma, showing multiple osteoblastic lesions: These are more radiodensethan the surrounding cancellous bone, in contrast to osteolytic lesions, which are less radiodense.

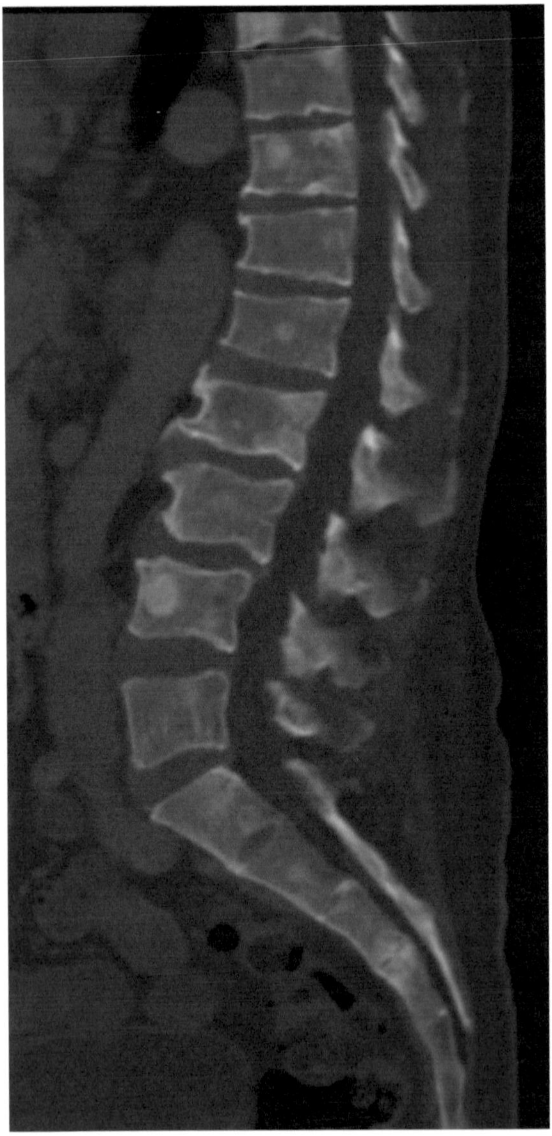

This image is by Mikael Häggström - Own work, CC0, https://commons.wikimedia.org/w/index.php?curid=56847744; https://en.wikipedia.org/wiki/Multiple_myeloma#/media/File:CT_of_osteoblastic_lesions_of_multiple_

myeloma.jpg. This file is made available under the Creative Commons CC0 1.0 Universal Public Domain Dedication. No changes were made to this image

In 2003 the IMG agreed on diagnostic criteria for symptomatic myeloma, asymptomatic myeloma, and MGUS, which was subsequently updated in 2009.

In 2014, the IMWG updated their criteria further to include biomarkers of malignancy. These biomarkers are >60% clonal plasma cells, a serum involved / uninvolved free light chain ratio ≥ 100 (the concentration of the involved free light chain must be ≥ 100 mg/l) and more than one focal lesion ≥ 5 mm by MRI. Together, these biomarkers and the previous criteria are known as myeloma-defining events (MDEs). A person must have >10 % clonal plasma cells and any MDE to be diagnosed with myeloma. The biomarker criteria were added so that people with smouldering myeloma at high risk of developing multiple myeloma could be diagnosed before organ damage occurred.

In multiple myeloma, staging helps with prognostication but does not guide treatment decisions. The Durie-Salmon staging system was used historically and was replaced by the International Staging System (ISS), published by the International Myeloma Working Group In 2005. The revised ISS (R-ISS) was published in 2015 and incorporates cytogenetics and lactate dehydrogenase (LDH).

Stage I: β2 microglobulin (β2M) < 3.5 mg/L, albumin ≥ 3.5 g/dL, normal cytogenetics, no elevated LDH

Stage II: Not classified under Stage I or Stage III

Stage III: β2M ≥ 5.5 mg/L and either elevated LDH or high-risk cytogenetics [t(4,14), t(14,16), and/or del(17p)]

Treatment is indicated in myeloma with symptoms. If there are no symptoms, but a paraprotein typical of myeloma and a diagnostic bone marrow appearance is present without end-organ damage, treatment is usually deferred or restricted to clinical trials. Treatment for multiple myeloma is focused on decreasing the clonal plasma cell population and consequently decrease the symptoms of disease.

Initial treatment of multiple myeloma depends on the person's age and other illnesses present.

The preferred treatment for those under the age of 65 is high-dose chemotherapy, commonly with bortezomib-based regimens, and lenalidomide–dexamethasone to be followed by a hematopoietic stem cell transplant. A 2016 study concluded that hematopoietic stem cell transplantion is the preferred treatment for multiple myeloma. There are two types of stem cell transplants to treat multiple myeloma. In autologous hematopoietic stem cell transplantation (ASCT), the patient's own stem cells are collected from the patient's own blood. The patient is then given high-dose chemotherapy, and the patient's stem cells are then transplanted back into the patient. The process is not curative, but does prolong overall survival and complete remission. In allogeneic hematopoietic stem cell transplantation, a healthy donor's hematopoietic stem cells are transplanted into the affected person. Allogenic hematopoietic stem cell transplantation has the potential to be curative, but is used in a very small percentage of people (and in the relapsed setting, not as part of initial treatment) since there is asignificant treatment-related mortality rate associated with allogeneic hematopietic stem cell transplantion.

People over age 65 and people with significant concurrent illnesses often cannot tolerate stem cell transplantation. For these people, the standard of care has been chemotherapy with melphalan and prednisone. Recent studies among this population suggest improved outcomes with new chemotherapy regimens, such as bortezomib and lenalidomide. Treatment with bortezomib, melphalan, and prednisone had an estimated overall survival of 83% at 30 months, lenalidomide plus low-dose dexamethasone an 82% survival at 2 years, and melphalan, prednisone, and lenalidomide had a 90% survival at 2 years.

There is support for continuous therapies with multiple drug combinations of the anti-myeloma drugs bortezomib, lenalidomide and thalidomide as initial treatment for transplant-ineligible multiple myeloma. Further clinical studies are required to determine the potential harms of these drugs and the effect on the person's quality of life. A 2009 review noted, "Deep venous thrombosis and pulmonary embolism are the major side effects of thalidomide and lenalidomide. Lenalidomide causes more myelosuppression, and thalidomide causes more sedation. Chemotherapy-induced peripheral neuropathy and thrombocytopenia are major side effects of bortezomib."

Treatment of related hyperviscosity syndrome with plasmapheresis may be required to prevent neurologic symptoms or kidney failure.

Most people, including those treated with an autologous hematopoietic stem cell transplant (ASCT), relapse after initial treatment. Maintenance therapy using a prolonged course of low-toxicity medications is often used to prevent relapse. A 2017 meta-analysis showed that post-ASCT maintenance therapy with lenalidomide improved progression-free survival and overall survival in people at standard risk. A 2012 clinical trial showed that people with intermediate- and high-risk disease benefit from a bortezomib-based maintenance regimen.

Relapse within the first 18 months of diagnosis is considered as functional high risk multiple myeloma. Depending on the person's condition, the prior treatment modalities used and the duration of remission, options for relapsed disease include retreatment with the original agent, use of other agents (such as melphalan, cyclophosphamide, thalidomide, or dexamethasone, alone or in combination), and a second ASCT.

Later in the course of the disease, it becomes refractory (resistant) to formerly effective treatment. This stage is referred to as relapsed/refractory multiple myeloma (RRMM). Treatment modalities that are commonly use to treat RRMM include dexamethasone, proteasome inhibitors (e.g. bortezomib and carfilzomib), immunomodulatory imide drugs (e.g. thalidomide, lenalidomide, and pomalidomide), and certain monoclonal antibodies (e.g. against CD38 and CD319). Survival expectancy has risen in recent years and new treatments are under development – such as **CAR T cell therapy**, as described in Sections 9.5 and 9.6 of this book.

Kidney failure in multiple myeloma can be acute (reversible) or chronic (irreversible). Acute kidney failure typically resolves when the calcium and paraprotein levels are brought under control. Treatment of chronic kidney failure is dependent on the type of kidney failure and may involve dialysis.

Bortezomib is a proteosome inhibitor. It works by inhibiting proteasomes, cellular complexes that break down proteins. Proteasomes are protein complexes which degrade unneeded or damaged proteins by proteolysis, a chemical reaction that breaks peptide bonds (Figures 26 and 27). Enzymes that help such reactions are called proteases.

Figure 26. Cartoon representation of a proteasome. Its active sites are sheltered inside the tube (blue). The caps (red; in this case, 11S regulatory particles) on the ends regulate entry into the destruction chamber, where the protein is degraded.

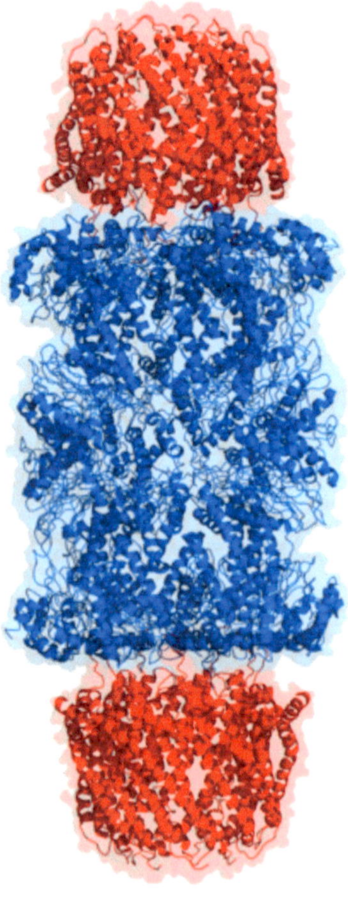

Figure 27. Top view of the proteasome shown in Figure 26.

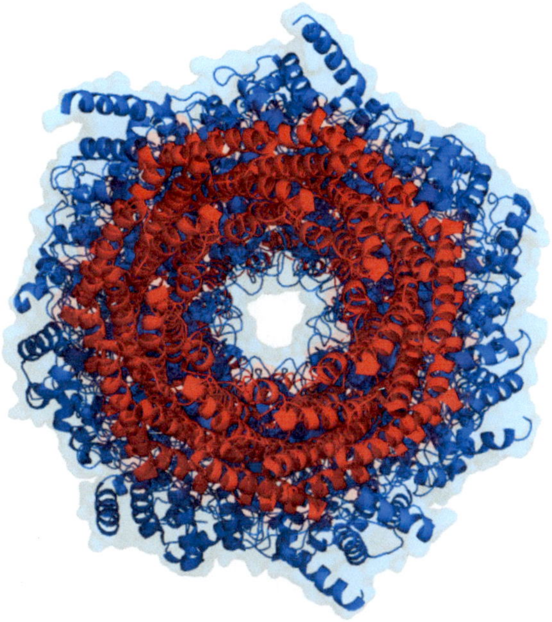

This image is by Thomas Splettstoesser (www.scistyle.com) - Based on atomic coordinates of PDB 1FNT, rendered with open source molecular visualization tool PyMol (www.pymol.org), CC BY-SA 3.0, https://commons.wikimedia.org/w/index.php?curid=1290290; https://en.wikipedia.org/wiki/Proteasome#/media/File:Proteaosome_1fnt_top.png. This file is licensed under the Creative Commons Attribution-Share Alike 3.0 Unported license. No changes were made to this image.

Proteasomes are part of a major mechanism by which cells regulate the concentration of particular proteins and degrade misfolded proteins. Proteins are tagged for degradation with a small protein called ubiquitin. The tagging reaction is catalyzed by enzymes called ubiquitin ligases. Once a protein is tagged with a single ubiquitin molecule, this is a signal to other ligases to attach additional ubiquitin molecules. The result is a polyubiquitin chain that is bound by the proteasome, allowing it to degrade the tagged protein. The degradation process yields peptides of about seven to eight amino acids long, which can then be further degraded into shorter amino acid sequences and used in synthesizing new proteins.

Proteasomes are located both in the nucleus and in the cytoplasm.

In structure, the proteasome is a cylindrical complex containing a "core" of four stacked rings forming a central pore. Each ring is composed of seven individual proteins. The inner two rings are made of seven β subunits that contain three to seven protease active sites. These sites are located on the interior surface of the rings, so that the target protein must enter the central pore before it is degraded. The outer two rings each contain seven α subunits whose function is to maintain a "gate" through which proteins enter the barrel. These α subunits are controlled by binding to "cap" structures or regulatory particles that recognize polyubiquitin tags attached to protein substrates and initiate the degradation process. The overall system of ubiquitination and proteasomal degradation is known as the ubiquitin–proteasome system.

Figure 28. Bortezomib bound to the core particle in a yeast proteasome. The bortezomib molecule is in the center colored by atom type (boron = pink, carbon = cyan, nitrogen = blue, oxygen = red), surrounded by the local protein surface. The blue patch is catalytic threonine residue whose activity is blocked by the presence of bortezomib.

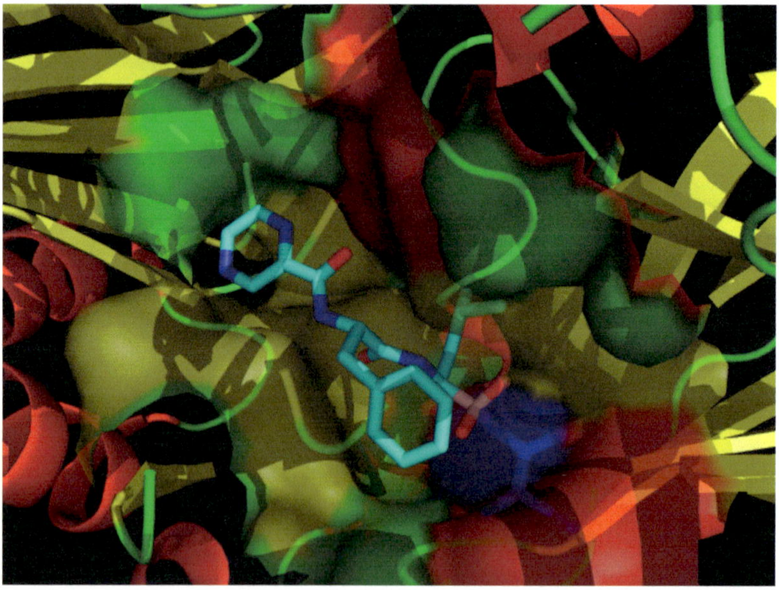

Thalidomide, lenalidomide and **pomalidomide** are immunomodulatory agents.

Thalidomide

Thalidomide is an immunomodulatory medication and works by a number of mechanisms, including stimulating T cells and decreasing TNF-α production. Thalidomide was first marketed in 1957 in West Germany, where it was available over the counter. When first released, thalidomide was promoted for anxiety, trouble sleeping, "tension", and morning sickness of pregnancy. While it was initially thought to be safe in pregnancy, concerns regarding birth defects arose until the medication was removed from the market in Europe in 1961. The total number of infants affected by use during pregnancy is estimated at 10,000, of which about 40% died around the time of birth. Those who survived had limb (Figure 29), eye, urinary tract, and heart problems.

Figure 29. Congenital malformation of the feet in a baby born to a mother who had taken thalidomide while pregnant.

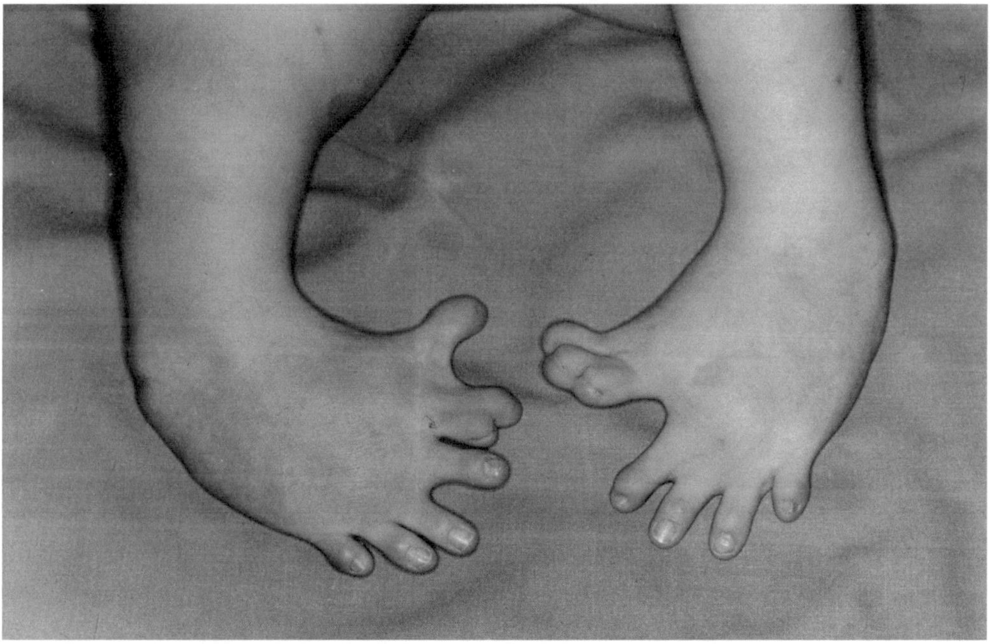

Lenalidomide

In vitro, lenalidomide has three main activities: a direct anti-tumor effect, inhibition of angiogenesis, and immunomodulation. In vivo, lenalidomide induces tumor cell apoptosis directly and indirectly by inhibition of bone marrow stromal cell support, by anti-angiogenic and anti-osteoclastogenic effects, and by immunomodulatory activity. Lenalidomide has a broad range of activities that can be exploited to treat many hematologic and solid cancers.Lenalidomide is related to thalidomide, which is known to be teratogenic. Tests in monkeys suggest that lenalidomide is likewise teratogenic.

Pomalidomide

Pomalidomide directly inhibits angiogenesis and myeloma cell growth. This dual effect is central to its activity in myeloma, rather than other pathways such as TNF alpha inhibition, since potent TNF inhibitors including rolipram and pentoxifylline do not inhibit myeloma cell growth or angiogenesis. Upregulation of interferon gamma, IL-2 and IL-10 as well as downregulation of IL-6 have been reported for pomalidomide. These changes may contribute to pomalidomide's anti-angiogenic and anti-myeloma activities. Because pomalidomide can cause harm to unborn babies when administered during pregnancy, women taking pomalidomide must not become pregnant.

Anti-CD38 monoclonal antibody

CD38, also known as cyclic ADP ribose hydrolase is a glycoprotein found on the surface of many immune cells (white blood cells), including CD4+, CD8+, B lymphocytes and natural killer cells. CD38 also functions in cell adhesion, signal transduction and calcium signaling. The CD38 protein is a marker of cell activation. It has been associated with HIV infection, leukemias, myelomas, solid tumors, type II diabetes mellitus and bone metabolism, as well as some genetically determined conditions.

Daratumumab (Darzalex) which targets CD38 has been used in treating multiple myeloma.

Figure 30. Space-filling model of the antigen-binding
fragment of daratumumab (teal/green) in complex with CD38 (pale pink).
Style made to resemble the Protein Data Bank's "Molecule of the Month" series, illustrated by Dr. David S. Goodsell of the Scripps Research Institute. Created using QuteMol (http://qutemol.sourceforge.net) and GIMP. Optimized with OptiPNG.

Figure 30. Space-filling model of the antigen-binding fragment of daratumumab.

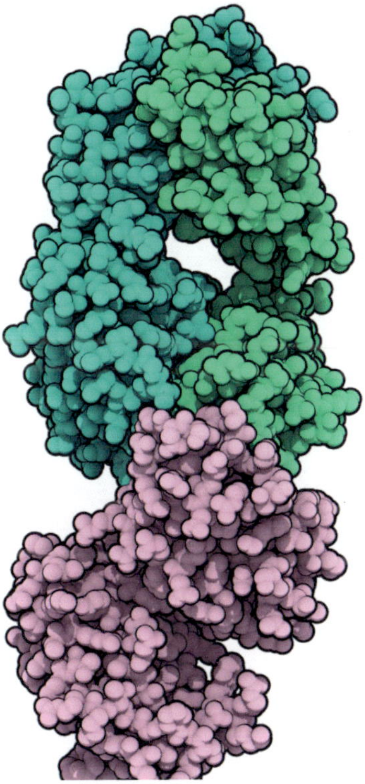

Several newer options are approved for the management of advanced disease: **belantamab mafodotin** — a monoclonal antibody against B cell maturation antigen (BCMA), also known as CD269, indicated for the treatment of adults with relapsed or refractory multiple myeloma who have received at least four prior therapies including an anti-CD38 monoclonal antibody, a proteasome inhibitor, and an immunomodulatory agent;

carfilzomib - a proteasome inhibitor that is indicated: as a single agent in people who have received one or more lines of therapy;

in combination with dexamethasone or with lenalidomide and dexamethasone in people who have received one to three lines of therapy;

daratumumab - a monoclonal antibody against CD38 that is indicated in people who have received at least three prior lines of therapy including a proteasome inhibitor and an immunomodulatory agent or who are double refractory to a proteasome inhibitor and an immunomodulatory agent;

elotuzumab - an immunostimulatory humanized monoclonal antibody against SLAMF7 (also known as CD319) indicated in combination with lenalidomide and dexamethasone in people who have received one to three prior therapies;

isatuximab - a monoclonal antibody against CD38 indicated in combination with pomalidomide and dexamethasone for the treatment of adults with multiple myeloma who have received at least two prior therapies including lenalidomide and a proteasome inhibitor;

ixazomib - an orally available proteasome inhibitor indicated in combination with lenalidomide and dexamethasone in people who have received at least one prior therapy;

panobinostat - an orally available histone deacetylase inhibitor used in combination with bortezomib and dexamethasone in people who have received at least two prior chemotherapy regimens, including bortezomib and an immunomodulatory agent;

selinexor - an orally available selective inhibitor of nuclear export indicated in combination with dexamethasone in people who have received at least four prior therapies and whose disease does not respond to at least two proteasome inhibitors, two immunomodulatory agents and an anti-CD38 monoclonal antibody;

idecabtagene vicleucel- the first cell-based gene therapy was approved by the USA FDA in 2021 for the treatment of adults with relapsed or refractory multiple myeloma who have received at least four prior therapies.

Hematopoietic stem cell transplantation

Hematopoietic stem cell transplantion can be used to treat multiple myeloma. Allogeneic hematopoietic stem cell transplants have a risk of a graft-versus-host-disease.

Cell-mediated gene therapy

Ciltacabtagene autoleucel (Carvykti) (a CAR T cell agent) was approved for medical use in the United States in February 2022. Ciltacabtagene autoleucel is indicated for the treatment of adults with relapsed or refractory multiple myeloma after four or more prior lines of therapy, including a proteasome inhibitor, an immunomodulatory agent and an anti-CD38 monoclonal antibody.

Other measures

In addition to direct treatment of the plasma cell proliferation, bisphosphonates (such as pamidronate or zoledronic acid) are routinely administered to prevent pathological fractures; they have also been observed to have a direct antitumor effect.

8. Introduction to CAR T cell therapies

The first successful form of cellular therapy was hematopoietic stem cell transplantation. This became part of mainstream medicine in the 1970s. Many other types of cellular therapy have been tried but none have been successful enough to be accepted as standard of care. CAR T cells are thus the second type of successful cell therapy. Their production, however, is, complex: first T cells have to be isolated from the blood and then they undergo a gene engineering process that results in their expressing a chimeric antigen receptor. This receptor is called “chimeric” because the total gene construct consists of at least three genes. First, there is the gene that encodes a receptor that recognises a protein present on the cell surface of the targeted disease. Attached to this are two other genes that, when the receptor engages with the protein, activate the T cell, resulting in specific destruction of the targeted cell. The T cells are transducted with a gene encoding the engineered CAR via a retroviral vector, typically either an integrating gamma retrovirus (RV) or a lentiviral (LV) vector. These vectors are now very safe due to a partial deletion of the U3 region. (The gene editing tool CRISPR/Cas9 has recently been used instead of retroviral vectors to integrate the CAR gene into specific sites in the genome of the T cells). Currently, these products are manufactured in biopharmaceutical good manufacturing process (GMP) facilities. Currently available CAR T cell therapies are thus customized for each individual patient, and are therefore very expensive – costing several hundred thousand dollars for a single infusion of the manufactured product. The reason they are so exciting, however, is their extraordinary efficacy in diseases resistant to the best available conventional treatment. Currently, FDA-approved CAR T cell therapies are available for the treatment of relapsed or refractory B cell acute lymphoblastic leukemia (ALL), relapsed or refractory B cell non-Hodgkin lymphomas, (NHL) and myeloma.

In the cell processing center, the transduced T cells are then expanded in large numbers. To drive their expansion, the T cells are typically treated with the T cell growth factor interleukin 2 (IL-2) and anti-CD3 antibodies.

Prior to the administration of the CAR T cells, the patient undergoes lymphodepletion chemotherapy. Fludarabine and cyclophosphamide are often used for lymphodepletion. The depletion of the number of circulating leukocytes in the patient upregulates the number of cytokines that are produced and reduces competition for resources, which helps to promote the expansion of the engineered CAR T cells after they are infused into the recipient.

Part of the CAR is located outside the T cell and part within the T cell. The part of the CAR that extends out from the cell’s surface is usually composed of fragments, or domains, of laboratory-manufactured antibodies. Which domains are used affects how well the receptor recognizes or binds to the antigen on tumor cells. The internal part of each CAR has signaling and co-stimulatory domains. These transmit signals into the cell after the receptor interacts with an antigen. The different domains that are used can affect the cells' overall function.

Chimeric antigen receptors combine many facets of normal T cell activation into a single protein. They link an extracellular antigen recognition domain to an intracellular signalling domain, which activates the T cell when an antigen is bound. CARs are composed of four regions: an antigen recognition domain, an extracellular hinge region, a transmembrane domain, and an intracellular T cell signaling domain (Figure 31).

Figure 31. The different components of a chimeric antigen receptor.

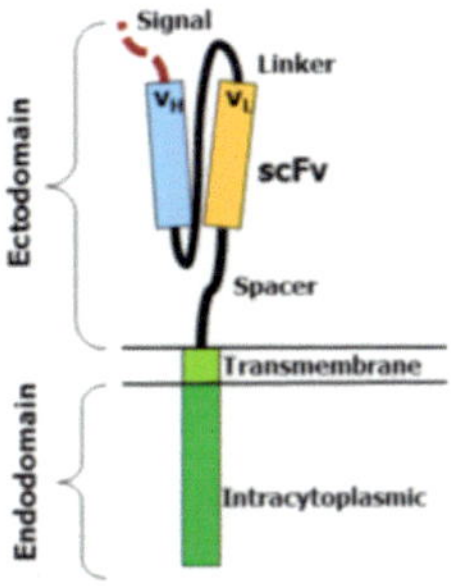

Antigen recognition domain

The antigen recognition domain is exposed to the outside of the cell, in the ectodomain portion of the receptor. It interacts with potential target molecules and is responsible for targeting the CAR T cell to any cell expressing a molecule for the receptor. The antigen recognition domain is typically derived from the variable regions of a monoclonal antibody linked together as a single-chain variable fragment (scFv). A scFv is a chimeric protein made up of the light (VL) and heavy

(VH) chains of immunoglobins, connected with a short linker peptide. These VL and VH regions are selected for their binding ability to the target antigen (such as CD19). The linker between the two chains consists of hydrophilic residues with stretches of glycine and serine in it for flexibility, as well as stretches of glutamate and lysine for added solubility. Single domain antibodies (e.g. VH, VHH) have been engineered and developed as antigen recognition domains in the CAR format due to their high transduction efficiency in T cells.

Hinge region

The hinge, also called a spacer, is a small structural domain that sits between the antigen recognition region and the cell's outer membrane. An ideal hinge enhances the flexibility of the scFv receptor head, reducing the spatial constraints between the CAR and its target antigen. This promotes antigen binding and synapse formation between the CAR T cells and their target cells. Hinge sequences are often based on membrane-proximal regions from other immune molecules including IgG, CD8, and CD28.

Transmembrane domain

The transmembrane domain is a structural component consisting of a hydrophobic alpha helix that spans the cell membrane. It anchors the CAR to the plasma membrane, bridging the extracellular hinge and antigen recognition domains with the intracellular signaling region. This domain is essential for the stability of the receptor as a whole. Generally, the transmembrane domain from the most membrane-proximal component of the endodomain is used, but different transmembrane domains result in different receptor stability.
The CD28 transmembrane domain is known to result in a highly expressed, stable receptor.

Using the CD3 zeta transmembrane domain is not recommended, as it can result in incorporation of the artificial T cell receptor (TCR) into the native TCR.

Intracellular T cell signaling domain

Figure 32. Depiction of first (1G), second (2G), and third (3G) generation chimeric antigen receptors with the scFv segments in green and the various intracellular TCR signaling components in red, blue and yellow.

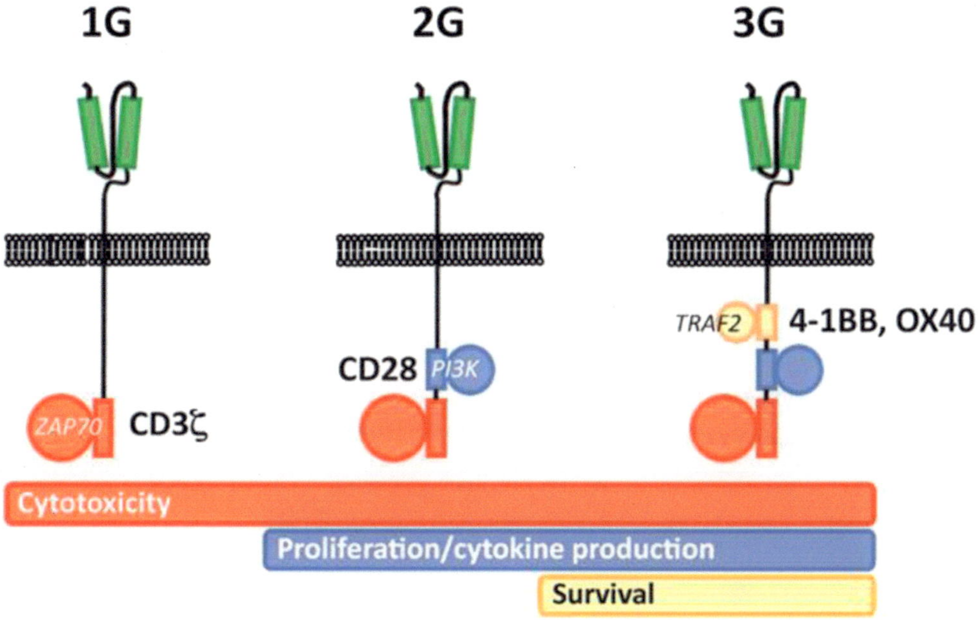

This image is by Monica Casucci and Attilio Bondanza - http://www.jcancer.org/v02p0378.htm, Public Domain, https://commons.wikimedia.org/w/index.php?curid=19265783; https://en.wikipedia.org/wiki/Chimeric_antigen_receptor_T_cell#/media/File:Depiction_of_3_generations_of_CARs.jpg. This work is in the public domain in the United States because it is a work prepared by an officer or employee of the United States Government as part of that person's official duties under the terms of Title 17, Chapter 1, Section 105 of the US Code. No changes were made to this image.

The intracellular T cell signaling domain lies in the receptor's endodomain, inside the cell. After an antigen is bound to the external antigen recognition domain, CAR receptors cluster together and transmit an activation signal. Then the internal cytoplasmic end of the receptor perpetuates signaling inside the T cell.

Normal T cell activation relies on the phosphorylation of immunoreceptor tyrosine-based activation motifs (ITAMs) present in the cytoplasmic domain of CD3 zeta. To mimic this process, CD3 zeta's cytoplasmic domain is commonly used as the main CAR endodomain component. Other ITAM-containing domains have also been tried, but are not as effective.

T cells also require co-stimulatory molecules in addition to CD3 signaling in order to persist after activation. For this reason, the endodomains of CAR receptors typically also include one or more chimeric domains from co-stimulatory proteins. Signaling domains from a wide variety of co-stimulatory molecules have been successfully tested, including CD28, CD27, CD134 (OX40), and CD137 (4-1BB).

The intracellular signaling domain used defines the generation of a CAR T cell. First generation CARs included only a CD3 zeta cytoplasmic domain. Second generation CARs added a co-stimulatory domain, like CD28 or 4-1BB. The involvement of these intracellular signaling domains improves T cell proliferation, cytokine secretion, resistance to apoptosis and in vivo persistence. Third generation CARs combine multiple co-stimulatory domains, such as CD28-41BB or CD28-OX40, to augment T cell activity. Preclinical data show that the third generation CARs exhibit improved effector functions and better in vivo persistence compared to second-generation CARs.

The CAR T cell therapies approved by FDA to date target CD19 on B cells or B cell maturation antigen (BCMA) on mature B cells and on myeloma cells.

The initial development of CAR T cell therapies focused largely on the most common cancer in children, acute lymphoblastic leukemia (ALL). More than 80% of children diagnosed with ALL that arises in B cells, the predominant type of pediatric ALL, will be cured by intensive chemotherapy. However, effective treatments have been limited for patients whose cancers return, or relapse, after chemotherapy or a hematopoietic stem cell transplant.

In 2017 the FDA approved tisagenlecleucel (Kymriah), the first CAR T cell therapy to be approved by the agency, based on clinical trials demonstrating it could eradicate cancer in children with relapsed ALL – an astonishing result.

CD19-targeted CAR T cells are also offering hope to adults and children with advanced aggressive B cell lymphomas. CAR T cells have become a frequently used therapy for several types of lymphoma. B-lymphocyte antigen CD19 (also known as CD19 molecule (Cluster of Differentiation 19), B-Lymphocyte Surface Antigen B4, T cell Surface Antigen Leu-12 and CVID3) is a transmembrane protein that is encoded by the gene CD19. In humans CD19 is expressed on all B lineage cells. Contrary to some early doubts, human plasma cells do express CD19. CD19 plays two major roles in human B cells: on the one hand, it acts as an adaptor protein to recruit cytoplasmic signaling proteins to the membrane; on the other, it works within the CD19/CD21 complex to decrease the threshold for B cell receptor signaling pathways. Due to its presence on all B cells, it is a biomarker for B lymphocyte development, lymphoma diagnosis and can be utilized as a target for leukemia immunotherapies.

Figure 33. 3D rendering of a human B cell.

This image is by Blausen Medical - BruceBlaus. When using this image in external sources it can be cited as: Blausen.com staff (2014). " Medical gallery of Blausen Medical 2014" WikiJournal of Medicine 1 (2). DOI:10.15347/wjm/2014.010. ISSN 2002-4436. CC BY-SA 4.0, https://commons.wikimedia.org/w/index.php?curid=56845139; https://en.wikipedia.org/wiki/B_cell#/media/File:Blausen_0624_Lymphocyte_B_cell_(crop).png. This file is licensed under the Creative Commons Attribution-Share Alike 4.0 International license. No chanes were made to this image

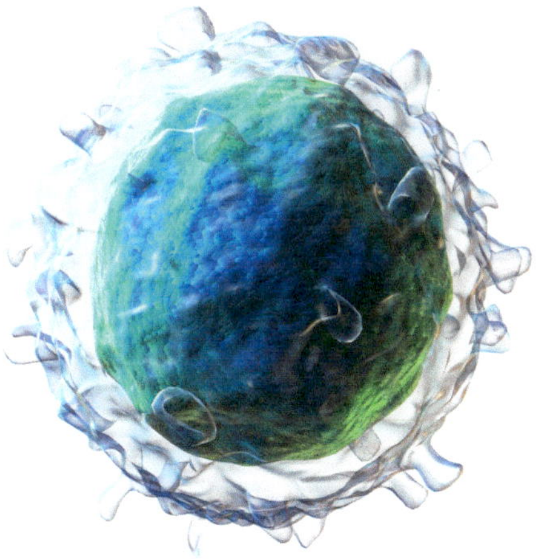

Figure 34. Transmission electronmicrograph of a human B cell. This image shows the mitochondria, a very large nucleus, and the tentacle-like cytoplasmic extensions which are used by the lymphocytes to move.

This image is by NIAID - Human B Lymphocyte, CC BY 2.0, https://commons.wikimedia.org/w/index.php?curid=62609476; https://en.wikipedia.org/wiki/B_cell#/media/File:Human_B_Lymphocyte_(28942386960).jpg.

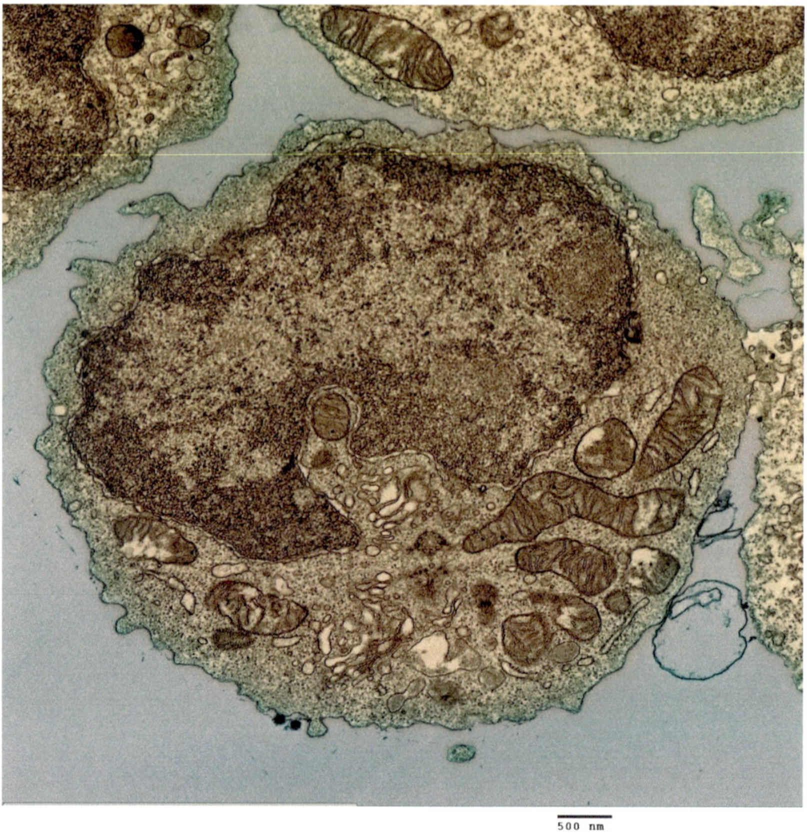

Like all cancer treatments, CAR T cell therapies can cause severe side effects. One of the most frequent and serious side effects is cytokine release syndrome (CRS). As part of their immune-related effects, T cells release cytokines - chemical messengers that help stimulate and direct the immune response. In the case of CRS, the infused T cells flood the bloodstream with cytokines, causing serious side effects. In some cases severe CRS can be fatal. In many patients, both children and adults, mild forms of CRS can be managed with standard supportive therapies, including corticosteroids. For more serious cases of CRS, tocilizumab (Actemra) can be effective. This drug blocks the activity of IL-6, a cytokine that is often secreted in large amounts by T cells and macrophages.

The other side effect of particular concern with CAR T cell therapies is neurologic effects, including severe confusion, seizure-like activity, and impaired speech. The precise cause of these neurologic side effects (also called immune effector cell–associated neurotoxicity syndrome, or ICANS) is still unclear. Tocilizumab does not seem to help with ICANS. Corticosteroids are currently the best treatment option for severe ICANS, particularly dexamethasone, which is better at penetrating the central nervous system than other corticosteroids.

Different ways of preventing CRS and ICANS are now under intense study. One approach is the prophylactic use of tocilizumab and low-dose corticosteroids. Other treatments for ICANS are being investigated. Smaller studies, for example, have found that anakinra (Kineret), which is used to treat rheumatoid arthritis, may help prevent severe ICANS in patients treated with CAR T cell therapies. Another idea for protecting against severe CRS and ICANS is to modify the CARs themselves. In a small clinical trial of adults with lymphoma, for example, patients treated with a "remodeled" CD-19-targeted CAR T cell developed at NCI had far fewer severe neurologic side effects than historically seen with the original form of the same CAR.

Research on CAR T cells is continuing at a swift pace, including hundreds of ongoing clinical trials. Part of this expansion is a product of researchers having identified additional antigens on tumor cells that might be good targets for CAR T cells.

Although CD19 and BCMA are the only antigens for which there are FDA-approved CAR T cell therapies, CAR T cell therapies have been developed that target other antigens commonly found in blood cancers, including therapies that target multiple antigens at one time.

9. Notes about Section 10.

In the following section (Section 10) it is important to state clearly that all the information from the FDA's approved label for each biologic (which is the public domain) is taken verbatim from the label. However, I have made some minor changes to the format of each label:

i. I have brought the "DESCRIPTION" and "MECHANISM OF ACTION" sections forward to be placed earlier, since how the drug works and what it is composed of, is key to understanding it.

iii. I have put other salient facts in **bold type** to emphasize them.

iv. I have not included all the tables detailing all of the side-effects of each of the six biologics, except for those relating to Kymriah, since the adverse event profile is similar for each of these six therapies.

v. I have also added some material in this section that is **not** in the FDA approval label in order to to illustrate certain points and to break up the many pages of words. *Please note that in these cases, I have put all such added text in [parentheses and italics].*

10. FDA-approved CAR T cell therapies

The USA FDA has approved six CAR T cell therapies for therapeutic use as of June 24th 2022 (Table 3).

Table 3. CAR T cell therapies FDA-approved for therapeutic use.

Generic name/	Brand name/ manufacturer	Target antigen	Targeted disease	Patient population
Tisagenlecleucel	Kymriah/ Novartis	CD19	B cell acute lymphoblastic leukemia (ALL). B cell non-Hodgkin lymphoma (NHL)	Children and young adults with refractory or relapsed (r/r) B cell ALL. Adults with r/r B cell NHL
Axicabtagene ciloleucel	Yescarta/Kite, a Gilead	CD19	B cell NHL	Adults with r/r B cell NHL.

	company		Follicular lymphoma	Adults with r/r follicular lymphoma
Brexucabtagene autoleucel	Tecartus/Kite, a Gilead company	CD19	Mantle cell lymphoma (MCL). B cell ALL	Adults with r/r MCL Adults with r/r B cell ALL
Lisocabtagene maraleucel	Breyanzi/Bristol Myers Squibb	CD19	B cell NHL	Adults with r/r B cell ALL
Idecabtagene vicleucel	Abecma/Bristol Myers Squibb	B cell maturation antigen (BCMA)	Multiple myeloma (MM)	Adults with r/r MM
Ciltacabtagene autoleucel	Carvikti/ Janssen Biotech	BCMA	MM	Adults with r/r MM

10.1. TISANGELECLEUCEL/KYMRIAH

DESCRIPTION

KYMRIAH (tisagenlecleucel) is a CD19-directed genetically modified autologous T cell immunotherapy comprised of autologous T cells that are genetically modified using a lentiviral vector to encode an **anti-CD19** chimeric antigen receptor (CAR). The CAR is comprised of a murine single-chain antibody fragment (scFv) specific for CD19, followed by a **CD8** hinge and transmembrane region that is fused to the intracellular signaling domains for **4-1BB (CD137) and CD3 zeta**. KYMRIAH is prepared from the patient's peripheral blood mononuclear cells, which are obtained via a standard leukapheresis procedure. The mononuclear cells are enriched for T cells, then transduced with the lentiviral vector containing the anti-CD19 CAR transgene, and activated with anti-CD3/CD28 antibody coated beads. The transduced T cells are expanded in cell culture, washed, and formulated into a suspension, which then is cryopreserved. The product must pass a sterility test before release for shipping as a frozen suspension in a patient-specific infusion bag(s). The product is thawed prior to administrationThe thawed product is a colorless to slightly yellow suspension of cells. In addition to T cells, other cell populations, including monocytes, NK cells, and B cells, may be present. The formulation contains 31.25% (v/v) of Plasma-Lyte A, 31.25% (v/v) of 5% Dextrose/0.45% sodium chloride, 10 % Dextran 40 (LMD)/5% Dextrose, 20% (v/v) of 25% Human Serum Albumin (HSA), and 7.5% (v/v) Cryoserv® dimethylsulfoxide (DMSO).

Pediatric and Young Adult r/r B-cell ALL

A single dose of KYMRIAH may contain up to 2.5 x 10^8 CAR-positive viable T cells provided in one to three patient-specific infusion bag(s). Based on the patient's weight reported at the time of leukapheresis, one of two possible dose ranges will be prepared for the patient:

- For patients 50 kg or less: 0.2 to 5.0 x 10^6 CAR-positive viable T cells per kg body weight

- For patients above 50 kg: 0.1 to 2.5 x 10^8 CAR-positive viable T cells.

Adult r/r DLBCL: A single dose of KYMRIAH may contain 0.6 to 6.0 x 10^8 CAR-positive viable T cells provided in one to three patient-specific infusion bag(s). The actual number of CAR-positive T cells in the product is reported on the Certificate of Analysis (CoA) that is shipped with KYMRIAH. The volume of CAR-positive viable T cells in an infusion bag ranges from 10 mL to 50 mL.

CLINICAL PHARMACOLOGY

Mechanism of action

KYMRIAH is a CD19-directed genetically modified autologous T cell immunotherapy which involves reprogramming a patient's own T cells with a transgene encoding a chimeric antigen receptor (CAR) to identify and eliminate CD19-expressing malignant and normal cells. The CAR is comprised of a murine single-chain antibody fragment which recognizes CD19 and is fused to intracellular signaling domains from

4-1BB (CD137) and CD3 zeta. The CD3 zeta component is critical for initiating T cell activation and antitumor activity, while 4-1BB enhances the expansion and persistence of KYMRIAH. Upon binding to CD19-expressing cells, the CAR transmits a signal to promote T cell expansion, activation, target cell elimination, and persistence of the KYMRIAH cells.

Pharmacokinetics/Cellular Kinetics Following infusion,

KYMRIAH exhibited an initial rapid expansion followed by a bi-exponential decline in both pediatric and young adult relapsed/refractory B-cell acute lymphoblastic leukemia (ALL) patients, and adult relapsed/refractory diffuse large B-cell lymphoma patients.

FULL PRESCRIBING INFORMATION

WARNING: CYTOKINE RELEASE SYNDROME AND NEUROLOGICAL TOXICITIES

• Cytokine Release Syndrome (CRS), including fatal or life-threatening reactions, occurred in patients receiving KYMRIAH. Do not administer KYMRIAH to patients with active infection or inflammatory disorders. Treat severe or life-threatening CRS with tocilizumab or tocilizumab and corticosteroids

• Neurological toxicities, which may be severe or life-threatening, can occur following treatment with KYMRIAH, including concurrently with CRS. Monitor for neurological events after treatment with KYMRIAH. Provide supportive care as needed

• KYMRIAH is available only through a restricted program under a Risk Evaluation and Mitigation Strategy (REMS) called the KYMRIAH REMS

INDICATIONS AND USAGE

KYMRIAH is a CD19-directed genetically modified autologous T cell immunotherapy indicated for the treatment of:

1.1 Pediatric and Young Adult Relapsed or Refractory (r/r) B-cell Acute Lymphoblastic Leukemia (ALL) Patients up to 25 years of age with B-cell precursor acute lymphoblastic leukemia (ALL) that is refractory or in second or later relapse.

1.2 Adult Relapsed or Refractory (r/r) Diffuse Large B-Cell Lymphoma (DLBCL) Adult patients with relapsed or refractory (r/r) large B-cell lymphoma after two or more lines of systemic therapy including diffuse large B-cell lymphoma (DLBCL) not otherwise specified, high grade B-cell lymphoma and DLBCL arising from follicular lymphoma.

Limitation of Use: KYMRIAH is not indicated for treatment of patients with primary central nervous system lymphoma.

DOSAGE AND ADMINISTRATION

For autologous use only. For intravenous use only.

2.1 Dosage in Pediatric and Young Adult Relapsed or Refractory (r/r) B-cell Acute Lymphoblastic Leukemia (ALL) KYMRIAH is provided as a single-dose for infusion containing a suspension of chimeric antigen receptor (CAR)-positive viable T cells. Based on the patient weight reported at the time of leukapheresis: – Patients 50 kg or less: administer 0.2 to 5.0 x 10^6 CAR-positive viable T cells per kg body weight – Patients above 50 kg: administer 0.1 to 2.5 x 10^8 CAR-positive viable T cells

2.2 Dosage in Adult Relapsed or Refractory (r/r) Diffuse Large B-cell lymphoma (DLBCL) KYMRIAH is provided as a single-dose for infusion containing a suspension of chimeric antigen receptor (CAR)-positive viable T cells. – For adult patients: administer 0.6 to 6.0 x 10^8 CAR-positive viable T cells

2.3 Administration

Preparing Patient for KYMRIAH Administration with Lymphodepletion – Confirm availability of KYMRIAH prior to starting the lymphodepleting regimen.

Pediatric and Young Adult Relapsed or Refractory (r/r) B-cell Acute Lymphoblastic Leukemia (ALL)

• Lymphodepleting chemotherapy: Fludarabine (30 mg/m^2 intravenous daily for 4 days) and cyclophosphamide (500 mg/m^2 intravenous daily for 2 days starting with the first dose of fludarabine). Infuse KYMRIAH 2 to 14 days after completion of the lymphodepleting chemotherapy.

Adult Relapsed or Refractory (r/r) Diffuse Large B-cell lymphoma (DLBCL)

• Lymphodepleting chemotherapy: Fludarabine (25 mg/m^2 i.v. daily for 3 days) and cyclophosphamide (250 mg/m^2 IV daily for 3 days starting with the first dose of fludarabine).

• Alternate lymphodepleting chemotherapy: bendamustine 90 mg/m^2 i.v. daily for 2 days if a patient experienced a previous Grade 4 hemorrhagic cystitis with cyclophosphamide or demonstrates resistance to a previous cyclophosphamide containing regimen.

• Infuse KYMRIAH 2 to 11 days after completion of the lymphodepleting chemotherapy.

• Lymphodepleting chemotherapy may be omitted if a patient's white blood cell (WBC) count is less than or equal to 1 x 10^9/L within 1 week prior to KYMRIAH infusion.

Preparation of KYMRIAH for Infusion and Administration

Delay the infusion of KYMRIAH if a patient has unresolved serious adverse reactions (including pulmonary reactions, cardiac reactions, or hypotension) from preceding chemotherapies, active uncontrolled infection, active graft-versus-host disease (GVHD), or worsening of leukemia burden following lymphodepleting chemotherapy

A KYMRIAH dose may be contained in one to three cryopreserved patient-specific infusion bag(s). Verify the number of bags received for the dose of KYMRIAH with the Certificate of Conformance (CoC) and Certificate of Analysis (CoA). Coordinate the timing of thaw of KYMRIAH and infusion in the following manner. Confirm the infusion time in advance, and adjust the start time for thaw so that KYMRIAH is available for infusion when the recipient is ready. If more than one bag has been received for the treatment dose, thaw 1 bag at a time. Wait to thaw/infuse the next bag until it is determined that the previous bag is safely administered.

Preparation of KYMRIAH for Infusion

1. Ensure tocilizumab and emergency equipment are available prior to infusion and during the recovery period.

2. Premedicate patient with acetaminophen and diphenhydramine or another H1-antihistamine approximately 30 to 60 minutes prior to KYMRIAH infusion. Avoid

prophylactic use of systemic corticosteroids, as it may interfere with the activity of KYMRIAH.

3. Confirm patient identity: Prior to KYMRIAH preparation, match the patient's identity with the patient identifiers on each KYMRIAH infusion bag(s). KYMRIAH is for autologous use only. Employ universal precautions to avoid potential transmission of infectious diseases when handling the product. Note: The patient identifier number may be preceded by the letters DIN or Aph ID.

Figure 35. KYMRIAH Infusion Bag

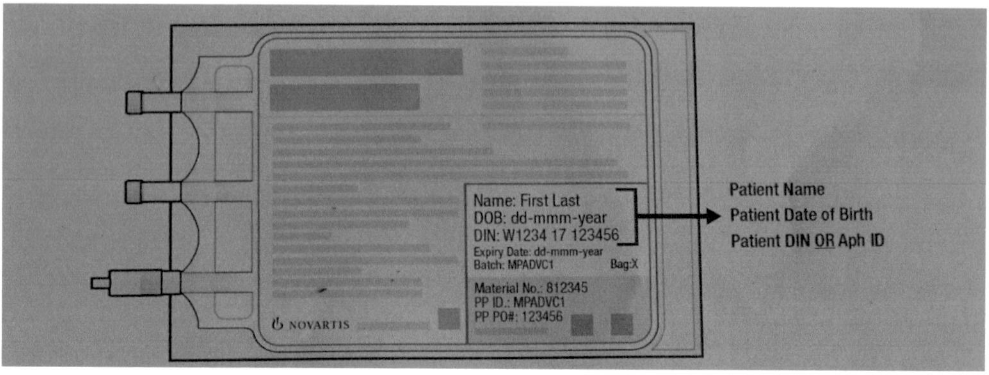

4. Inspect the infusion bag(s) for any breaks or cracks prior to thawing. If a bag is compromised, do not infuse the contents. Call Novartis at 1-844-4KYMRIAH.

5. Place the infusion bag inside a second, sterile bag in case of a leak and to protect ports from contamination.

6. Thaw each infusion bag one at a time at 37°C using either a water bath or dry thaw method until there is no visible ice in the infusion bag. Remove bag from thawing device immediately; do not store product bag at 37°C. Once the infusion bag has been thawed and is at room temperature (20°C to 25°C), it should be infused within 30 minutes. Do not wash, spin down, and/or resuspend KYMRIAH in new media prior to infusion.

7. Inspect the contents of the thawed infusion bag for any visible cell clumps. If visible cell clumps remain, gently mix the contents of the bag. Small clumps of cellular material should disperse with gentle manual mixing. Do not infuse KYMRIAH if clumps are not dispersed, the infusion bag is damaged or leaking, or otherwise appears to be compromised. Call Novartis at 1-844-4KYMRIAH. Administration

8. Confirm the patient's identity with the patient identifiers on the infusion bag.

9. Administer KYMRIAH as an intravenous infusion at 10 mL to 20 mL per minute, adjusted as appropriate for smaller children and smaller volumes. The volume in the infusion bag ranges from 10 mL to 50 mL. Do NOT use a leukocyte-depleting filter. If more than one bag is being infused for the treatment dose, wait to thaw/infuse the next bag until it is determined that the previous bag is safely administered. - Prime the tubing prior to infusion with normal saline. - Infuse all contents of the infusion bag. - Rinse the infusion bag with 10 mL to 30 mL normal saline while maintaining a closed tubing system to assure as many cells as possible are infused into the patient. - Cells from all the bag(s) must be infused to complete a single dose. KYMRIAH contains human cells genetically modified with a lentivirus. Follow local biosafety guidelines applicable for handling and disposal of such products.

Monitoring - Administer KYMRIAH at a certified healthcare facility. Monitor patients 2-3 times during the first week following KYMRIAH infusion at the certified healthcare facility for signs and symptoms of CRS and neurologic toxicities

Instruct patients to remain within proximity of the certified healthcare facility for at least 4 weeks following infusion.

Management of Severe Adverse Reactions

Cytokine release syndrome (CRS). *[Please also see Appendix 11.2].*

Table 4. An overview of treatment of cytokine release syndrome.

CRS severity	Management
Prodromal syndrome: low grade fever, fatigue, anorexia	Observe in person, exclude infection, administer antibiotics per local guidelines of neutropenic; provide symptomatic relief
CRS requiring mild intervention (one	Administer antipyretics, oxygen,

or more of the following): high fever, hypoxia, mild hypertension	intravenous fluids and/or low-dose vasopressors as needed
CRS requiring moderate to aggressive intervention (one or more of the following): hemodynamic instability despite intravenous fluids and vasopressor support, worsening respiratory distress including pulmonary infiltrates, oxygen requirement including high-flow oxygen and/or need for mechanical ventilation, rapid clinical deterioration	• Administer high-dose or multiple vasopressors, oxygen, mechanical ventilation and/or other supportive care as needed • Administer tocilizumab - patient weight less than 30kg: 12 mg/kg intravenously over1 hour - patient weight greater than or equal to 30 kg: 8 mg/kg intravenously over 1 hour (maximum dose 800 mg) Repeat tocilizumab as needed at a minimum interval of 8 hours if there is no clinical improvement. If no response to second dose of tocilizumab, consider a third dose of tocilizumab or pursue alternative measures for treatment of CRS. Limit to a maximum total of 4 tocilizumab doses. • If no clinical improvement within 12 to 18 hours of the first tocilizumab dose, or worsening at any time, administer methylprednisolone 2 mg/kg as an initial dose, then 2 mg/kg per day until vasopressors and high flow oxygen are no longer needed, then taper.

Please note that the treatment of CRS after Kymriah administration is also shown in Table 13.

[Tocilizumab is a humanized monoclonal antibody against the interleukin-6 receptor (IL-6R). Interleukin 6 (IL-6) is a cytokine that plays an important role in immune response and is implicated in the pathogenesis of many diseases including CRS. The most common adverse effects observed in clinical trials were upper respiratory tract infections (more than 10% of patients), nasopharyngitis (common cold), headache, and high blood pressure (at least 5%). The enzyme alanine transaminase was also elevated in at least 5% of patients, but in most cases without symptoms. Elevated total cholesterol levels were common. Among the less common side effects are dizziness, various infections, as well as reactions of the skin and mucosae such as mild rashes, gastritis and mouth ulcers. Rare but severe reactions are gastrointestinal perforations (0.26% in six months) and anaphylaxis (0.2%). In June 2021, the U.S. Food and Drug Administration issued an emergency use authorization for tocilizumab for the treatment of COVID-19 in hospitalized people aged two years of age and older who are receiving systemic corticosteroids and require supplemental oxygen, non-invasive or invasive mechanical ventilation, or extracorporeal membrane oxygenation

Figure 36. Structure of the IL6R protein.

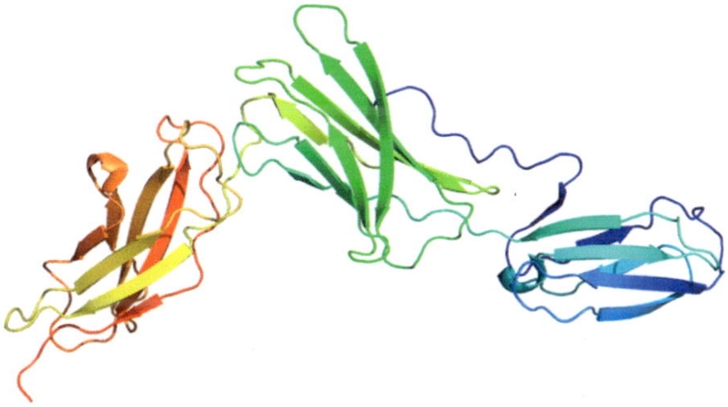

This image is by Emw - Own work, CC BY-SA 3.0, https://commons.wikimedia.org/w/index.php?curid=8820135; https://en.wikipedia.org/wiki/Interleukin-6_receptor#/media/File:Protein_IL6R_PDB_1n26.png. This file is licensed under the Creative Commons Attribution-Share Alike 3.0 Unported license. No changes were made to this image).

Figure 37. Crystal structure of the hexameric human IL-6/IL-6 alpha receptor/gp130 complex.

This image is by By Jawahar Swaminathan and MSD staff at the European Bioinformatics Institute - http://www.ebi.ac.uk/pdbe-srv/view/images/entry/1p9m600.png, displayed on http://www.ebi.ac.uk/pdbe-srv/view/entry/1p9m/summary, Public Domain, https://commons.wikimedia.org/w/index.php?curid=5911932; https://en.wikipedia.org/wiki/Interleukin-6_receptor#/media/File:PDB_1p9m_EBI.jpg. This image has been released into the public domain by its creator and original copyright holder. (http://www.ebi.ac.uk/)].

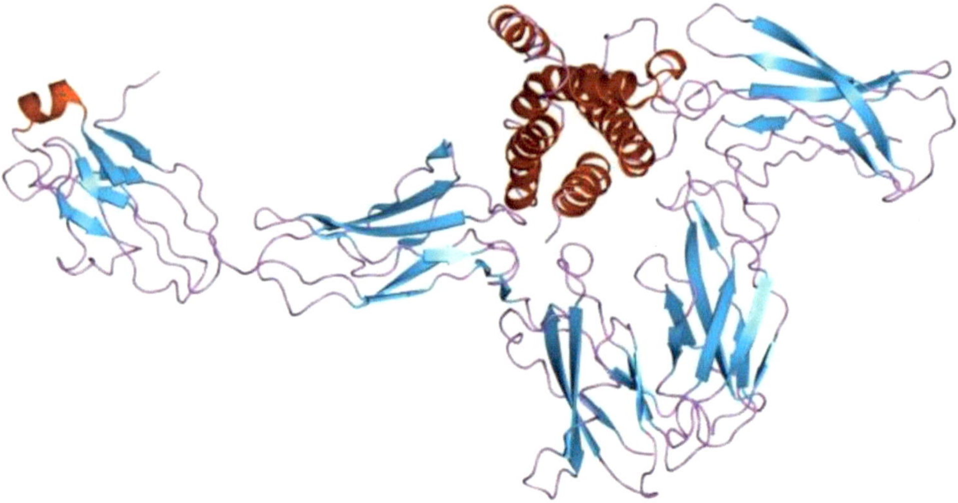

DOSAGE FORMS AND STRENGTHS

Pediatric and Young Adult r/r B-cell ALL (up to 25 years of age): A single dose of KYMRIAH contains 0.2 to 5.0 x 10^6 CAR-positive viable T cells per kg of body weight for patients 50 kg and below or 0.1 to 2.5 x 10^8 CAR-positive viable T cells for patients above 50 kg, suspended in one to three patient-specific infusion bag(s). Adult r/r DLBCL: A single dose of KYMRIAH contains 0.6 to 6.0 x 10^8 CAR-positive viable T cells, which may be suspended in one to three patient-specific infusion bag(s). See the CoA for actual cell count. The volume in the infusion bag ranges from 10 mL to 50 mL.

CONTRAINDICATIONS: None.

WARNINGS AND PRECAUTIONS

1. **Cytokine Release Syndrome (CRS)** *[Please also see Appendix 11.2].*

CRS, including fatal or life-threatening reactions, occurred following treatment with KYMRIAH. CRS occurred in 54 (79%) of the 68 pediatric and young adult patients with r/r ALL and 78 (74%) of the 106 adult patients with r/r DLBCL receiving KYMRIAH, including ≥ Grade 3 (Penn grading system1) in 49% of patients with r/r ALL and in 23% of patients with r/r DLBCL. The median time to onset was 3 days (range: 1-51), and in only two patients was onset after Day 10. The median time to resolution of CRS was 8 days (range: 1-36). Of the 54 patients with r/r ALL who had CRS, 27 (50%) received tocilizumab. Seven (13%) patients received two doses of tocilizumab, 3 (6%) patients received three doses of tocilizumab, and 14 (26%) patients received addition of corticosteroids (e.g., methylprednisolone). Of the 78 patients with r/r DLBCL who had CRS, 16 (21%) received systemic tocilizumab or corticosteroids. Six (8%) patients received a single dose of tocilizumab, 10 (13%) patients received two doses of tocilizumab, and 10 (13%) patients received corticosteroids in addition to tocilizumab. Two patients with r/r DLBCL received corticosteroids for CRS without concomitant tocilizumab, and two patients received corticosteroids for persistent neurotoxicity after resolution of CRS. Five deaths occurred within 30 days of KYMRIAH infusion. One patient with r/r ALL died with CRS and progressive leukemia, and one patient had resolving CRS with **abdominal compartment syndrome** *[see below and Appendix 11.6],* coagulopathy, and renal failure when an intracranial hemorrhage occurred. Of the 3 r/r DLBCL patients who died within 30 days of infusion, all had CRS in the setting of stable to progressive underlying disease, one of whom developed bowel necrosis. Among patients with CRS, key manifestations include fever (92% in r/r ALL and r/r DLBCL), hypotension (67% in r/r ALL; 47% in r/r DLBCL), hypoxia (20% in r/r ALL; 35% in r/r DLBCL) and tachycardia (30% in r/r ALL; 14% in r/r DLBCL). CRS may be associated with hepatic, renal, and cardiac dysfunction, and coagulopathy.

[Abdominal compartment syndrome occurs when tissue fluid within the peritoneal and retroperitoneal space (either edema, retroperitoneal blood or free fluid in the abdomen) accumulates in such large volumes that the abdominal wall compliance threshold is crossed and the abdomen can no longer stretch. Once the

abdominal wall can no longer expand, any further fluid leaking into the tissue results in fairly rapid rises in the pressure within the closed space. Initially this increase in pressure does not cause organ failure but does prevent organs from working properly – this is called intra-abdominal hypertension and is defined as a pressure over 12 mmHg in adults. ACS is defined by a sustained IAP (intra-abdominal pressure) above 20 mmHg with new-onset or progressive organ failure. Severe organ dysfunction syndrome: These pressure measurements are relative. Small children get into trouble and develop compartment syndromes at much lower pressures while young previously healthy athletic individuals may tolerate an abdominal pressure of 20 mmHg very well. The underlying cause of the disease process is capillary permeability caused by the systemic inflammatory response syndrome (SIRS) that occurs in every critically ill patient. SIRS leads to leakage of fluid out of the capillary beds into the interstitial space in the entire body with a profound amount of this fluid leaking into the gut wall, mesentery and retroperitoneal tissue].

Delay the infusion of KYMRIAH after lymphodepleting chemotherapy if the patient has unresolved serious adverse reactions from preceding chemotherapies (including pulmonary toxicity, cardiac toxicity, or hypotension), active uncontrolled infection, active graft- versus-host disease (GVHD), or worsening of leukemia burden. Ensure that two doses of tocilizumab are available on site prior to infusion of KYMRIAH. Monitor patients for signs or symptoms of CRS for at least 4 weeks after treatment with KYMRIAH. Counsel patients to seek immediate medical attention should signs or symptoms of CRS occur at any time. At the first sign of CRS, immediately evaluate patient for hospitalization and institute treatment with supportive care, tocilizumab and/or corticosteroids as indicated. Risk factors for severe CRS in the pediatric and young adult r/r B-cell ALL population are high pre-infusion tumor burden (greater than 50% blasts in bone marrow), uncontrolled or accelerating tumor burden following lymphodepleting chemotherapy, active infections, and/or inflammatory processes. Risk factors for developing severe CRS in adult r/r DLBCL are not known.

2. Neurological Toxicities

Neurological toxicities including severe or life-threatening reactions, occurred in 49 (72%) of the 68 patients with r/r ALL and 62 (58%) of the 106 patients with r/r DLBCL following treatment with KYMRIAH, including ≥ Grade 3 in 21% of patients with r/r ALL and 18% of patients with r/r DLBCL. Among patients who had a neurological toxicity, 88% occurred within 8 weeks following KYMRIAH infusion. Median time to the first event was 6 days from infusion (range: 1-359), and the median duration was 6 days for patients with r/r ALL and 14 days for patients with r/r DLBCL. Resolution occurred within 3 weeks in 79% of patients with r/r ALL and 61% of patients with r/r DLBCL. Encephalopathy lasting up to 50 days was noted. The onset of neurological toxicity can be concurrent with CRS, following resolution of CRS or in the absence of CRS. The most common neurological toxicities observed with KYMRIAH include headache (37% in r/r ALL; 21% in r/r DLBCL), encephalopathy (34% in r/r ALL; 16% in r/r DLBCL), delirium (21% in r/r ALL; 6% in r/r DLBCL), anxiety (13% in r/r ALL; 9% in r/r DLBCL), sleep disorders (10% in r/r ALL; 9% in r/r DLBCL), dizziness (6% in r/r ALL; 11% in r/r DLBCL), tremor (9% in r/r ALL; 7% r/r DLBCL) and peripheral neuropathy (4% in r/r ALL; 8% in r/r DLBCL). Other manifestations included seizures, mutism and aphasia. Monitor patients for neurological events and exclude other causes for neurological symptoms. Provide supportive care as needed for KYMRIAH-associated neurological events.

KYMRIAH REMS to mitigate cytokine release syndrome and neurological toxicities

Because of the risk of CRS and neurological toxicities, KYMRIAH is available only through a restricted program under a Risk Evaluation and Mitigation Strategy (REMS) called the KYMRIAH REMS.

The required components of the KYMRIAH REMS are:

• Healthcare facilities that dispense and administer KYMRIAH must be enrolled and comply with the REMS requirements. Certified healthcare facilities must have on-site, immediate access to tocilizumab, and ensure that a minimum of two doses of tocilizumab are available for each patient for administration within 2 hours after KYMRIAH infusion, if needed for treatment of CRS.

• Certified healthcare facilities must ensure that healthcare providers who prescribe, dispense or administer KYMRIAH are trained about the management of CRS and neurological toxicities. Further information is available at www.kymriah-rems.com or 1-844-4KYMRIAH.

Hypersensitivity reactions

Allergic reactions may occur with infusion of KYMRIAH. Serious hypersensitivity reactions, including anaphylaxis, may be due to the dimethyl sulfoxide (DMSO) or dextran 40 in KYMRIAH.

Serious infections

Infections, including life-threatening or fatal infections, occurred in 95 (55%) of 174 patients with r/r ALL or r/r DLBCL after KYMRIAH infusion. Fifty-eight patients (33%) experienced Grade ≥ 3 infections, including fatal infections in 2 patients (3%) with r/r ALL and 1 patient (1%) with r/r DLBCL. Prior to KYMRIAH infusion, infection prophylaxis should follow local guidelines. Patients with active uncontrolled infection should not start KYMRIAH treatment until the infection is resolved. Monitor patients for signs and symptoms of infection after treatment with KYMRIAH and treat appropriately.

Febrile neutropenia (≥ Grade 3) was also observed in 37% of patients with r/r ALL and 17% of patients with r/r DLBCL after KYMRIAH infusion and may be concurrent with CRS. In the event of febrile neutropenia, evaluate for infection and manage with broad spectrum antibiotics, fluids and other supportive care as medically indicated.

Viral reactivation

Hepatitis B virus (HBV) reactivation, in some cases resulting in fulminant hepatitis, hepatic failure and death, can occur in patients treated with drugs directed against B cells. Perform screening for HBV, HCV, and HIV in accordance with clinical guidelines before collection of cells for manufacturing.

(Figure 38. Ground glass hepatocytes as seen in a chronic hepatitis B liver biopsy. H&E stain.

This image is by Nephron - Own work, CC BY-SA 3.0, https://commons.wikimedia.org/w/index.php?curid=7789677; https://en.wikipedia.org/wiki/Hepatitis_B#/media/File:Ground_glass_hepatocytes_hig

h_mag_cropped.jpg. This file is licensed under the Creative Commons Attribution-Share Alike 3.0 Unported license. No changes were made to this image).

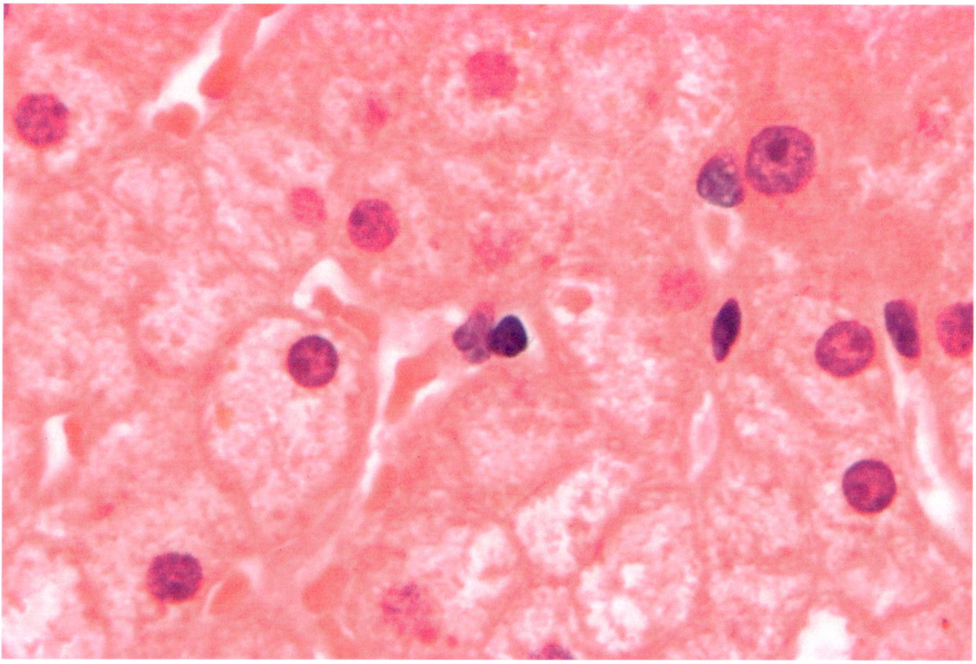

Prolonged cytopenias

Patients may exhibit cytopenias for several weeks following lymphodepleting chemotherapy and KYMRIAH infusion. In the ELIANA study (Study 1), ≥ Grade 3 cytopenias not resolved by Day 28 following KYMRIAH treatment included neutropenia (40%), and thrombocytopenia (27%) among 52 responding patients. At 56 days following KYMRIAH, 17% and 12% of responding patients had ≥ Grade 3 neutropenia or thrombocytopenia respectively. In the JULIET study (Study 2), ≥ Grade 3 cytopenias not resolved by Day 28 following KYMRIAH treatment included thrombocytopenia (40%) and neutropenia (25%) among 106 treated patients. Prolonged neutropenia has been associated with increased risk of infection. Myeloid growth factors, particularly GMCSF, are not recommended during the first 3 weeks after KYMRIAH infusion or until CRS has resolved.

Hypogammaglobulinemia

Hypogammaglobulinemia and agammaglobulinemia (IgG) related to B cell aplasia can occur in patients with a complete remission (CR) after KYMRIAH infusion. Hypogammaglobulinemia was reported in 43% of patients treated with KYMRIAH for r/r ALL and 14% of patients with r/r DLBCL. Monitor immunoglobulin levels after treatment with KYMRIAH and manage using infection precautions, antibiotic prophylaxis and immunoglobulin replacement standard guidelines.

Immunization with live vaccines

The safety of immunization with live viral vaccines during or following KYMRIAH treatment has not been studied. Vaccination with live virus vaccines is not recommended for at least 6 weeks prior to the start of lymphodepleting chemotherapy, during KYMRIAH treatment, and until immune recovery following treatment with KYMRIAH. Pregnant women who have received KYMRIAH may have hypogammaglobulinemia. Assess immunoglobulin levels in newborns of mothers treated with KYMRIAH.

Secondary malignancies

Patients treated with KYMRIAH may develop secondary malignancies or recurrence of their cancer. Monitor life-long for secondary malignancies. In the event that a secondary malignancy occurs, contact Novartis Pharmaceuticals Corporation at 1-844-4KYMRIAH to obtain instructions on patient samples to collect for testing.

Effects on ability to drive and use machines

Due to the potential for neurological events, including altered mental status or seizures, patients receiving KYMRIAH are at risk for altered or decreased consciousness or coordination in the 8 weeks following KYMRIAH infusion. Advise patients to refrain from driving and engaging in hazardous occupations or activities, such as operating heavy or potentially dangerous machinery, during this initial period.

ADVERSE REACTIONS

The most common adverse reactions (> 20%) were cytokine release syndrome (79%), hypogammaglobulinemia (43%), infections -pathogen unspecified (41%), pyrexia (40%), decreased appetite (37%), headache (37%), encephalopathy (34%), hypotension (31%), bleeding episodes (31%), tachycardia (26%), nausea (26%), diarrhea (26%), vomiting (26%), viral infectious disorders (26%), hypoxia (24%), fatigue (25%), acute kidney injury (24%), edema (21%), cough (21%), and delirium (21%). The adverse reactions with greater or equal to 10% incidence for any Grade are as follows:

Table 5. Selected adverse reactions any time after infusion (≥ 10%). Following treatment with Kymriah in pediatric and young adult r/r b-cell ALL (N = 68). Please note that the ***italics*** text in Table 4 and the footnotes to Table 4 are used in the FDA package insert.

Adverse reaction	**All grades (%)**	**Grades 3 or higher (%)**
Blood and lymphatic system disorders:		
Febrile Neutropenia	37	37
Cardiac disorders		
Tachycardia[a]	26	4
Gastrointestinal disorders:		
Nausea	26	3
Diarrhea	26	1
Vomiting	26	1
Constipation	18	0
Abdominal pain[b]	16	3
General disorders and administration site conditions:		
Pyrexia	40	15
Fatigue[c]	25	0
Edema[d]	21	1
Chills	10	0

Pain[e]	18	3
Infections and infestations:		
Infections - pathogen unspecified	41	16
Viral infectious disorders	26	18
Bacterial infectious disorders	19	13
Fungal infectious disorders	13	7
Investigations:		
International normalized ratio increased	13	0
Metabolism and nutrition disorders:		
Decreased appetite	37	15
Fluid overload	10	7
Musculoskeletal and connective tissue disorders:		
Myalgia	15	0
Arthralgia	12	1
Back pain	10	3

Nervous system disorders:		
Headache[g]	37	3
Encephalopathy[h]	34	10
Psychiatric disorders:	21	4
Delirium[i]	13	3
Anxiety	10	0
Sleep disorders[j]		
Respiratory, thoracic and mediastinal disorders:	24	18
Hypoxia	21	0
Cough[l]	16	12
Dyspnea[m]	16	10
Pulmonary edema	12	6
Tachypnea	10	4
Pleural effusion	10	0
Nasal congestion		
Skin and subcutaneous tissue disorders:	16	1
Rash[n]		
Vascular disorders:	31	22
Hypotension	19	6
Hypertension		

[a]*Tachycardia includes tachycardia and sinus tachycardia.*

[b]*Abdominal pain includes abdominal pain, abdominal pain upper.*

[c]*Fatigue includes fatigue and malaise.*

[d]*Edema includes face edema, generalised edema, localised edema, edema peripheral.*

[e]*Pain includes pain and pain in the extremity.*

[f]*Hypogammaglobulinemia includes hypogammaglobulinemia, immunoglobulins decreased, blood immunoglobulin G decreased, blood immunoglobulin A decreased, blood immunoglobulin M decreased.*

[g]*Headache includes headache and migraine.*

[h]*Encephalopathy includes encephalopathy, cognitive disorder, confusional state, depressed level of consciousness, disturbance in attention, lethargy, mental status changes, somnolence, and automatism.*

[i]*Delirium includes delirium, agitation, hallucination, hallucination visual, irritability, restlessness.*

[j]*Sleep disorders includes sleep disorder, insomnia and nightmare.*

[k]*Acute kidney injury includes acute kidney injury, anuria, azotemia, renal failure, renal tubular dysfunction, renal tubular necrosis, and blood creatinine increased.*

[l]*Cough includes cough and productive cough.*

[m]*Dyspnea includes dyspnea and respiratory distress, respiratory failure.*

[n]*Rash includes rash, rash maculo-papular, rash papular, and rash pruritic.*

Additional important adverse reactions that did not meet the threshold criteria for inclusion in Table 4 were:

Blood and lymphatic system disorders: disseminated intravascular coagulation (9%); histiocytosis lymphocytic hemophagocytosis (7%); coagulopathy (6%); Grade 3 and Grade 4 hypofibrinogenemia with Grade 3 and 4 CRS (16%).

Cardiac disorders: cardiac arrest (4%), cardiac failure (7%).

Gastrointestinal disorders: abdominal compartment syndrome (1%).

General disorders and administration site conditions: multiple organ dysfunction syndrome (3%).

Immune system disorders: graft-versus-host disease (1%).

Investigations: activated partial thromboplastin time prolonged (6%).

Nervous system: tremor (9%), dizziness (6%), seizure (3%), speech disorders[a] (3%), motor dysfunction[b] including muscle spasms (1%)

Respiratory, thoracic, and mediastinal disorders: respiratory distress (6%), respiratory failure (6%), acute respiratory distress syndrome (4%), oropharyngeal pain (6%).

Metabolism and nutrition disorders: tumor lysis syndrome (6%).

Vascular disorders: capillary leak syndrome (3%), thrombosis (3%)

Eye disorders: visual impairment (3%)

[a]Speech disorder includes aphasia and dysarthria. [b]Motor dysfunction includes muscle spasms.

[Some of the above disorders are described further below: This information is ***not*** *included in the FDA package insert and thus, as per my note in Section 8, they are placed in parentheses and written in italics.*

*[**Hemophagocytic lymphohistiocytosis** (HLH), also known as haemophagocytic lymphohistiocytosis (British spelling), and hemophagocytic or haemophagocytic syndrome, is an uncommon hematologic disorder seen more often in children than in adults. It is a life-threatening disease of severe hyperinflammation caused by uncontrolled proliferation of activated lymphocytes and macrophages, characterised by proliferation of morphologically benign lymphocytes and macrophages that secrete high amounts of inflammatory cytokines. It is classified as one of the cytokine storm syndromes. There are inherited and non-inherited (acquired) causes of hemophagocytic lymphohistiocytosis (HLH).*

Figure 39. Light microscopic image of bone marrow showing stromal macrophages containing numerous red blood cells in their cytoplasm.

This image is by Jon salisbury at English Wikipedia - Transferred from en.wikipedia to Commons. Public Domain, https://commons.wikimedia.org/w/index.php?curid=11557969; https://en.wikipedia.org/wiki/Hemophagocytic_lymphohistiocytosis#/media/File:Haemophagocytic_lymphohistiocytosis_Bone_marrow.JPG. This work has been released into the public domain by its author, Jon salisbury at English Wikipedia. No changes were made to this image).

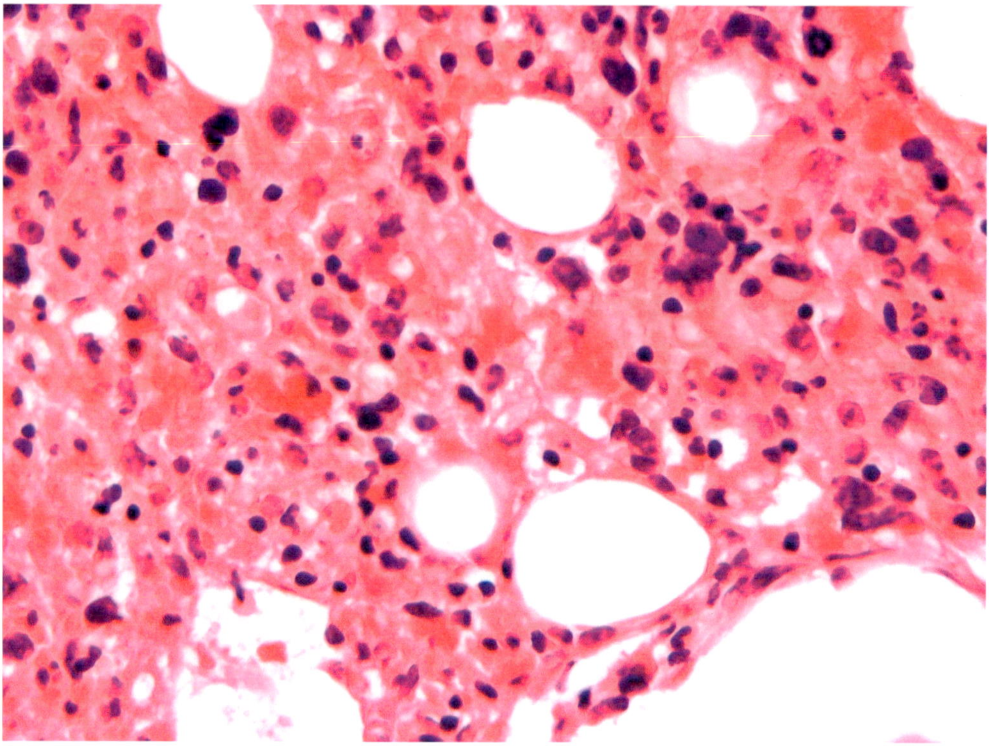

(Hypogammaglobulinemia

Hypogammaglobulinemia is a situation with the immune system in which not enough gamma globulins are produced in the blood. This results in a lower antibody count, which impairs the immune system, increasing risk of infection. Hypogammaglobulinemia may result from a variety of primary genetic immune system defects, such as common variable immunodeficiency, or it may be caused by secondary effects such as medication, blood cancer, or poor nutrition, or loss of gamma globulins in urine, as in nonselective glomerular proteinuria. Patients with hypogammaglobulinemia have reduced immune function; important considerations include avoiding use of live vaccines, and take precautionary measures when traveling to regions with endemic disease or poor sanitation such as receiving immunizations, taking antibiotics abroad, drinking only safe or boiled water, arranging appropriate medical cover in advance of travel, and ensuring continuation of any immunoglobulin infusions needed).

(Capillary leak syndrome.

Capillary leak syndrome is characterized by the escape of blood plasma through capillary walls, from the blood circulatory system to surrounding tissues, muscle compartments, organs or body cavities. It is a phenomenon most commonly witnessed in sepsis, and less frequently in autoimmune diseases, ***differentiation syndrome, engraftment syndrome****, hemophagocytic lymphohistiocytosis [see above], the* ***ovarian hyperstimulation syndrome****, viral hemorrhagic fevers, and snakebite and ricin poisoning. Pharmaceuticals, including the chemotherapy medications gemcitabine and tagraxofusp, as well as certain interleukins and monoclonal antibodies, can also cause capillary leaks. These conditions and factors are sources of secondary capillary leak syndrome.*

(Differentiation syndrome

Differentiation syndrome, formerly known as Retinoic acid syndrome (RAS), is a potentially life-threatening complication observed in people with acute promyelocytic leukemia (APML) and first thought to be specifically associated with all-trans retinoic acid (ATRA) (also known as tretinoin) treatment. Subsequently, so-called RAS was recognized in APML patients who had been treated with another highly efficacious drug, arsenic trioxide, and yet did not appear in patients treated with tretinoin for other disorders. These facts and others support the notion that RAS depends on the presence of the malignant promyelocytes. This has led to the growing deprecation of the term 'retinoic acid syndrome' and to an increasing use of the term differentiation syndrome to signify this APML treatment complication.

(Engraftment syndrome

Engraftment syndrome (ES) is an early complication of hematopoietic stem cell transplantation (HSCT) that occurs around neutrophil engraftment time and is attributed to the sudden cytokine discharge associated with robust engraftment of transplanted cells. The secreted cytokines cause a clinical picture suggestive of an exaggerated inflammatory response. This complication has been described both in autologous and allogeneic transplantation.

The diagnostic clinical features include the presence of two or more of the following symptoms usually 96 hours before neutrophil engraftment time: 1. fever of unknown origin (38.0-38.5 °C) with no detectable infectious agent or other cause, 2. erythematous skin rash not related to drug reactions or viral infection (usually covering >25% of the body surface), 3. weight gain of 2.5-5% (above baseline of admission) and albumin drop to 90% of pretransplant levels, and 4. pulmonary symptoms with dyspnea, hypoxia and pulmonary infiltrates on a chest X-ray (excluding infection, thromboembolism, pulmonary hemorrhage, fluid overload, or cardiac causes). Though hepatic dysfunction, renal insufficiency and transient encephalopathy have been described in adults, they have not been reported as common findings in pediatric practice.

Risk Factors include;1. High cell doses infused on day 0, 2. Prompt increase in white blood cell (WBC) counts, 3. Autologous peripheral blood as stem cell source, and 4. Autoimmune disease as an underlying condition.

Differential diagnosis and early recognition are particularly important since corticosteroids have a critical role in the reversal of symptoms and management of the condition.

The prognosis is usually good with early corticosteroid use, and complete resolution is seen in 1-5 days in >80% of cases. Otherwise, this complication occasionally may lead to increased morbidity and mortality if not managed appropriately and timely.

ES is associated with increased length of hospitalization. It may be problematic since it can resemble cutaneous acute graft-versus-host disease (aGvHD) or be complicated by capillary leak syndrome and noncardiogenic pulmonary edema. Rarely, ES can mimic aGvHD by affecting the liver and gastrointestinal tract. It has been shown that patients who develop ES receive empirical antifungal therapy more frequently than patients who do not, most likely due to persistent fever. Patients undergoing autologous HSCT for multiple sclerosis who develop ES may experience transient worsening of neurological symptoms. In pediatric patients, ES is also associated with increased transfusion requirements, need for parenteral nutrition and increased risk of critical care requirement

Corticosteroids also have a role in the prevention of ES.

(Multiple organ dysfunction syndrome

Multiple dysfunction syndrome is the presence of altered organ function in acutely ill patients such that homeostasis cannot be maintained without intervention. It usually involves two or more organ systems. It calls for an immediate intervention. Although Irwin and Rippe cautioned in 2005 that the use of "multiple organ failure" or "multisystem organ failure" should be avoided, both Harrison's (2015) and Cecil's (2012) medical textbooks still use the terms "multi-organ failure" and "multiple organ failure" in several chapters and do not use "multiple organ dysfunction syndrome" at all.

The condition results from infection, injury (accident, surgery), hypoperfusion and hypermetabolism. The primary cause triggers an uncontrolled inflammatory response.

Sepsis is the most common cause of multiple organ dysfunction syndrome and may result in septic shock. In the absence of infection, a sepsis-like disorder is termed systemic inflammatory response syndrome (SIRS). Both SIRS and sepsis could ultimately progress to multiple organ dysfunction syndrome. However, in one-third of the patients no primary focus can be found. Multiple organ dysfunction syndrome is well established as the final stage of a continuum: SIRS + infection → sepsis → severe sepsis → Multiple organ dysfunction syndrome.

At present, there is no drug or device that can reverse organ failure that has been judged by the health care team to be medically and/or surgically irreversible (organ function can recover, at least to a degree, in patients whose organs are very dysfunctional, where the patient has not died, and some organs, like the liver or the skin, can regenerate better than others),- with the possible exception of single or multiple organ transplants or the use of artificial organs or organ parts, in certain candidates in specific situations. Therapy, therefore, is usually mostly limited to supportive care, i.e. safeguarding hemodynamics, and respiration. Maintaining adequate tissue oxygenation is a principal target. Starting enteral nutrition within 36 hours of admission to an intensive care unit has reduced infectious complications.

Mortality, though it has lessened to a limited degree, at least in high income countries with timely access to initial and tertiary care, varies where the chance of survival is diminished as the number of organs involved increases. Mortality in MODS from septic shock (which itself has a mortality of 25-50%), and from multiple traumas, especially if not rapidly treated, appear to be especially severe. If more than one organ system is affected, the mortality rate is higher, and this is especially the case when five or more systems or organs are affected. Old age is a risk factor in and of itself, and immunocompromised patients, such as with cancer or HIV/AIDS or recipients of organ transplants, are at risk. Earlier and aggressive treatment, the use of experimental treatments, or at least modern tools such as ventilators, ECMO, dialysis, bypass, and transplantation, especially at a trauma center, may improve outcomes in certain cases, but this depends in part on speedy and affordable access to high-quality care. Measurements of lactate, cytokines, albumin and other proteins, urea, blood oxygen and carbon dioxide levels, insulin, and blood sugar, adequate hydration, constant monitoring of vital signs, good communication within and between facilities and staff, and adequate staffing, training, and charting are important in MODS.

(Tumor lysis syndrome

Tumor lysis syndrome (TLS) is a group of metabolic abnormalities that can occur as a complication from the treatment of cancer, where large amounts of tumor cells are lysed from the treatment, releasing their contents into the bloodstream. This occurs most commonly after the treatment of lymphomas and leukemias and in particular when treating non-Hodgkin's lymphoma (NHL), acute myeloid leukemia (AML), and acute lymphoblastic leukemia. This is a potentially fatal complication and patients at increased risk for TLS should be closely monitored while receiving chemotherapy and should receive preventive measures and treatments TLS can also occur on its own (while not being treated with chemotherapy) although this is less common.

Tumor lysis syndrome is characterized by hyperkalemia, hyperphosphatemia, hypocalcemia), hyperuricemia and higher than normal levels of blood urea nitrogen (BUN). These changes in blood electrolytes and metabolites are a result of the release of cellular contents of dying cells into the bloodstream. In this respect, TLS is analogous to rhabdomyolysis, with comparable mechanism and blood chemistry effects but with a different cause. In TLS, the breakdown occurs after cytotoxic therapy or from cancers with high cell turnover and tumor proliferation rates. The metabolic abnormalities seen in tumor lysis syndrome can ultimately result in serious complications such as acute uric acid nephropathy, acute kidney failure, seizures, cardiac arrhythmias, and death.

It can be prevented by prophylactically ensuring good renal output with administration of intravenous fluids and a loop diuretic together with rasburicase to help clear uric acid from the blood. Mild hyperkalemia without symptoms can be treated with a loop diuretic and sodium polystirene, while a temporizing agent such as rapid acting insulin (in conjunction with glucose) and an agent to stabilize cardiac membranes such as calcium carbonate may be given in cases of severe hyperkalemia. For symptoms due to hypocalcemia (e.g. seizures) patients can be treated with calcium gluconate. Tumor lysis patients may ultimately also require renal replacement therapy such as through hemodialysis if indicated.

(Graft-versus-host disease.

Graft-versus-host disease (GvHD) is a syndrome, characterized by inflammation in different organs, most commonly associated with hematopoietic stem cell transplants. T cells of the donor's immune system which remain within the donated tissue (the graft) recognize the recipient (the host) as foreign (non-self). The T cells present within the transplanted tissue then attack the recipient's body's cells, which leads to GvHD. This should not be confused with a transplant rejection, which occurs when the immune system of the transplant recipient rejects the transplanted tissue. GvHD occurs when the donor's immune system's T cells reject the recipient. GvHD can also occur after a blood transfusion if the blood products used have not been irradiated or treated with an approved pathogen reduction system).

(Ovarian hyperstimulation syndrome.

Ovarian hyperstimulation syndrome (OHSS) is a medical condition that can occur in some women who take fertility medication to stimulate egg growth, and in other women in very rare cases. Most cases are mild, but rarely the condition is severe and can lead to serious illness or death. Symptoms can be mild, moderate, or severe. Mild symptoms include abdominal bloating and feeling of fullness, nausea, diarrhea, and slight weight gain. Moderate symptoms include excessive weight gain (weight gain of greater than 2 pounds per day), increased abdominal girth, vomiting, diarrhea, darker urine, decreased urine output, excessive thirst, and skin and/or hair feeling dry (in addition to mild symptoms). Severe symptoms are fullness/bloating above the waist, shortness of breath, pleural effusion, urination significantly darker or has ceased, calf and chest pains, marked abdominal bloating or distention, and lower abdominal pains (in addition to mild and moderate symptoms).

The central feature of clinically significant OHSS is the development of vascular hyperpermeability and the resulting shift of fluids into the third space. As hCG causes the ovary to undergo extensive luteinization, large amounts of estrogens, progesterone, and local cytokines are released. It is almost certain that vascular endothelial growth factor (VEGF) is a key substance that induces vascular hyperpermeability, making local capillaries "leaky", leading to a shift of fluids from the intravascular system to the abdominal and pleural cavity. Supraphysiologic production of VEGF from many follicles under the prolonged effect of hCG appears to be the specific key process underlying OHSS. Thus, while the woman accumulates fluid in the third space, primarily in the form of ascites, she actually becomes hypovolemic and is at risk for respiratory, circulatory (such as arterial thromboembolism since blood is now thicker), and renal problems. Women who are pregnant sustain the ovarian luteinization process through the production of hCG)].

Laboratory abnormalities

Table 6. Selected other laboratory abnormalities worsening (>10%) from baseline grade 0-2 to grade 3 – 4 following treatment with KYMRIAH in pediatric and young adult patients with r/r B cell ALL based on CTCAE[a] (N = 68).

	Grade 3-4 (%)
Increased aspartate transaminase	28
Hypokalemia	27
Increased Alanine Aminotransferase	21
Increased bilirubin	21
Hypophosphatemia	19

[a]CTCAE = Common Terminology Criteria for Adverse Events version 4.03

Table 7. Prolonged cytopenias following treatment with KYMRIAK in pediatric and young adult patients with r/r B cell ALL.

Prolonged cytopenia	N = 52 (%) Day 28	N = 52 (%) Day 56
Prolonged neutropenia[a]	40	17
Prolonged thrombocytopenia[a]	27	12

[a] ≥ Grade 3 observed within 14 days after Day 28 or Day 56 in responding patients

Use of KYMTIA in adult r/r Diffuse Large B-cell Lymphoma (DLBCL)

In the JULIET study (Study 2) 106 adults with r/r DLBCL received a single intravenous dose of KYMRIAH. The most common adverse reactions (incidence > 20%) were cytokine release syndrome, infections-pathogen unspecified, diarrhea, nausea, pyrexia, fatigue, hypotension, edema and headache.

The study population characteristics were: median age of 56 years (range: 22 to 76 years), 79% DLBCL; a median of 3 prior lines of therapy (range: 1-6), 49% had a prior autologous hematopoietic stem cell transplantation, and 33% had received prior radiation therapy. Ninety-nine patients (93%) received lymphodepleting chemotherapy prior to KYMRIAH, that included fludarabine (n = 77) or bendamustine (n = 22).

The adverse reactions with greater than or equal to 10% incidence for any Grade are summarized in Table 7 below.

Table 8. Selected adverse reactions any time after infusion reported in ≥ 10% following treatment with

KYMRIAH in adult r/r DLBCL (N = 106)

Adverse reaction	All grades (%)	Grade 3 or higher
Blood and lymphatic system disorders:		

Febrile Neutropenia	17	17
Cardiac disorders: [a]Tachycardia	 13	 3
Gastrointestinal disorders: Diarrhea Nausea Constipation	 31 27 16	 1 1 1
General disorders and administration site conditions: Pyrexia [b]Fatigue [c]Edema [d]Pain Chills	 34 26 23 15 13	 6 7 2 3 0
Immune system disorders: Cytokine release syndrome [e]Hypogammaglobulinemia	 74 14	 23 4
Infections and infestations: Infections-pathogen unspecified	 42	 25
Investigations: Weight decreased	 11	 3
Metabolism and nutrition disorders: Decreased appetite	 12	 4
Musculoskeletal and connective tissue disorders: Arthralgia	 10	 0
Nervous system disorders:	21	0

[f]Headache [g]Encephalopathy [h]Dizziness	16 11	11 1
Renal and Urinary Disorders: [i]Acute kidney injury	17	6
Thoracic, respiratory and mediastinal disorders: [j]Cough [k]Dyspnea	19 18	0 6
Vascular disorders: [l]Hypotension	26	8

[a]Tachycardia includes tachycardia and sinus tachycardia.

(Sinus tachycardia.

In adults, sinus tachycardia is defined as a heart rate greater than 100 beats/min (bpm). The normal resting heart rate is 60–90 bpm in an average adult. Normal heart rate varies with age and level of fitness, from infants having faster heart rates (110-150 bpm) and the elderly having slower heart rates.

Tachycardia is often asymptomatic. It is often a resulting symptom of a primary disease state and can be an indication of the severity of a disease. If the heart rate is too high, cardiac output may fall due to the markedly reduced ventricular filling time. Rapid rates, though they may be compensating for ischemia elsewhere, increase myocardial oxygen demand and reduce coronary blood flow, thus precipitating an ischemic heart or valvular disease).

Figure 40. ECG of a 29-year-old female with sinus tachycardia. Heart rate 125 bpm QT/QTc 316/456 ms.

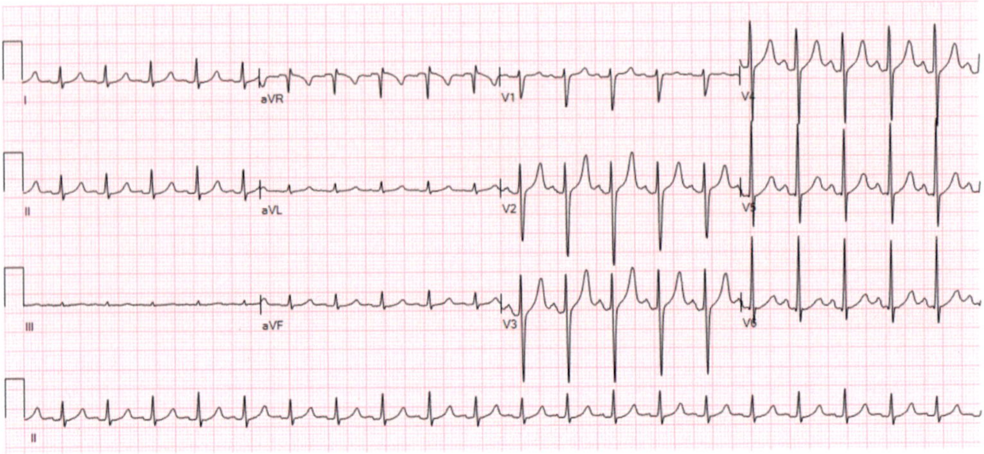

This image is by Ewingdo - Own work, CC BY-SA 4.0, https://commons.wikimedia.org/w/index.php?curid=96414277; https://en.wikipedia.org/wiki/Sinus_tachycardia#/media/File:ECG_Sinus_Tachycardia_125_bpm.jpg. This file is licensed under the Creative Commons Attribution-Share Alike 4.0 International license. No changes were made to this image).

[b]Fatigue includes fatigue and malaise.

[c]Edema includes face edema, generalised edema, localized edema, edema peripheral, peripheral swelling.

[d]Pain includes pain and pain in the extremity.

[e]Hypogammaglobulinemia includes blood immunoglobulin G decreased, immunoglobulins decreased and hypogammaglobulinemia.

[f]Headache includes headache and migraine.

[g]Encephalopathy includes encephalopathy, cognitive disorder, confusional state, disturbance in attention, lethargy, mental status changes, somnolence, memory impairment, metabolic encephalopathy and thinking abnormal.

[h]Dizziness includes dizziness, presyncope, and syncope.

[i]Acute kidney injury includes acute kidney injury and blood creatinine increased.

[j]Cough includes cough, productive cough, and upper-airway cough syndrome.

[k]Dyspnea includes dyspnea, dyspnea exertional, respiratory distress, and respiratory failure.

[l]Hypotension includes hypotension and orthostatic hypotension.

Additional important adverse reactions that did not meet the threshold criteria for inclusion in Table 7 were:

Blood and lymphatic system disorders: disseminated intravascular coagulation (3%), pancytopenia (2%), histiocytosis hematophagic (1%)

Cardiac Disorders: arrhythmia[a] (6%)

Gastrointestinal disorders: vomiting (9%), abdominal pain[b] (9%), anal incontinence (1%)

General disorders and administration site conditions: asthenia (7%), multiple organ dysfunction syndrome (3%)

Infections and infestations: fungal infectious disorders (9%), viral infectious disorders (9%), bacterial infectious disorders (9%)

Musculoskeletal and connective tissue disorders: myalgia (7%), back pain (6%)

Nervous System: peripheral neuropathy[c] (8%), motor dysfunction[d] (6%), speech disorder[e] (3%), seizure[f] (3%), ischemic cerebral infarction (1%), tremor (7%), ataxia (2%)

Psychiatric disorders: anxiety (9%), delirium[g] (6%), sleep disorders[h] (9%)

Respiratory, thoracic, and mediastinal disorders: hypoxia (8%), oropharyngeal pain[i] (8%), pleural effusion (5%) pulmonary edema[j] (3%)

[Pulmonary edema. Pulmonary edema, also known as pulmonary congestion, is excessive liquid accumulation in the tissue and air spaces (usually alveoli) of the lungs. It leads to impaired gas exchange and may cause hypoxemia and respiratory failure.

Figure 41. Pulmonary edema in CT-scan coronal MPR.

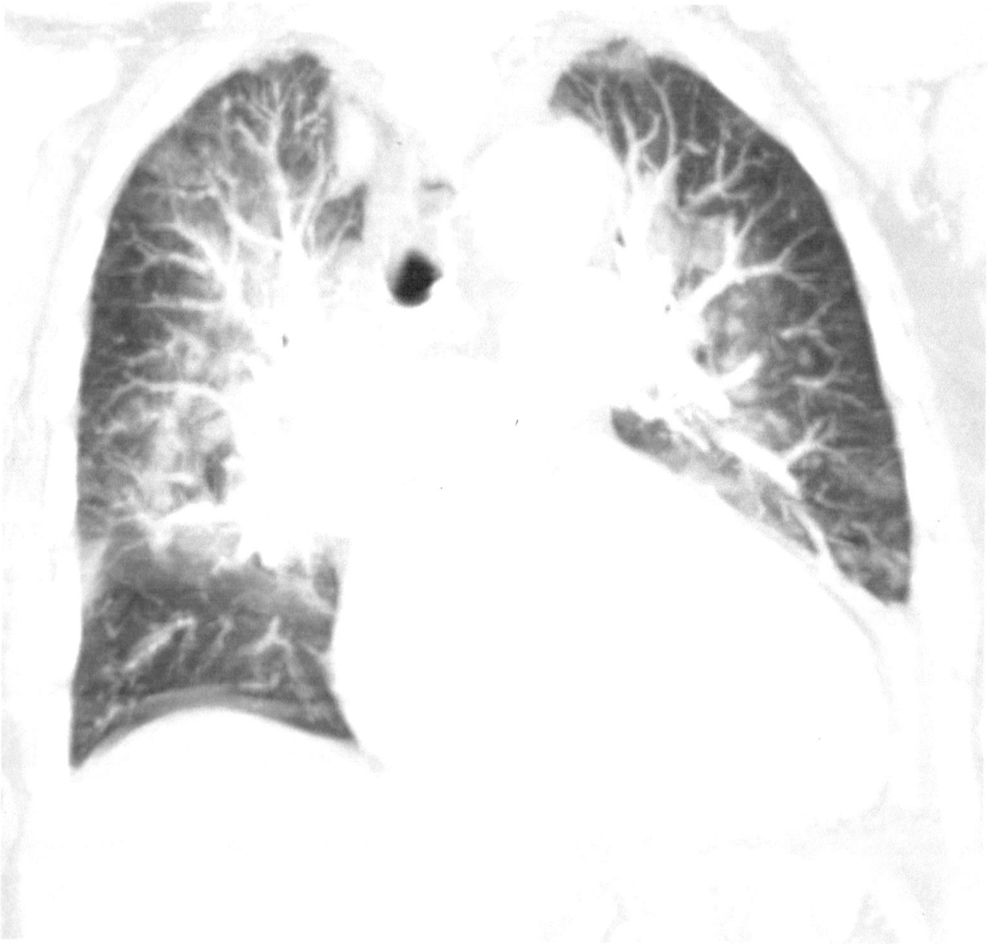

This image is by Hellerhoff - Own work, CC BY-SA 3.0, https://commons.wikimedia.org/w/index.php?curid=12228135; https://en.wikipedia.org/wiki/Pulmonary_edema#/media/File:18-01-Lungenoedem_CT_coronar.png. This file is licensed under the Creative Commons Attribution-Share Alike 3.0 Unported license. No changes were made to this image].

Metabolism and nutrition disorders: fluid overload (3%), tumor lysis syndrome (1%)

Vascular disorders: thrombosis[k] (7%), hypertension (2%), capillary leak syndrome (1%)

Skin and subcutaneous tissue disorders: rash[l] (8%), dermatitis[m] (4%)

Eye disorders: visual impairment[n] (7%).

[a]Arrhythmia includes atrial fibrillation, supraventricular tachycardia, ventricular extrasystoles.

[Figure 42. ECG showing normal sinus rhythm on the top tracing and atrial fibrillation on the lower tracing.

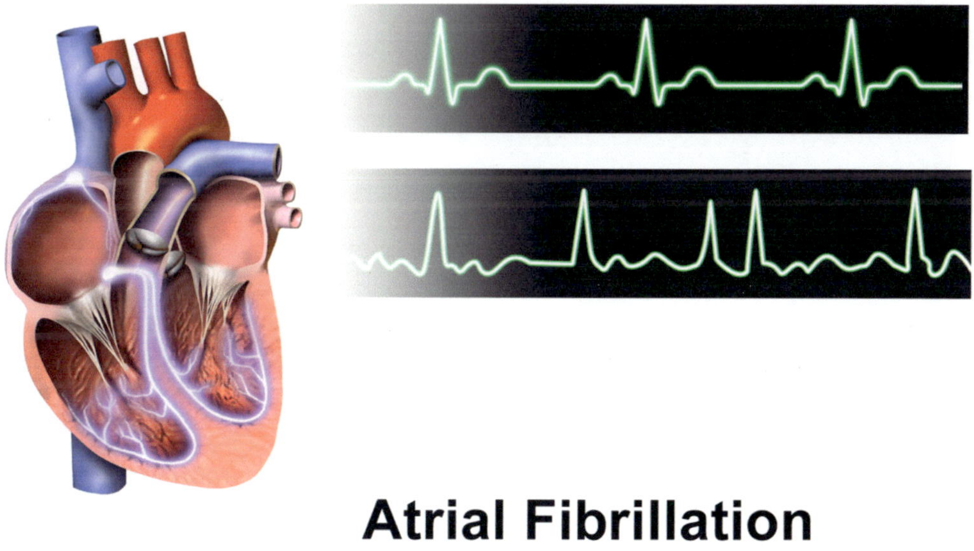

[Figure 43. Supraventricular tachycardia.

Supraventricular tachycardia (SVT) is an umbrella term for fast heart rhythms arising from the upper part of the heart. This is in contrast to the other group of fast heart rhythms - ventricular tachycardia, which start within the lower chambers of the heart. There are four main types of SVT: atrial fibrillation, atrial flutter, paroxysmal supraventricular tachycardia (PSVT), and Wolff–Parkinson–White syndrome.

Figure 43. Lead II (2) ECG (EKG) tracing of supraventricular tachycardia (SVT) in a 40 year old male.

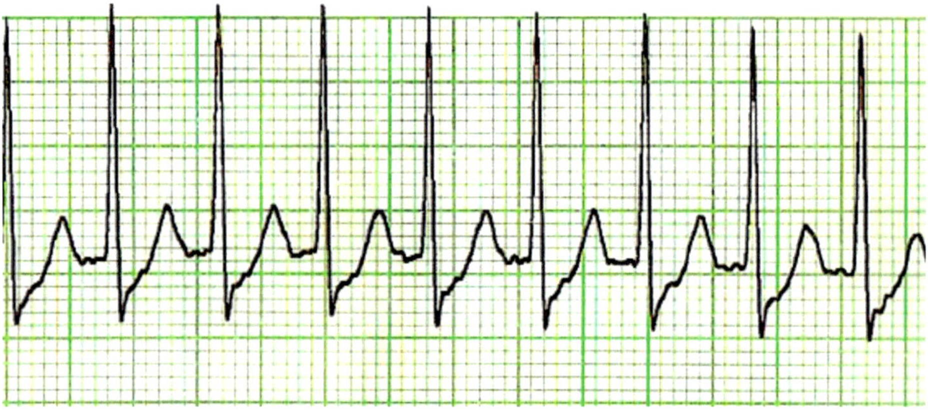

[Figure 44. Ventricular extrasystole.

A premature ventricular contraction (PVC) is a common event where the heartbeat is initiated by Purkinje fibers in the ventricles rather than by the sinoatrial node. PVCs may cause no symptoms or may be perceived as a "skipped beat" or felt as palpitations in the chest. PVCs do not usually pose any danger. PVCs are also known as premature ventricular complex, ventricular premature contraction (complex or complexes) (VPC), ventricular premature beat (VPB), ventricular extrasystole (VES). In Figure 45, two ventricular extrasystoles are indicated by the arrows

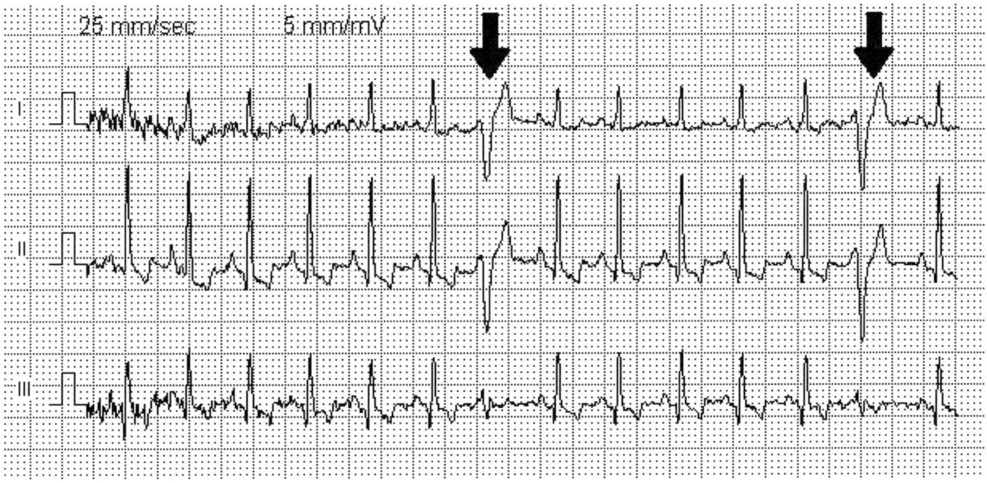

[b]Abdominal pain includes abdominal pain and abdominal pain upper.

[c]Peripheral Neuropathy includes paraethesia, hypoaesthesia, hyperaesthesia, peripheral sensory neuropathy, and neuropathy peripheral.

[d]Motor dysfunction includes muscle spasms, muscle twitching, myoclonus and myopathy.

[e]Speech disorder includes speech disorder, aphasia.

[f]Seizure includes PTs seizure and status epilepticus.

[g]Delirium includes delirium, agitation, and irritability.

[h]Sleep disorders includes sleep disorder, insomnia and nightmare.

[i]Oropharyngeal pain includes oral pain and oropharyngeal pain.

[j]Pulmonary edema includes acute pulmonary edema and pulmonary edema.

[k]Thrombosis includes deep vein thrombosis, embolism, pulmonary embolism, thrombosis, vena cava thrombosis, and venous thrombosis.

[l]Rash includes rash, rash maculo-papular, rash papular and rash pruritic.

[m]Dermatitis includes dermatitis, dermatitis acneiform and dermatitis contact.

[n]Visual impairment includes vision blurred and visual impairment.

[Inferior vena cava thrombosis is a very rare constellation of symptoms resulting from either an obstruction, or stenosis of the inferior vena cava. It can be caused by physical invasion or compression by a pathological process or by thrombosis within the vein itself. It can present with a wide variety of signs and symptoms but the commonest is edema of the lower extremities (peripheral edema), caused by an increase in the venous blood pressure.

Superior vena cava syndrome (SVCS), is a group of symptoms caused by obstruction of the superior vena cava. Characteristic features are edema (swelling due to excess fluid) of the face and arms and development of swollen collateral veins on the front of the chest wall. Shortness of breath and coughing are quite common symptoms;

Figure 46. Thrombosis of the superior vena cava (arrow) caused by an indwelling central venous catheter which caused superior vena cava syndrome.

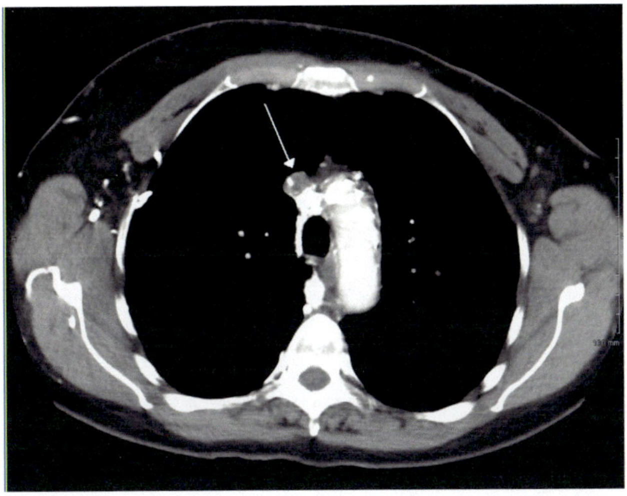

This image is by James Heilman, MD - Own work, CC BY-SA 3.0, https://commons.wikimedia.org/w/index.php?curid=15376784; https://en.wikipedia.org/wiki/Superior_vena_cava_syndrome#/media/File:SVCsyndrome.png. This file is licensed under the Creative Commons Attribution-Share Alike 3.0 Unported license. No changes were made to this image.

[Figure 47. Deep vein thrombosis, indicated by swelling of the right leg (arrow), is a risk factor for pulmonary embolism.

This image is by James Heilman, MD - Own work, CC BY-SA 3.0, https://commons.wikimedia.org/w/index.php?curid=9444797; https://en.wikipedia.org/wiki/Pulmonary_embolism#/media/File:Deep_vein_thrombosis_of_the_right_leg.jpg. This file is licensed under the Creative Commons Attribution-Share Alike 3.0 Unported license. No changes were made to this image.

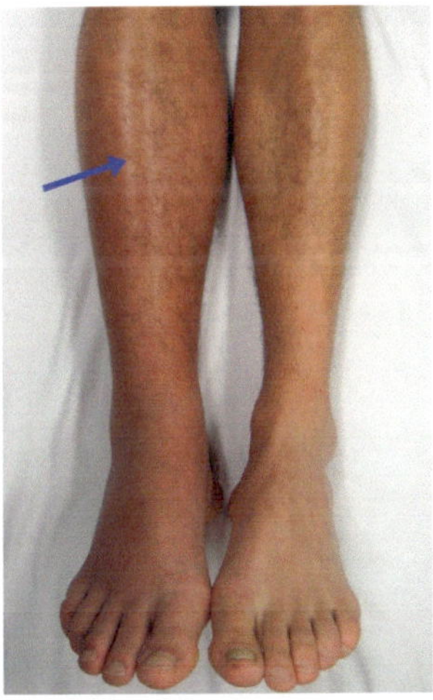

[Figure 48. Pulmonary embolism: a large saddle embolus seen in the pulmonary artery (white arrows).

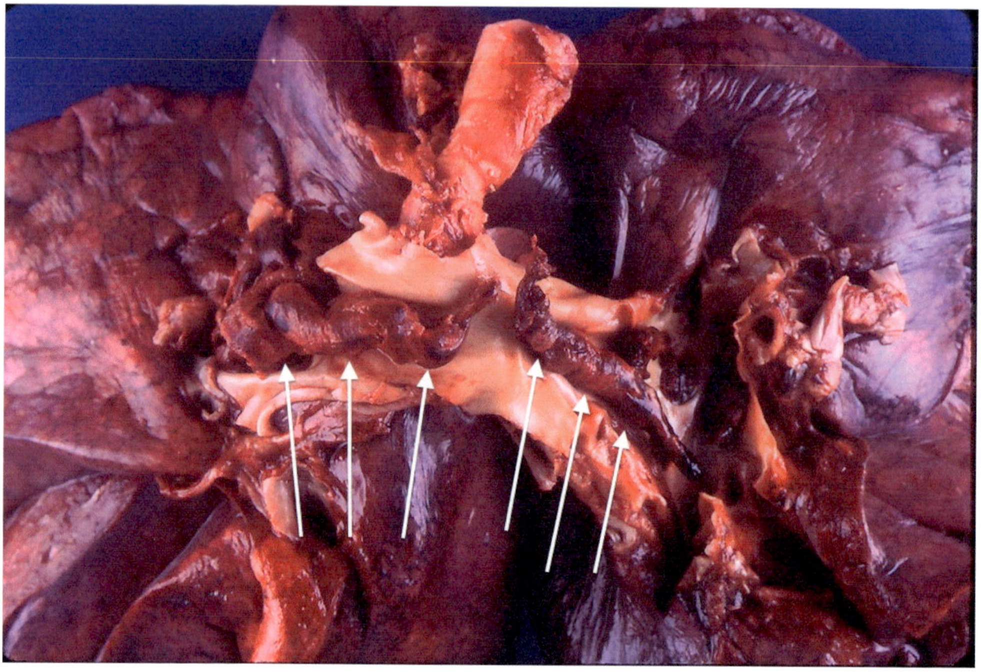

This image is by Bakerstmd - Own work, CC BY-SA 4.0, https://commons.wikimedia.org/w/index.php?curid=39263792; https://en.wikipedia.org/wiki/Pulmonary_embolism#/media/File:Saddle_thromboembolus_wArrows.jpg . This file is licensed under the Creative Commons Attribution-Share Alike 4.0 International license. No changes were made to this image].

Laboratory abnormalities

Selected laboratory abnormalities worsening from baseline Grade 0-2 to Grade 3-4 are shown in Table 8.

Table 9. Grade 3 or 4 laboratory abnormalities occurring in > 10% of patients following KYMRIAH infusion in adult r/r DLBCL patients based on CTCAE[a]. N = 106.

Laboratory parameter	Grade 3 or 4 (%)
Hematology	

Lymphopenia	94
Neutropenia	81
Leukopenia	77
Anemia	58
Thrombocytopenia	54
Biochemistry	
Hypophosphatemia	24
Hypokalemia	12
Hyponatremia	11

[a]CTCAE = Common Terminology Criteria for Adverse Events version 4.

Immunogenicity

In clinical studies, humoral immunogenicity of KYMRIAH was measured by determination of anti-murine CAR19 antibodies (anti-mCAR19) in serum pre- and post-administration. The majority of patients, 86% in ELIANA (Study 1) and 91.4% in JULIET (Study 2) tested positive for pre-dose anti-mCAR19 antibodies prior to KYMRIAH infusion; Treatment induced anti-mCAR19 antibodies were detected in 5% of the patients in JULIET. However, the pre-existing and treatment-induced antibodies were not associated with an impact on clinical response and did not have an impact on the initial expansion and persistence of KYMRIAH. Persistence of KYMRIAH was similar between patients with positive post-infusion anti-mCAR19 antibodies compared with patients with negative post-infusion anti-mCAR19 antibodies. There is no evidence that the presence of pre-existing and treatment-induced anti-mCAR19 antibodies impact the safety or effectiveness of KYMRIAH. T cell immunogenicity responses were not observed in adult r/r DLBCL patients.

DRUG INTERACTIONS

HIV and the lentivirus used to make KYMRIAH have limited, short spans of identical genetic material (RNA). Therefore, some commercial HIV nucleic acid test (NATs) tests may yield false-positive results in patients who have received KYMRIAH.

USE IN SPECIFIC POPULATIONS

Pregnancy

Risk summary

There are no available data with KYMRIAH use in pregnant women. No animal reproductive and developmental toxicity studies have been conducted with KYMRIAH to assess whether it can cause fetal harm when administered to a pregnant woman. It is not known if KYMRIAH has the potential to be transferred to the fetus. Based on the mechanism of action, if the transduced cells cross the placenta, they may cause fetal toxicity, including B-cell lymphocytopenia. Therefore, KYMRIAH is not recommended for women who are pregnant, and pregnancy after KYMRIAH administration should be discussed with the treating physician. Report pregnancies to Novartis Pharmaceuticals Corporation at 1-888-669-6682. In the U.S. general population, the estimated background risk of major birth defects and miscarriage in clinically recognized pregnancies is 2%-4% and 15%-20%, respectively.

Lactation

Risk summary

There is no information regarding the presence of KYMRIAH in human milk, the effect on the breastfed infant, and the effects on milk production. The developmental and health benefits of breastfeeding should be considered along with the mother's clinical need for KYMRIAH and any potential adverse effects on the breastfed infant from KYMRIAH or from the underlying maternal condition.

Females and Males of Reproductive Potential

Pregnancy testing

Pregnancy status of females with reproductive potential should be verified. Sexually-active females of reproductive potential should have a pregnancy test prior to starting treatment with KYMRIAH.

Contraception

See the prescribing information for fludarabine and cyclophosphamide for information on the need for effective contraception in patients who receive the lymphodepleting chemotherapy. There are insufficient exposure data to provide a recommendation concerning duration of contraception following treatment with KYMRIAH.

Infertility

There are no data on the effect of KYMRIAH on fertility.

Pediatric use

The safety and efficacy of KYMRIAH have been established in pediatric patients with r/r B-cell ALL. Use of KYMRIAH is supported by a single-arm trial that included 52 pediatric patients with r/r B-cell precursor ALL in the following age groups: 33 children (age 3 years to less than 12 years) and 19 adolescents (age 12 years to less than 17 years). No differences in efficacy or safety were observed between the different age subgroups or in comparison to the young adults in the trial. The safety and efficacy of KYMRIAH in pediatric patients with relapsed or refractory DLBCL has not been established.

Geriatric use

The safety and effectiveness of KYMRIAH have not been established in geriatric patients with r/r B-cell ALL. Clinical studies of KYMRIAH did not include sufficient numbers of subjects aged 65 and over to determine whether they respond differently from younger subjects.

CLINICAL STUDIES

Relapsed or refractory (r/r) B-cell acute lymphoblastic leukemia (ALL)

The efficacy of KYMRIAH in pediatric and young adults with r/r B-cell precursor ALL was evaluated in an open-label, multicenter single-arm trial (ELIANA, NCT02228096). In total, 107 patients were screened, 88 were enrolled, 68 were treated, and 63 were evaluable for efficacy. Nine percent of the enrolled patients did not receive the product due to manufacturing failure. The 63 evaluable patients included 35 males and 28 females of median age 12 years (range: 3-23 years). Seventy-three percent of patients were White, 10% were Asian, and 17% were of other races. Six (10%) had primary refractory disease, 30 (48%) had one prior stem cell transplant, 5 patients (8%) had two stem cell transplants. Treatment consisted of lymphodepleting chemotherapy (fludarabine 30 mg/m^2 daily for 4 days and cyclophosphamide 500 mg/m^2 daily for 2 days) followed by a single dose of KYMRIAH. Of the 22 patients who had a WBC count < 1000/μL, 20 received lymphodepleting chemotherapy prior to KYMRIAH while 2 received KYMRIAH infusion without lymphodepleting chemotherapy. Fifty-three patients received bridging chemotherapy between time of enrollment and lymphodepleting chemotherapy. The efficacy of KYMRIAH was established on the basis of complete remission (CR) within 3 months after infusion, the duration of CR, and proportion of patients with CR and minimal residual disease (MRD) < 0.01% by flow cytometry (MRD-negative) are shown in Table 10**). Among the 63 infused patients, 52 (83%) achieved CR/CRi, all of which were minimal residual disease (MRD)-negative.** With a median follow-up of 4.8 months from response, the median duration of CR/CRi was not reached (range: 1.2 to 14.1+ months). Median time to onset of CR/CRi was 29 days with onset of CR/CRi between 26 and 31 days for 50/52 (96%) responders. The stem cell transplantation rate among those who achieved CR/CRi was 12% (6/52).

Table 10. Efficacy results in pediatric and young adult patients with r/r B-cell ALL Results. N = 63.

Results	**N = 63**
CR/Cri[1,2]	52 (83%)
95% CI	71%, 91%
	p<0.0001
CR[3]	40 (63%)
Cri[4]	12 (19%)
CR or CRi with MRD-negative bone marrow[5,6]	52 (83%)
95% CI	71%, 91%
	p<0.0001
Duration of remission[7]	N = 52
Median (months)	Not reached
95% CI	7.5, Not reached[8]

[1]CR/CRi was calculated based on all patients who received KYMRIAH and completed at least 3 months follow-up, or discontinued earlier prior to the data cut-

off. Requires remission status to be maintained for at least 28 days without clinical evidence of relapse.

[2]The null hypothesis of CR/CRi less than or equal to 20% was rejected.

[3]CR (complete remission) was defined as less than 5% of blasts in the bone marrow, no evidence of extramedullary disease, and full recovery of peripheral blood counts (platelets greater than 100,000/microliter and absolute neutrophil counts [ANC] greater than 1,000/microliter) without blood transfusion.

[4]CRi (complete remission with incomplete blood count recovery) was defined as less than 5% of blasts in the bone marrow, no evidence of extramedullary disease, and without full recovery of peripheral blood counts with or without blood transfusion.
[5]MRD (minimal residual disease) negative was defined as MRD by flow cytometry less than 0.01%.

[6]The null hypothesis of MRD-negative remission rate less than or equal to 15% was rejected.

[7]DOR (duration of remission) was defined as time since onset of CR or CRi to relapse or death due to underlying cancer, whichever is earlier, censoring for new cancer therapy including stem cell transplantation (N = 52).

[8]Not estimable.

Use of KYMRIAH in adult relapsed or refractory (r/r) diffuse large B-cell lymphoma (DLBCL)

The efficacy and safety of KYMRIAH was evaluated in an open-label, multicenter, single-arm trial (JULIET; NCT02445248). Eligible patients were ≥ 18 years of age with relapsed or refractory DLBCL, who received ≥ 2 lines of chemotherapy, including rituximab and anthracycline, or relapsed following autologous hematopoietic stem cell transplantation (HSCT). The study excluded patients with active central nervous system malignancy, prior allogenic HSCT, an ECOG performance status ≥ 2, a creatinine clearance < 60, alanine aminotransferase > 5 times normal, cardiac ejection fraction < 45%, or absolute lymphocyte concentration less than 300/µL. Following 2 to 11 days after completion of lymphodepleting (LD) chemotherapy consisting of either fludarabine (25 mg/m^2 i.v. daily for 3 days) and cyclophosphamide (250 mg/m^2 i.v. daily for 3 days starting with the first dose of fludarabine) or bendamustine (90 mg/m^2 i.v. daily for 2 days), KYMRIAH was administered as a single intravenous infusion. Bridging chemotherapy between leukapheresis and LD chemotherapy was permitted to control disease burden. LD chemotherapy could be omitted if the white blood cell count was < 1000 cells/μL. The major efficacy outcome measures were objective response rate per Lugano criteria [2014] as assessed by an independent review committee and duration of response. Of the 160 patients enrolled, 106 patients received tisagenlecleucel, including 92 patients who received product manufactured in the U.S. and were followed for at least 3 months or discontinued earlier. Eleven out of 160 patients enrolled did not receive tisagenlecleucel due to manufacturing failure. Thirty-eight other patients did not receive tisagenlecleucel, primarily due to death (n = 16), physician decision (n = 16), and adverse events (n = 3). Of the 92 patients receiving KYMRIAH, 90% received physician's choice of bridging chemotherapy in the interval between start of screening and KYMRIAH infusion, among whom the median number of bridging chemotherapy regimens was 1 (range: 1 to 5) with 83% of patients receiving ≤ 2 regimens. A retrospectively identified sub-group of 68 patients was evaluable for the major efficacy outcome measures. Patients included in this sub-group had either had no bridging chemotherapy, or had imaging that showed measurable disease after completion of bridging chemotherapy, prior to KYMRIAH infusion. Of the 24 patients not included, 8 had no evidence of disease at baseline prior to KYMRIAH infusion, 15 did not have baseline imaging following bridging chemotherapy, and 1 was excluded because of initial misclassification of a neuroendocrine tumor as DLBCL. Among the efficacy evaluable population of 68 patients, the baseline characteristics were: median age 56 years (range: 22 to 74 years); 71% male; 90% White, 4% Asian, and 3% Black or African American; 78% had primary DLBCL not otherwise specified (NOS) and 22% had DLBCL following transformation from follicular lymphoma, of whom 17% were identified as high grade; and 44% had undergone prior autologous HSCT. The median number of prior therapies was 3 (range: 1 to 6), 56% had refractory disease and 44% relapsed after their last therapy. Ninety percent of patients received lymphodepleting chemotherapy (66% of patients received fludarabine and 24% received bendamustine) and 10% did not receive any LD chemotherapy. The median time from leukapheresis and cryopreservation to KYMRIAH infusion was 113 days (range: 47 to 196 days). The median dose was 3.5 × 10^8 CAR-positive viable T cells (range: 1.0 to 5.2 × 10^8 cells). Seventy-three percent of patients received KYMRIAH in an inpatient setting. Efficacy was established on the basis of complete response (CR) rate and duration of response (DOR), as determined by an independent review committee (Table 9 and Table 10). **The median time to first response to KYMRIAH (CR or PR) was 0.9 months (range: 0.7 to 3.3 months). The median duration of response was not reached.** Response durations were longer in patients who achieved CR, as compared to patients with a best response of partial response (PR) (Table 10). Of the 22 patients who experienced a CR, 9 achieved this status by 1 month, 12 more by month 3, and the last by month 6 after KYMRIAH infusion.

Table 11. Response rates in relapsed or refractory DLBCL in the Juliet study.

Response rate	**N = 68**
Overall response rate (ORR) (CR+PR), n (%)	34 (50)
(95% CI)	(37.6%, 62.4%)
Complete response rate n (%)	22 (32%)
(95% CI)	(21.5%, 44.8%)
Partial response rate n (%)	12 (18%)
(95% CI)	(9.5%, 28.8%)

Table 12. Duration of response[a] (months) in relapsed or refractory DLBCL in the JULIET Study.

Duration of response	**Results**
Overall DOR for responders (months)	N = 64
Median DOR[a,b]	NE
(95% CI)	(5.1, NE)
Range[c]	(0.03+ – 11.3+)
Median Follow-up (95% CI)[b]	9.4 (7.9, 10.8)
DOR if BOR is CR	N = 22
Median DOR[a,b]	NE
(95% CI)	(10.0, NE)
Range[c]	(1.5+ – 11.3+)
DOR if BOR is PR	N = 12
Median DOR[a,b]	3.4
(95% CI)	(1.0, NE)
Range[c]	(0.03+ – 11.3+)

Abbreviations used in Table 10:

CR, complete response; DOR, duration of response: DOR measured from date of first objective response to date of progression or death from relapse. NE, not estimable, PR, partial response

[a]Among all responders.

[b]Kaplan-Meier estimate in months

[c]A + sign indicates a censored value

[Author's comments:

B cell ALL: a complete remission rate (including no evidence of minimal residual disease by flow cytometry) is remarkable in relapsed or refractory B cell ALL.

DLBCL: a complete remission rate of 32% in relapsed or refractory DLBCL is also striking, especially given that fact that the duration of remission was not yet evaluable with a range of 0.03+ to 11.3+ months].

10.2. AXICABTAGENE CILOLEUCEL/YESCARTA

[Author's comment:

Current similarities between tisangelecleucel/Kymriah and axicabtagene ciloleucel/Yescarta are that

1. Both target CD19.

2. Both are FDA-approved for adults with relapsed or refractory (r/r) diffuse B cell non-Hodgkin lymphomas.

Current differences between the two are that

1. *Kymriah is approved for children and young adults with r/r B cell ALL, whereas Yescarta is not.*
2. *Yescarta is approved for r/r follicular lymphoma, whereas Kymriah is not.*
3. *The co-stimulatory domains used in Kymriah are CD137 and CD3 zeta, whereas those used in Yescarta are CD28 and CD3 zeta.*

Many other aspects of the two drugs are similar – for example, the toxicities - and will not be repeated in full for Yescarta

Full details on Yescarta are in the FDA insert package at

https://www.fda.gov/media/108377/download].

WARNING: CYTOKINE RELEASE SYNDROME and NEUROLOGIC TOXICITIES

• Cytokine Release Syndrome (CRS), including fatal or life-threatening reactions, occurred in patients receiving YESCARTA. Do not administer YESCARTA to patients with active infection or inflammatory disorders. Treat severe or life-threatening CRS with tocilizumab or tocilizumab and corticosteroids.

• Neurologic toxicities, including fatal or life-threatening reactions, occurred in patients receiving YESCARTA, including concurrently with CRS or after CRS resolution. Monitor for neurologic toxicities after treatment with YESCARTA. Provide supportive care and/or corticosteroids as needed.

• YESCARTA is available only through a restricted program under a Risk Evaluation and Mitigation Strategy (REMS) called the YESCARTA and TECARTUS REMS Program.

INDICATIONS AND USAGE

1.1. Large B-cell Lymphoma YESCARTA is indicated for the treatment of:

• Adult patients with large B-cell lymphoma that is refractory to first-line chemoimmunotherapy or that relapses within 12 months of first-line chemoimmunotherapy.

• Adult patients with relapsed or refractory large B-cell lymphoma after two or more lines of systemic therapy, including diffuse large B-cell lymphoma (DLBCL) not otherwise specified, primary mediastinal large B-cell lymphoma, high grade B-cell lymphoma, and DLBCL arising from follicular lymphoma. Limitations of Use: YESCARTA is not indicated for the treatment of patients with primary central nervous system lymphoma.

1.2. Follicular Lymphoma

YESCARTA is indicated for the treatment of adult patients with relapsed or refractory follicular lymphoma (FL) after two or more lines of systemic therapy. This indication is approved under accelerated approval based on response rate. Continued approval for this indication may be contingent upon verification and description of clinical benefit in confirmatory trial(s).

DESCRIPTION

YESCARTA (axicabtagene ciloleucel) is a CD19-directed genetically modified autologous T cell immunotherapy. To prepare YESCARTA, a patient's own T cells are harvested and genetically modified ex vivo by retroviral transduction to express a chimeric antigen receptor (CAR) comprising a murine **anti-CD19** single chain variable fragment (scFv) linked to **CD28 and CD3 zeta** co-stimulatory domains. The anti-CD19 CAR T cells are expanded and infused back into the patient, where they can recognize and eliminate CD19-expressing target cells. YESCARTA is prepared from the patient's peripheral blood mononuclear cells, which are obtained via a standard leukapheresis procedure. The mononuclear cells are enriched for T cells and activated with anti-CD3 antibody in the presence of IL-2, then transduced with the replication incompetent retroviral vector containing the anti-CD19 CAR transgene. The transduced T cells are expanded in cell culture, washed, formulated into a suspension, and cryopreserved. The product must pass a sterility test before release for shipping as a frozen suspension in a patient-specific infusion bag. The product is thawed prior to infusion. In addition to T cells, YESCARTA may contain NK and NK-T cells. The formulation contains 5% dimethyl sulfoxide (DMSO) and 2.5% albumin (human).

CLINICAL PHARMACOLOGY

Mechanism of Action

YESCARTA, a CD19-directed genetically modified autologous T cell immunotherapy, binds to CD19-expressing cancer cells and normal B cells. Studies demonstrated that following anti-CD19 CAR T cell engagement with CD19-expressing target cells, the CD28 and CD3 zeta co-stimulatory domains activate downstream signaling cascades that lead to T cell activation, proliferation, acquisition of effector functions and secretion of inflammatory cytokines and chemokines. This sequence of events leads to killing of CD19-expressing cells.

DOSAGE AND ADMINISTRATION

For autologous use only. For intravenous use only.

Dose

Each single infusion bag of YESCARTA contains a suspension of chimeric antigen receptor (CAR)-positive T cells in approximately 68 mL. The target dose is 2×10^6 CAR-positive viable T cells per kg body weight, with a maximum of 2×10^8 CAR-positive viable T cells.

Administration

YESCARTA is for autologous use only. The patient's identity must match the patient identifiers on the YESCARTA cassette and infusion bag. Do not infuse YESCARTA if the information on the patient-specific label does not match the intended patient.

WARNING: CYTOKINE RELEASE SYNDROME and NEUROLOGIC TOXICITIES • Cytokine Release Syndrome (CRS), including fatal or life-threatening reactions, occurred in patients receiving YESCARTA. Do not administer YESCARTA to patients with active infection or inflammatory disorders. Treat severe or life-threatening CRS with tocilizumab or tocilizumab and corticosteroids.

• Neurologic toxicities, including fatal or life-threatening reactions, occurred in patients receiving YESCARTA, including concurrently with CRS or after CRS resolution. Monitor for neurologic toxicities after treatment with YESCARTA. Provide supportive care and/or corticosteroids as needed.

• YESCARTA is available only through a restricted program under a Risk Evaluation and Mitigation Strategy (REMS) called the YESCARTA and TECARTUS REMS Program

Preparing the patient for YESCARTA infusion

Confirm availability of YESCARTA prior to starting the lymphodepleting regimen.
Pre-treatment

• Administer a lymphodepleting chemotherapy regimen of cyclophosphamide 500 mg/m^2 intravenously and fludarabine 30 mg/m^2 intravenously on the fifth, fourth, and third day before infusion of YESCARTA.

Premedication

• Administer acetaminophen 650 mg PO and diphenhydramine 12.5 mg intravenously or PO approximately 1 hour before YESCARTA infusion.

• Consider the use of prophylactic corticosteroid in patients after weighing the potential benefits and risks.

Preparation of YESCARTA for infusion

Coordinate the timing of YESCARTA thaw and infusion. Confirm the infusion time in advance, and adjust the start time of YESCARTA thaw such that it will be available for infusion when the patient is ready.

• Confirm patient identity: Prior to YESCARTA preparation, match the patient's identity with the patient identifiers on the YESCARTA cassette.

• Do not remove the YESCARTA product bag from the cassette if the information on the patient-specific label does not match the intended patient.

• Once patient identification is confirmed, remove the YESCARTA product bag from the cassette and check that the patient information on the cassette label matches the bag label.

• Inspect the product bag for any breaches of container integrity such as breaks or cracks before thawing. If the bag is compromised, follow the local guidelines (or call Kite at 1-844-454-KITE).

• Place the infusion bag inside a second sterile bag per local guidelines.

• Thaw YESCARTA at approximately 37°C using either a water bath or dry thaw method until there is no visible ice in the infusion bag. Gently mix the contents of the bag to disperse clumps of cellular material. If visible cell clumps remain continue to gently mix the contents of the bag. Small clumps of cellular material should disperse with gentle manual mixing. Do not wash, spin down, and/or re-suspend YESCARTA in new medium prior to infusion.

• Once thawed, YESCARTA may be stored at room temperature (20°C to 25°C) for up to 3 hours.

Administration

• For autologous use only.

• Ensure that tocilizumab and emergency equipment are available prior to infusion and during the recovery period.

• Do NOT use a leukodepleting filter.

• Central venous access is recommended for the infusion of YESCARTA.

• Confirm the patient's identity matches the patient identifiers on the YESCARTA product bag.

• Prime the tubing with normal saline prior to infusion.

• Infuse the entire contents of the YESCARTA bag within 30 minutes by either gravity or a peristaltic pump. YESCARTA is stable at room temperature for up to 3 hours after thaw.

• Gently agitate the product bag during YESCARTA infusion to prevent cell clumping.

• After the entire content of the product bag is infused, rinse the tubing with normal saline at the same infusion rate to ensure all product is delivered. YESCARTA contains human blood cells that are genetically modified with replication incompetent retroviral vector. Follow universal precautions and local biosafety guidelines for handling and disposal to avoid potential transmission of infectious diseases.

Monitoring

• Administer YESCARTA at a certified healthcare facility.

• Monitor patients at least daily for 7 days at the certified healthcare facility following infusion for signs and symptoms of CRS and neurologic toxicities.

• Instruct patients to remain within proximity of the certified healthcare facility for at least 4 weeks following infusion.

Management of severe adverse reactions

Cytokine release syndrome

Identify CRS based on clinical presentation. Evaluate for and treat other causes of fever, hypoxia, and hypotension. If CRS is suspected, manage according to the recommendations in Table 13. Patients who experience Grade 2 or higher CRS (e.g., hypotension not responsive to fluids, or hypoxia requiring supplemental oxygenation) should be monitored with continuous cardiac telemetry and pulse oximetry. For patients experiencing severe CRS, consider performing an echocardiogram to assess cardiac function. For severe or life-threatening CRS, consider intensive-care supportive therapy.

Table 13. CRS grading and management guidance.

CRS Grade[a]	Tocilizumab	Corticosteroids
Grade 1: Symptoms require symptomatic treatment only (e.g., fever, nausea, fatigue, headache, myalgia, malaise).	If symptoms (e.g., fever) not improving after 24 hours, consider managing as Grade 2.	If not improving after 3 days, administer one dose of dexamethasone 10 mg intravenously.
Grade 2: Symptoms require and respond to moderate intervention. Oxygen requirement less than 40% FiO2 or hypotension responsive to fluids or low-dose of one vasopressor or Grade 2 organ toxicity[b].	Administer tocilizumab[c] 8 mg/kg intravenously over 1 hour (not to exceed 800 mg). If no clinical improvement in the signs and symptoms of CRS after the first dose, repeat tocilizumab every 8 hours as needed. Limit to a maximum of 3 doses in a 24- hour period; maximum total of 4 doses. If improving, discontinue tocilizumab.	Administer dexamethasone 10 mg intravenously once daily. If improving, manage as Grade 1 above and continue corticosteroids until the severity is Grade 1 or less, then quickly taper as clinically appropriate. If not improving, manage as appropriate grade below.
Grade 3: Symptoms require and respond to aggressive intervention. Oxygen requirement greater than or equal to 40% FiO2 or hypotension requiring high-dose or multiple vasopressors or Grade 3 organ toxicity or Grade 4 transaminitis.	Per Grade 2. If improving, manage as appropriate grade above.	Dexamethasone 10 mg intravenously three times a day. If improving, manage as appropriate grade above and continue corticosteroids until the severity is Grade 1 or less, then quickly taper as clinically appropriate. If not improving, manage as Grade 4.
Grade 4: Life-threatening symptoms. Requirements for ventilator support, continuous veno-venous hemodialysis (CVVHD) or Grade 4 organ toxicity (excluding transaminitis).	Per Grade 2. If improving, manage as appropriate grade above.	Administer methylprednisolone 1000 mg intravenously once per day for 3 days. If improving, manage as appropriate grade above and continue corticosteroids until the severity is Grade 1 or less, then taper as clinically appropriate. If not improving, consider methylprednisolone 1000

		mg 2-3 times a day or alternate therapy[d]

[a]Lee et al. 2014.

[b]Refer to Table 13 for management of neurologic toxicity.

[c]Refer to tocilizumab Prescribing Information for details.

[d]Alternate therapy includes (but is not limited to): anakinra, siltuximab, ruxolitinib, cyclophosphamide, IVIG and ATG

Neurological toxicity

Monitor patients for signs and symptoms of neurologic toxicity/immune effector cell-associated neurotoxicity syndrome (ICANS) (Table 14). Rule out other causes of neurologic symptoms. Patients who experience Grade 2 or higher neurologic toxicities/ICANS should be monitored with continuous cardiac telemetry and pulse oximetry. Provide intensive care supportive therapy for severe or life-threatening neurologic toxicities. Consider levetiracetam for seizure prophylaxis for any grade of neurologic toxicities.

Table 14. Neurologic toxicity/ICANS grading and management guidance.

Grading Assessment[a]	Concurrent CRS	No Concurrent CRS
Grade 1	Administer tocilizumab per Table 13 for management of Grade 1 CRS. In addition, administer one dose of dexamethasone 10 mg intravenously. If not improving after 2 days, repeat dexamethasone 10 mg intravenously.	Administer one dose of dexamethasone 10 mg intravenously. If not improving after 2 days, repeat dexamethasone 10 mg intravenously
	Consider levetiracetam for seizure prophylaxis	Consider levetiracetam for seizure prophylaxis
Grade 2	Administer tocilizumab per Table 13 for management of Grade 2 CRS. In addition, administer dexamethasone 10 mg intravenously four times a day. If improving, continue corticosteroids	Administer dexamethasone 10 mg intravenously four times a day. If improving, continue corticosteroids until the severity is Grade 1 or less, then quickly taper as clinically appropriate. If not

	until the severity is Grade 1 or less, then quickly taper as clinically appropriate. If not improving, manage as appropriate grade below	improving, manage as appropriate grade below
	Consider levetiracetam for seizure prophylaxis.	Consider levetiracetam for seizure prophylaxis.
Grade 3	Administer tocilizumab per Table 13 for management of Grade 2 CRS. In addition, administer methylprednisolone 1000 mg intravenously once daily. If improving, manage as appropriate grade above and continue corticosteroids until the severity is Grade 1 or less, then taper as clinically appropriate. If not improving, manage as Grade 4.	Administer methylprednisolone 1000 mg intravenously once daily. If improving, manage as appropriate grade above and continue corticosteroids until the severity is Grade 1 or less, then taper as clinically appropriate. If not improving, manage as Grade 4.
	Consider levetiracetam for seizure prophylaxis.	Consider levetiracetam for seizure prophylaxis.
Grade 4	Administer tocilizumab per Table 13 for management of Grade 2 CRS. In addition, administer methylprednisolone 1000 mg intravenously twice per day. If improving, manage as appropriate grade above and continue corticosteroids until the severity is Grade 1 or less, then taper as clinically appropriate. If not improving, consider 1000 mg of methylprednisolone intravenously 3 times a day or alternate therapy[b]	Administer methylprednisolone 1000 mg intravenously twice per day. If improving, manage as appropriate grade above and continue corticosteroids until the severity is Grade 1 or less, then taper as clinically appropriate. If not improving, consider 1000 mg of methylprednisolone intravenously 3 times a day or alternate therapy
	Consider levetiracetam for seizure prophylaxis.	Consider levetiracetam for seizure prophylaxis.

[Levetiracetam is a medication used to treat epilepsy. It is used for partial-onset, myoclonic, or tonic–clonic seizures and is taken either by mouth as an immediate or extended release formulation or by injection into a vein.

Common side effects of levetiracetam include sleepiness, dizziness, feeling tired, and aggression. Severe side effects may include psychosis, suicide, and allergic reactions such as Stevens–Johnson syndrome or anaphylaxis. It is unclear if levetiracetam is safe for use during pregnancy and breastfeeding. Levetiracetam is the S-enantiomer of etiracetam. Its mechanism of action is not yet clear].

DOSAGE FORMS AND STRENGTHS

YESCARTA is available as a cell suspension for infusion. A single dose of YESCARTA contains 2×10^6 CAR-positive viable T cells per kg of body weight (or maximum of 2×10^8 CAR-positive viable T cells for patients 100 kg and above) in approximately 68 mL suspension in an infusion bag.

CONTRAINDICATIONS: none.

WARNINGS AND PRECAUTIONS

Cytokine Release Syndrome (CRS), including fatal or life-threatening reactions, occurred following treatment with YESCARTA. CRS occurred in 90% (379/422) of patients with non-Hodgkin lymphoma (NHL) receiving YESCARTA, including ≥ Grade 3 (Lee grading system) CRS in 9%. CRS occurred in 93% (256/276) of patients with large B-cell lymphoma (LBCL), including ≥ Grade 3 CRS in 9%. Among patients with LBCL who died after receiving YESCARTA, four had ongoing CRS events at the time of death. For patients with LBCL in ZUMA-1 *[trial],* the median time to onset of CRS was 2 days following infusion (range: 1 to12 days) and the median duration of CRS was 7 days (range: 2 to 58 days). For patients with LBCL in ZUMA-7, the median time to onset of CRS was 3 days following infusion (range: 1 to 10 days) and the median duration was 7 days (range: 2 to 43 days). CRS occurred in 84% (123/146) of patients with indolent non-Hodgkin lymphoma (iNHL) in ZUMA-5, including ≥ Grade 3 CRS in 8%. Among patients with iNHL who died after receiving YESCARTA, one patient had an ongoing CRS event at the time of death. The median time to onset of CRS was 4 days (range: 1 to 20 days) and the median duration was 6 days (range: 1 to 27 days) for patients with iNHL. Key manifestations of CRS (≥ 10%) in all patients combined included fever (85%), hypotension (40%), tachycardia (32%), chills (22%), hypoxia (20%), headache (15%), and fatigue (12%). Serious events that may be associated with CRS include, cardiac arrhythmias (including atrial fibrillation and ventricular tachycardia), renal insufficiency, cardiac failure, respiratory failure, cardiac arrest, capillary leak syndrome, multi-organ failure, and hemophagocytic lymphohistiocytosis/macrophage activation syndrome (HLH/MAS).

The impact of tocilizumab and/or corticosteroids on the incidence and severity of CRS was assessed in two subsequent cohorts of LBCL patients in ZUMA-1. Among patients who received tocilizumab and/or corticosteroids for ongoing Grade 1 events, CRS occurred in 93% (38/41), including 2% (1/41) with Grade 3 CRS; no patients experienced a Grade 4 or 5 event. The median time to onset of CRS was 2 days (range: 1 to 8 days) and the median duration of CRS was 7 days (range: 2 to 16 days). Prophylactic treatment with corticosteroids was administered to a cohort of 39 patients for 3 days beginning on the day of infusion of YESCARTA. Thirty-one of the 39 patients (79%) developed CRS at which point the patients were managed with tocilizumab and/or therapeutic doses of corticosteroids with no patients developing Grade 3 or higher CRS. The median time to onset of CRS was 5 days (range: 1 to 15 days) and the median duration of CRS was 4 days (range: 1 to 10 days). Although there is no known mechanistic explanation, consider the risk and benefits of prophylactic corticosteroids in the context of pre-existing comorbidities for the individual patient and the potential for the risk of Grade 4 and prolonged neurologic toxicities. Ensure that 2 doses of tocilizumab are available prior to infusion of YESCARTA. Monitor patients at least daily for 7 days at the certified healthcare facility following infusion for signs and symptoms of CRS. Monitor patients for signs or symptoms of CRS for 4 weeks after infusion. Counsel patients to seek immediate medical attention should signs or symptoms of CRS occur at any time. At the first sign of CRS, institute treatment with supportive care, tocilizumab, or tocilizumab and corticosteroids as indicated.

Neurologic toxicities

Neurologic toxicities (including ICANS) that were fatal or life-threatening occurred following treatment with YESCARTA. Neurologic toxicities occurred in 78% (330/422) of patients with NHL receiving YESCARTA, including ≥ Grade 3 cases in 25%. Neurologic toxicities occurred in 87% (94/108) of patients with LBCL in ZUMA-1, including ≥ Grade 3 cases in 31% and in 74% (124/168) of patients in ZUMA-7 including ≥ Grade 3 cases in 25%. The median time to onset was 4 days (range: 1 to 43 days) and the median duration was 17 days in patients with LBCL in ZUMA-1. The median time to onset for neurologic toxicity was 5 days (range: 1 to 133 days) and median duration was 15 days in patients with LBCL in ZUMA-7. Neurologic toxicities occurred in 77% (112/146) of patients with iNHL, including ≥ Grade 3 in 21%. The median time to onset was 6 days (range: 1 to 79 days) and the median duration was 16 days. Ninety-eight percent of all neurologic toxicities in patients with LBCL and 99% of all neurologic toxicities in patients with iNHL occurred within the first 8 weeks of YESCARTA infusion. Neurologic toxicities occurred within the first 7 days of YESCARTA infusion in 87% of affected patients with LBCL and 74% of affected patients with iNHL. The most common neurologic toxicities (≥ 10%) in all patients combined included encephalopathy (50%), headache (43%), tremor (29%), dizziness (21%), aphasia (17%), delirium (15%), and insomnia (10%). Prolonged encephalopathy lasting up to 173 days was noted. Serious events including aphasia, leukoencephalopathy, dysarthria, lethargy, and seizures occurred with YESCARTA. Fatal and serious cases of cerebral edema and encephalopathy, including late-onset encephalopathy, have occurred in patients treated with YESCARTA.

The impact of tocilizumab and/or corticosteroids on the incidence and severity of neurologic toxicities was assessed in two subsequent cohorts of LBCL patients in ZUMA-1. Among patients who received corticosteroids at the onset of Grade 1 toxicities (see Table 14), neurologic toxicities occurred in 78% (32/41) and 20% (8/41) had Grade 3 neurologic toxicities; no patients experienced a Grade 4 or 5 event. The median time to onset of neurologic toxicities was 6 days (range: 1 to 93 days) with a median duration of 8 days (range: 1 to 144 days). Prophylactic treatment with corticosteroids was administered to a cohort of 39 patients for 3 days beginning on the day of infusion of YESCARTA. Of these 39 patients, 85% (33/39) developed neurologic toxicities; 8% (3/39) developed Grade 3 and 5% (2/39) developed Grade 4 neurologic toxicities. The median time to onset of neurological toxicities was 6 days (range: 1 to 274 days) with a median duration of 12 days (range: 1 to 107 days). **Prophylactic corticosteroids for management of CRS and neurologic toxicities may result in higher grade of neurologic toxicities or prolongation of neurologic toxicities, delay the onset and decrease the duration of CRS** *[author's bolding].* Monitor patients at least daily for 7 days at the certified healthcare facility following infusion for signs and symptoms of neurologic toxicities. Monitor patients for signs or symptoms of neurologic toxicities for 4 weeks after infusion and treat promptly.

YESCARTA and TECARTUS REMS Program

Because of the risk of CRS and neurologic toxicities, YESCARTA is available only through a restricted program under a Risk Evaluation and Mitigation Strategy (REMS) called the YESCARTA and TECARTUS REMS Program. The required components of the YESCARTA and TECARTUS REMS Program are:

• Healthcare facilities that dispense and administer YESCARTA must be enrolled and comply with the REMS requirements. Certified healthcare facilities must have on-site, immediate access to tocilizumab, and ensure that a minimum of 2 doses of tocilizumab are available for each patient for infusion within 2 hours after YESCARTA infusion, if needed for treatment of CRS.

• Certified healthcare facilities must ensure that healthcare providers who prescribe, dispense, or administer YESCARTA are trained about the management of CRS and neurologic toxicities. Further information is available at www.YescartaTecartusREMS.com or 1-844-454-KITE (5483).

Hypersensitivity reactions

Allergic reactions may occur with the infusion of YESCARTA. Serious hypersensitivity reactions, including anaphylaxis, may be due to dimethyl sulfoxide (DMSO) or residual gentamicin in YESCARTA.

Serious infections

Severe or life-threatening infections occurred in patients after YESCARTA infusion. Infections (all grades) occurred in 45% of patients with NHL. Grade 3 or higher infections occurred in 17% of patients, including Grade 3 or higher infections with an unspecified pathogen in 12%, bacterial infections in 5%, viral infections in 3%, and fungal infections in 1%. YESCARTA should not be administered to patients with clinically significant active systemic infections. Monitor patients for signs and symptoms of infection before and after YESCARTA infusion and treat appropriately. Administer prophylactic antimicrobials according to local guidelines. Febrile neutropenia was observed in 36% of patients with NHL after YESCARTA infusion and may be concurrent with CRS. In the event of febrile neutropenia, evaluate for infection and manage with broad-spectrum antibiotics, fluids, and other supportive care as medically indicated.

In immunosuppressed patients, including those who have received YESCARTA, life-threatening and fatal opportunistic infections including disseminated fungal infections (e.g., candida sepsis *[Figures 49 and 50]* and aspergillus infections *[Figure 51 and 52])* and viral reactivation (e.g., human herpes virus-6 [HHV-6] *[Figures 53 and 54]* encephalitis and JC virus progressive multifocal leukoencephalopathy [PML] *[Figure 55]*) have been reported. The possibility of HHV-6 encephalitis and PML should be considered in immunosuppressed patients with neurologic events and appropriate diagnostic evaluations should be performed.

[Figure 49. Agar plate showing growth of colonies of Candida albicans.

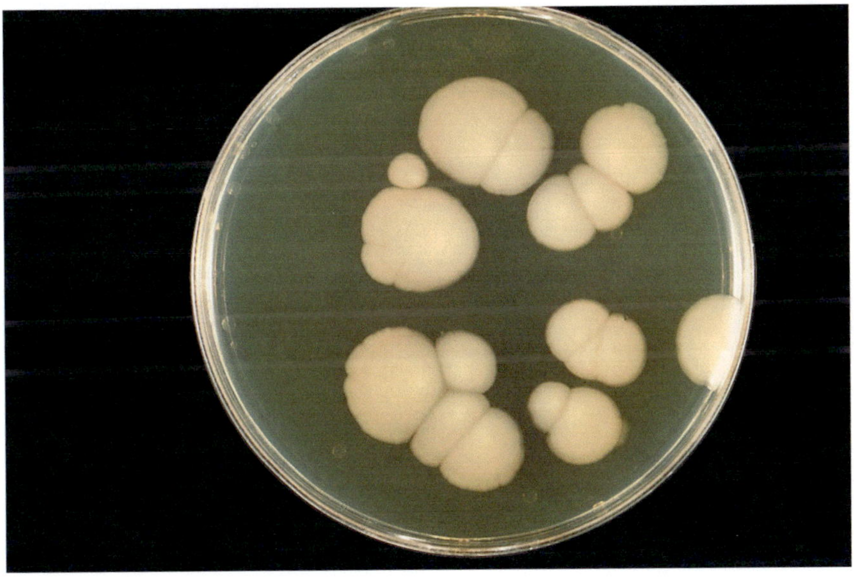

This image is by CDC/Dr. William Kaplan - This media comes from the Centers for Disease Control and Prevention's Public Health Image Library (PHIL), with identification number #3192. https://commons.wikimedia.org/w/index.php?curid=760343; https://en.wikipedia.org/wiki/Candidiasis#/media/File:Candida_albicans_PHIL_3192_lores.jpg. This image is a work of the Centers for Disease Control and Prevention, part of the United States Department of Health and Human Services, taken or made as part of an employee's official duties. As a work of the U.S. federal government, the image is in the public domain. No changes were made to this image.

Figure 50. Micrograph of esophageal candidiasis showing hyphae, biopsy specimen, PAS stain.

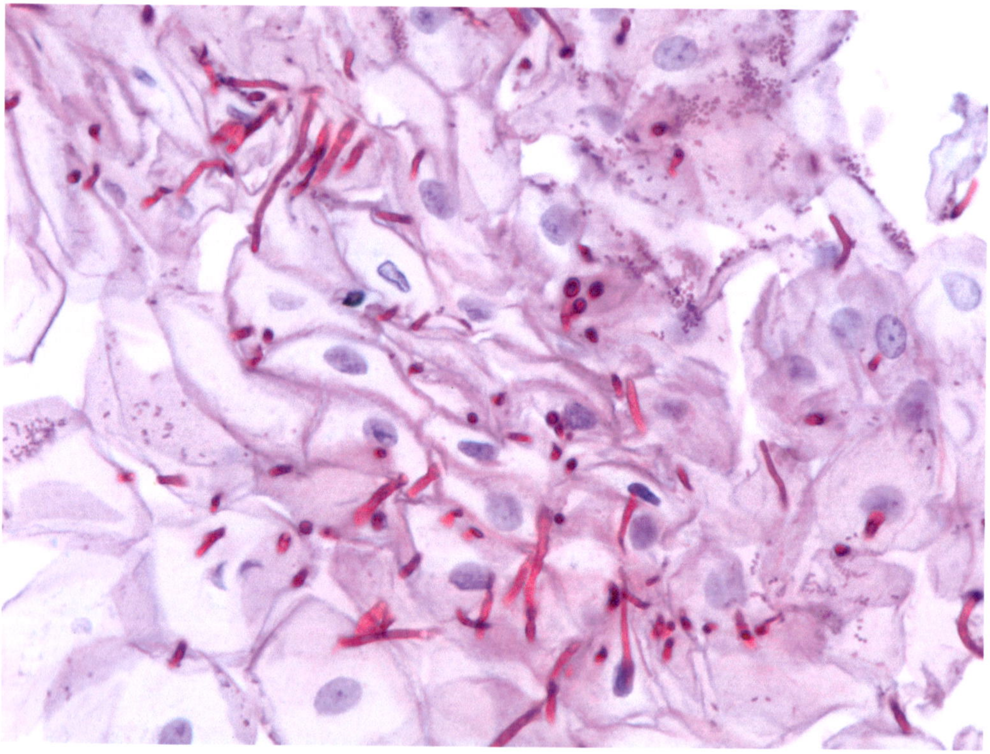

This image is by KGH - Personal collection of histopathologic slides, CC BY-SA 3.0, https://commons.wikimedia.org/w/index.php?curid=445262; https://en.wikipedia.org/wiki/Candidiasis#/media/File:Esophageal_candidiasis_(2)_PAS_stain.jpg. This file is licensed under the Creative Commons Attribution-Share Alike 3.0 Unported license. No changes were made to this image.

Figure 51. A scan of Aspergillus taken at 235 magnifications under a scanning electron microscope.

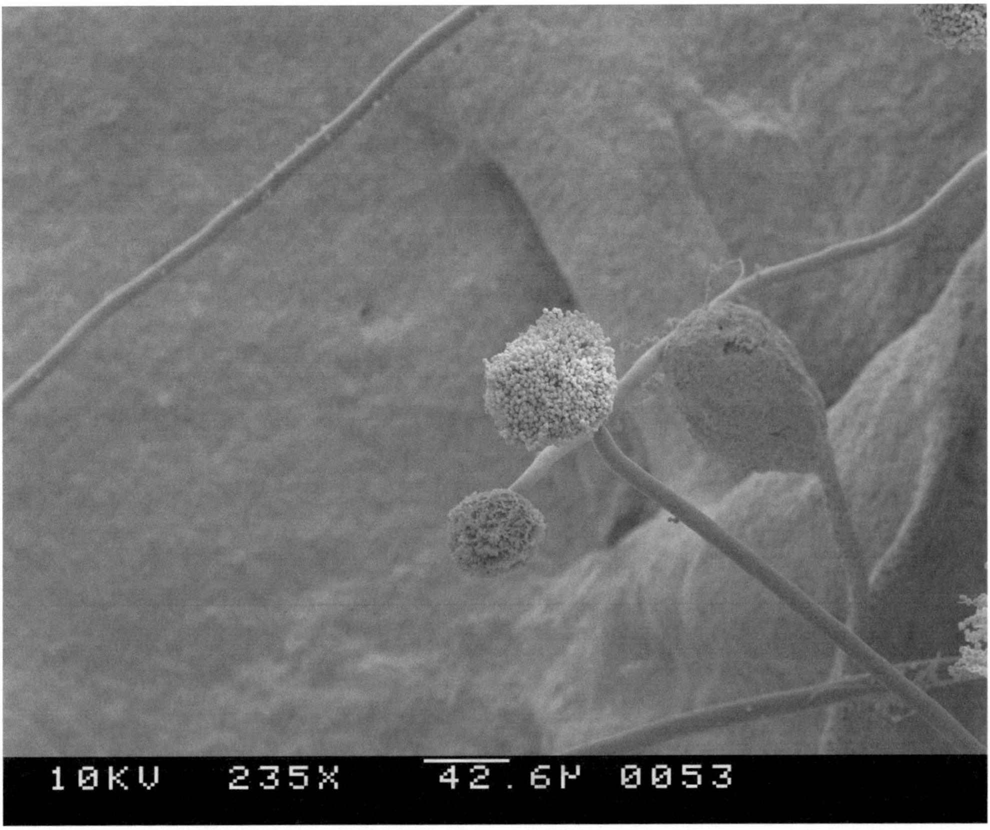

This image is by MWolfin - Own work, CC0, https://commons.wikimedia.org/w/index.php?curid=9646505; https://en.wikipedia.org/wiki/Aspergillus#/media/File:Aspergillus_235_mags_3X3_copy.jpeg. This file is made available under the Creative Commons CC0 1.0 Universal Public Domain Dedication. No changes were made to this image.

Figure 52. Pulmonary aspergillosis. Aspergillus hyphae have a uniform thickness and typically branch at a 45 degree angle.

This image is by Nephron - Own work, CC BY-SA 3.0, https://commons.wikimedia.org/w/index.php?curid=9097954; https://en.wikipedia.org/wiki/Aspergillus#/media/File:Pulmonary_aspergillosis.jpg. This file is licensed under the Creative Commons Attribution-Share Alike 3.0 Unported license. No changes were made to this image.

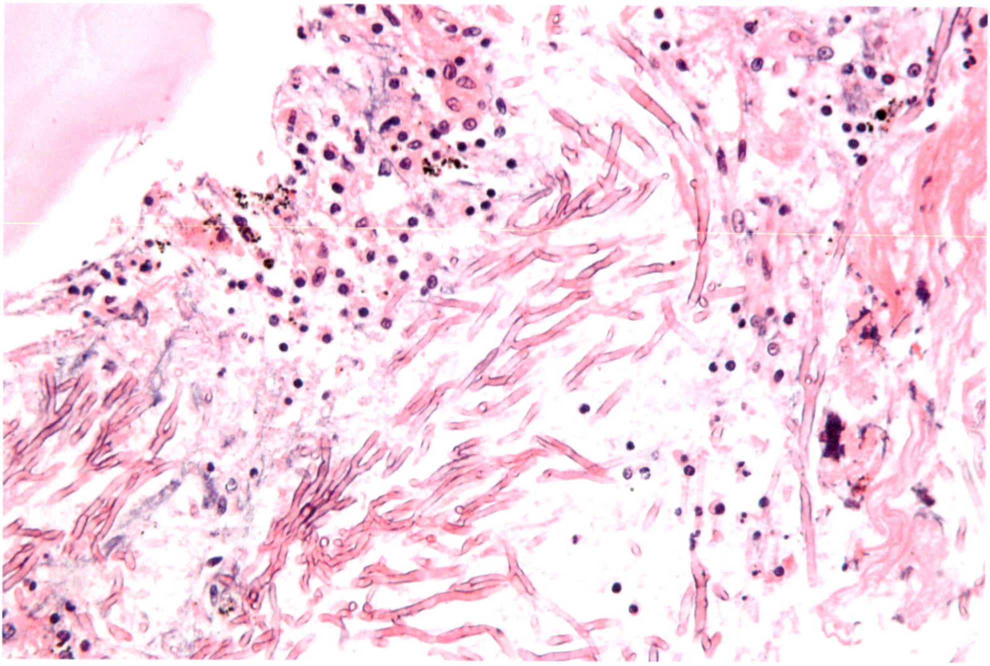

Figure 53. An electron micrograph of HHV-6 also includes a labeled insert of the mature virus particle.

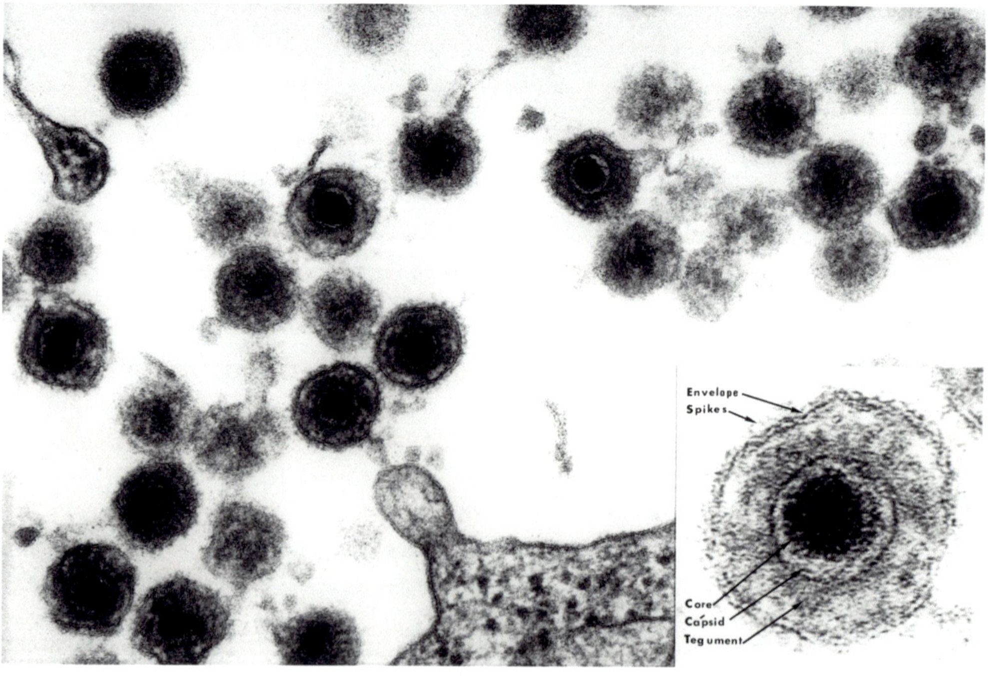

This image is by Bernard Kramarsky (Photographer) - This image was released by the <a href="https://en.wikipedia.org/wiki/National_Cancer_Institute" class="extiw" title="en:National Cancer Institute">National Cancer Institute</a>, an agency part of the <a href="https://en.wikipedia.org/wiki/National_Institutes_of_Health" https://en.wikipedia.org/wiki/Human_herpesvirus_6#/media/File:Hhv-6_(1).jpg; This work has been released into the public domain by its author, Bernard Kramarsky (Photographer). This image is a work of the National Institutes of Health, part of the United States Department of Health and Human Services, taken or made as part of an employee's official duties. As a work of the U.S. federal government, the image is in the public domain. No changes were made to this image.

Figure . Histological slide of the human herpes virus-6 showing infected cells, with inclusion bodies in both the nucleus and the cytoplasm. The slide is stained with H&E.

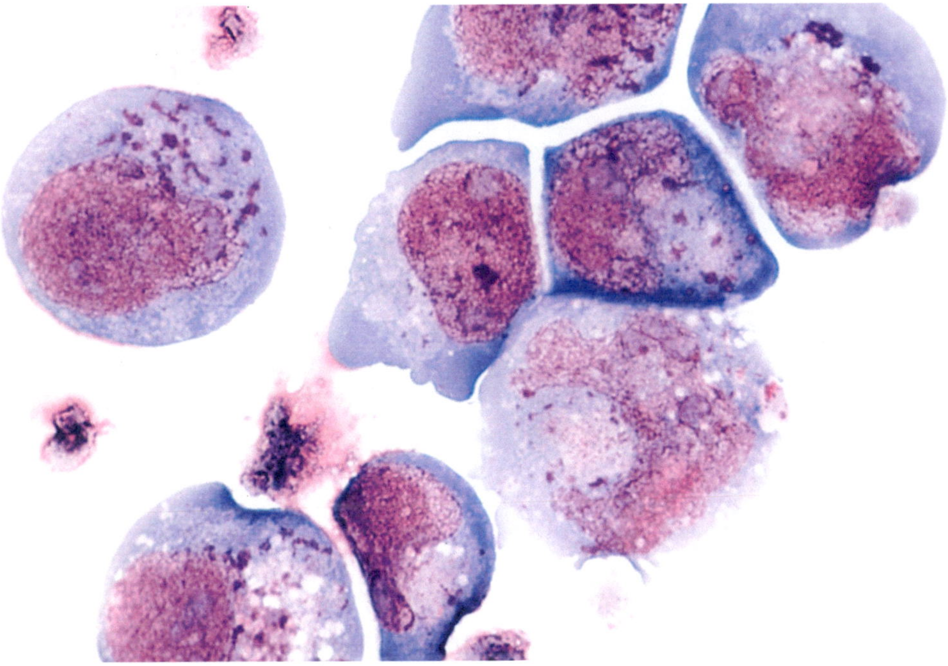

This image is by Unknown photographer - This image was released by the National Cancer Institute, an agency part of the National Institutes of Health, with the ID 2252 (image) (next)., Public Domain, https://commons.wikimedia.org/w/index.php?curid=24061203. https://en.wikipedia.org/wiki/Human_herpesvirus_6#/media/File:Inclusion_bodies.jpg. This image is a work of the National Institutes of Health, part of the United States Department of Health and Human Services, taken or made as part of an employee's official duties. As a work of the U.S. federal government, the image is in the public domain. No changes were made to this image.

Figure 55. CT brain scan of a person with JC virus-mediated progressive multifocal leukoencephalopathy (PML). CT of the brain in PML reveals hypodense lesions of the affected white matter.

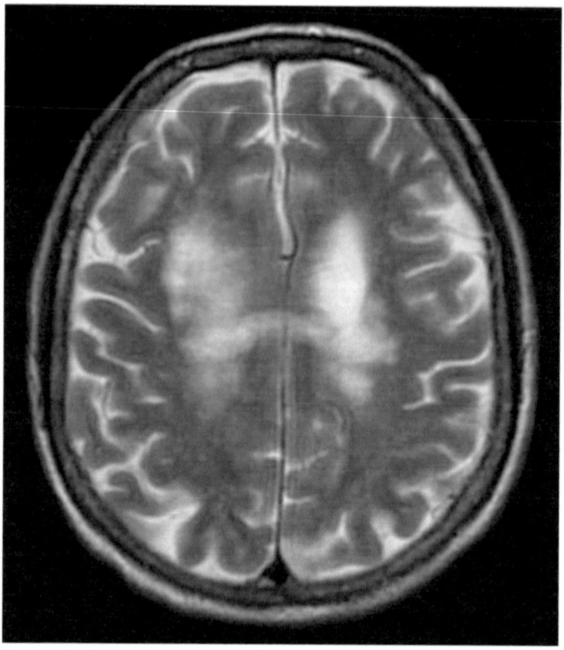

Hepatitis B virus reactivation

Hepatitis B virus (HBV) reactivation, in some cases resulting in fulminant hepatitis, hepatic failure, and death, has occurred in patients treated with drugs directed against B cells, including YESCARTA. Perform screening for HBV, HCV, and HIV and management in accordance with clinical guidelines before collection of cells for manufacturing.

[Figure 56. This electron micrograph reveals the presence of hepatitis-B virus HBV "Dane particles", or virions. These particles measure 42nm in their overall diameter, and contain a DNA-based core that is 27nm in diameter.

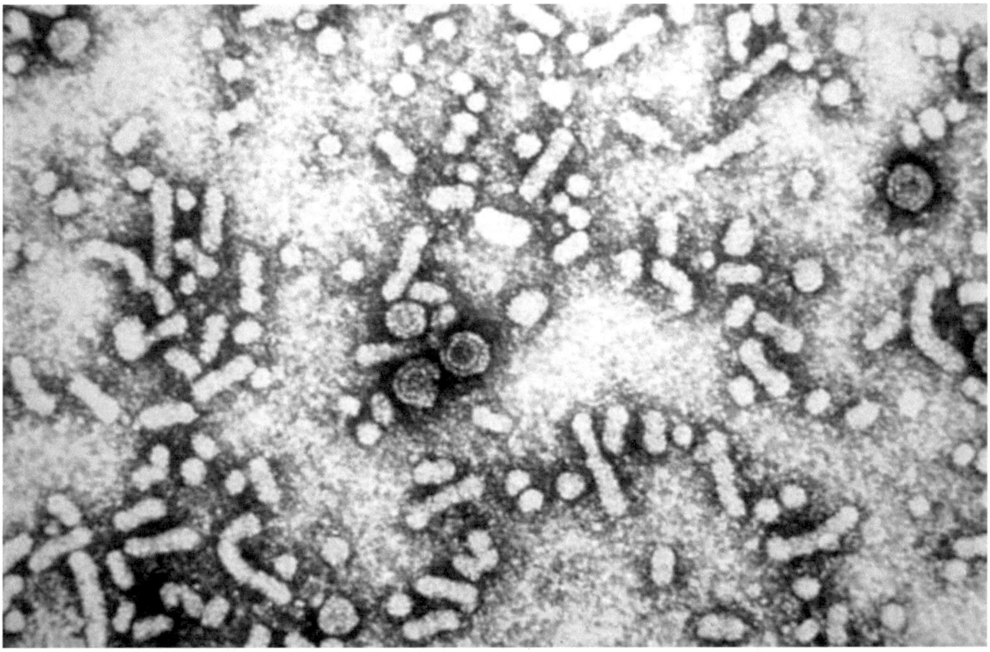

This image is by CDC - This media comes from the Centers for Disease Control and Prevention's Public Health Image Library (PHIL), with identification number #5631. Public Domain, https://commons.wikimedia.org/w/index.php?curid=9023749; https://en.wikipedia.org/wiki/Hepatitis_B#/media/File:Hepatitis-B_virions.jpg. This image is a work of the Centers for Disease Control and Prevention, part of the United States Department of Health and Human Services, taken or made as part of an employee's official duties. As a work of the U.S. federal government, the image is in the public domain. No changes were made to this image].

Prolonged cytopenias

Patients may exhibit cytopenias for several weeks following lymphodepleting chemotherapy and YESCARTA infusion. Grade 3 or higher cytopenias not resolved by Day 30 following YESCARTA infusion occurred in 39% of all patients with NHL and included neutropenia (33%), thrombocytopenia (13%), and anemia (8%). Monitor blood counts after YESCARTA infusion.

Hypogammaglobulinemia

B cell aplasia and hypogammaglobulinemia can occur in patients receiving treatment with YESCARTA. Hypogammaglobulinemia was reported as an adverse reaction in 14% of all patients with NHL. Monitor immunoglobulin levels after treatment with

YESCARTA and manage using infection precautions, antibiotic prophylaxis, and immunoglobulin replacement. The safety of immunization with live viral vaccines during or following YESCARTA treatment has not been studied. Vaccination with live virus vaccines is not recommended for at least 6 weeks prior to the start of lymphodepleting chemotherapy, during YESCARTA treatment, and until immune recovery following treatment with YESCARTA.

Secondary malignancies

Patients treated with YESCARTA may develop secondary malignancies. Monitor life-long for secondary malignancies. In the event that a secondary malignancy occurs, contact Kite at 1-844-454-KITE (5483) to obtain instructions on patient samples to collect for testing.

Effects on ability to drive and use machines

Due to the potential for neurologic events, including altered mental status or seizures, patients receiving YESCARTA are at risk for altered or decreased consciousness or coordination in the 8 weeks following YESCARTA infusion. Advise patients to refrain from driving and engaging in hazardous occupations or activities, such as operating heavy or potentially dangerous machinery, during this initial period.

Clinical trials experience

The most common non-laboratory adverse reactions to YESCARTA (incidence ≥ 20%) included fever, CRS, fatigue, hypotension, encephalopathy, tachycardia, diarrhea, headache, musculoskeletal pain, nausea, febrile neutropenia, chills, cough, infection with unspecified pathogen, dizziness, tremor, decreased appetite, edema, hypoxia, abdominal pain, aphasia, constipation, and vomiting. Serious adverse reactions occurred in 50% of patients. The most common serious adverse reactions (> 5%) included CRS, fever, encephalopathy, hypotension, infection with unspecified pathogen, and pneumonia. Fatal adverse reactions occurred in 2% of patients. The most common (≥ 10%) Grade 3 or higher non-laboratory adverse reactions included febrile neutropenia, encephalopathy, and hypotension. Sixty-seven percent (112/168) of patients received tocilizumab after infusion of YESCARTA.

Other clinically important adverse reactions that occurred in less than 10% of patients treated with YESCARTA include the following:

• Blood and lymphatic system disorders: coagulopathy (9%)

• Cardiac disorders: cardiac failure (1%)

• Eye Disorders: visual impairment (7%)

• Infections and infestations: pneumonia (8%), sepsis (4%)

• Nervous system disorders: ataxia (6%), seizure (3%), myoclonus (2%), facial paralysis (2%), paresis (2%)

• Respiratory, thoracic and mediastinal disorders: dyspnea (8%), pleural effusion (6%), respiratory failure (2%)

• Vascular disorders: hypertension (9%), thrombosis (7%).

Table 15. Grade 3 or 4 Laboratory Abnormalities Occurring in ≥ 10% of Patients in ZUMA-7 Following Treatment with YESCARTA[1] (N = 168)

Laboratory abnormality	**Grades 3 or 4 (%)**
Leukocyte decrease	96
Neutrophil decrease	94
Lymphocyte decrease	94
Hemoglobin decrease	40
Platelet decrease	26
Sodium decrease	12
Glucose increase	11

[1]Baseline lab values were assessed prior to lymphodepleting chemotherapy.

Immunogenicity

YESCARTA has the potential to induce anti-product antibodies. The immunogenicity of YESCARTA has been evaluated using an enzyme-linked immunosorbent assay (ELISA) for the detection of binding antibodies against FMC63, the originating antibody of the anti-CD19 CAR. Eleven patients (4%) tested positive for pre-dose anti-FMC63 antibodies at baseline in ZUMA-7 and ZUMA-1, and one patient (1%)

who had a negative test result at baseline had a positive test result post administration of YESCARTA in the screening ELISA in ZUMA-7. In ZUMA-5, 19 patients (13%) were antibody-positive at baseline, and 3 patients (2%) who had negative test results at baseline had positive test results post administration of YESCARTA in the screening ELISA. Results of a confirmatory cell-based assay, leveraging a properly folded and expressed extracellular portion of the CAR (ScFv, hinge and linker) demonstrated that all patients treated with YESCARTA that had a positive result in the screening ELISA were antibody negative at all time points tested. There is no evidence that the kinetics of initial expansion and persistence of YESCARTA, or the safety or effectiveness of YESCARTA, was altered in these patients.

USE IN SPECIFIC POPULATIONS

Pregnancy

Risk summary

There are no available data with YESCARTA use in pregnant women. No animal reproductive and developmental toxicity studies have been conducted with YESCARTA to assess whether it can cause fetal harm when administered to a pregnant woman. It is not known if YESCARTA has the potential to be transferred to the fetus. Based on the mechanism of action, if the transduced cells cross the placenta, they may cause fetal toxicity, including B-cell lymphocytopenia. Therefore, YESCARTA is not recommended for women who are pregnant, and pregnancy after YESCARTA infusion should be discussed with the treating physician. In the U.S. general population, the estimated background risk of major birth defects and miscarriage in clinically recognized pregnancies is 2% - 4% and 15% - 20%, respectively.

Lactation

Risk summary

There is no information regarding the presence of YESCARTA in human milk, the effect on the breastfed infant, and the effects on milk production. The developmental and health benefits of breastfeeding should be considered along with the mother's clinical need for YESCARTA and any potential adverse effects on the breastfed infant from YESCARTA or from the underlying maternal condition.

Females and males of reproductive potential

Pregnancy testing

Pregnancy status of females with reproductive potential should be verified. Sexually active females of reproductive potential should have a pregnancy test prior to starting treatment with YESCARTA.

Contraception

See the prescribing information for fludarabine and cyclophosphamide for information on the need for effective contraception in patients who receive the lymphodepleting chemotherapy. There are insufficient exposure data to provide a recommendation concerning duration of contraception following treatment with YESCARTA.

Infertility

There are no data on the effect of YESCARTA on fertility.

Pediatric use

The safety and efficacy of YESCARTA have not been established in pediatric patients.

Geriatric use

Of the 422 patients with NHL who received YESCARTA in clinical trials, 127 patients (30%) were 65 years of age and older. No clinically important differences in safety or effectiveness were observed between patients aged 65 years and older and younger patients.

CLINICAL STUDIES

Relapsed or refractory large B cell lymphoma.

In the ZUMA-7 trial the primary efficacy measure was event-free survival (EFS) as determined by an independent review committee. Efficacy is summarized in Table 16. The estimated EFS rate at 18 months was 41.5% [95% CI: 34.2, 48.6] in the YESCARTA arm and 17.0% [95% CI: 11.8, 23.0] in the standard therapy arm.

Table 16. Efficacy results for Yescarta in r/r diffuse large B cell lymphoma.

Outcome[a]	YESCARTA (N = 180)[e]	Standard Therapy (N = 179)
Event-free survival[b]		
Number of events, n (%)	108 (60)	144 (80)
Median, months [95% CI][c]	8.3 [4.5, 15.8]	2.0 [1.6, 2.8]
Stratified hazard ratio [95% CI]	0.40 [0.31, 0.51]	0.40 [0.31, 0.51]
Stratified log-rank p-value	<0.0001	<0.0001
Best Objective Response Rate, % [95% CI]	83 [77, 88]	50 [43, 58]
Difference in ORR, % [95% CI]	33 [23, 42]	33 [23, 42]
Stratified p-value[d]	<0.0001	<0.0001
Complete remission rate, % [95% CI]	65 [58, 72]	32 [26, 40]
Partial remission rate, % [95% CI]	18 [13, 25]	18 [13, 24]
Progression-Free Survival		
Number of events, n (%)	93 (52)	81 (45)
Median, months [95% CI] [c]	14.9 [7.2, NE]	5.0 [3.4, 8.5]
Stratified hazard ratio [95% CI]	0.56 [0.41, 0.76]	0.56 [0.41, 0.76]

CI, confidence interval; NE, not estimable.

[a]Per the International Working Group Lugano Classification (Cheson 2014), as assessed by the independent review committee.

[b]EFS is defined as time from randomization to the earliest date of disease progression or relapse, best response of stable disease up to and including the Day 150 assessment, commencement of new lymphoma therapy, or death from any cause.

[c]Kaplan-Meier estimate.

[d]Per Cochran-Mantel-Haenszel method. For all stratified analyses, stratification was based on response to first-line therapy (primary refractory, vs relapse within 6

months of first-line therapy vs relapse within > 6 but ≤ 12 months) and second-line age-adjusted International Prognostic Index.

[e]Two recipients of non-conformal product are included in the efficacy analysis.

[Author's comments:

The EFS of 8.3 vs 2.0 months, the CR rate of 65% vs 32% and the PFS of 14.9 vs 5 months, all in favour of Yescarta, are impressive].

Relapsed or refractory follicular lymphoma (FL)

The efficacy of Yescarta in FL is based on a single-arm, open-label, multicenter trial (ZUMA-5; NCT03105336) that evaluated a single infusion of YESCARTA in adult patients with relapsed or refractory FL after two or more lines of systemic therapy, including the combination of an anti-CD20 monoclonal antibody and an alkylating agent. The study excluded patients with active or serious infections, transformed lymphoma or other aggressive lymphomas, prior allogeneic HSCT, or any history of CNS lymphoma or CNS disorders.

Of 123 patients with FL who underwent leukapheresis, 120 received YESCARTA. Of the remaining three patients (2%) who were not treated, one was ineligible due to thrombocytopenia, one went into remission prior to initiating lymphodepletion, and one died of cardiac arrest. There were no manufacturing failures. Of the 120 patients with FL infused with YESCARTA, the 81 consecutive patients included in the primary efficacy analysis had at least 9 months of potential follow-up from date of first response. Among the 81 patients with FL included in the primary efficacy analysis, the median age was 62 years (range: 34 to 79 years), 46% were female, 93% were white, 4% were black, and 3% were Asian. The median number of prior systemic therapies was 3 (range: 2 to 9), with 32% having 2 prior lines, 22% having 3 prior lines, and 46% having ≥ 4 prior lines. Thirty-one percent had received a PI3K inhibitor, 72% had progression within 6 months of the most recent regimen, and 56% had progression within 24 months of initiating their first anti-CD20 combination therapy. Between leukapheresis and administration of YESCARTA, one patient (1%) in the primary efficacy analysis received bridging therapy.

Among the 81 patients included in the primary efficacy analysis, the median time from leukapheresis to product delivery was 17 days (range 13 to 33 days) and leukapheresis to product infusion was 27 days (range 19 to 250 days). The median dose of YESCARTA was 2.0×10^6 CAR T cells/kg (range 1.3 to 2.1×10^6 CAR T cells/kg). All treated patients received YESCARTA infusion on day 0 and were hospitalized until at least day 7. Efficacy was established on the basis of objective response rate and duration of response (DOR) as determined by an independent review committee (Table 17 and Table 18). The median time to response in the primary efficacy population was 1.0 month (range: 0.8 to 3.1 months).

Table 17. Response rate in patients with relapsed or refractory FL in ZUMA-5.

	Primary efficacy analysis (N = 81)	All leukapheresed patients (N = 123)
Objective response rate[a] , n (95% CI)	74 (91%) (83, 96)	110 (89%) (83, 94)
Complete remission[b] , n (95% CI)	49 (60%) (49, 71)	76 (62%) (53, 70)
Partial remission, n (95% CI)	25 (31%) (21, 42)	34 (28%) (20, 36)

CI, confidence interval.

[a]Per the International Working Group Lugano Classification (Cheson 2014), as assessed by the independent review committee.

[b]Complete remission required documentation of a negative bone marrow biopsy after treatment, in patients who did not have a negative bone marrow biopsy between their most recent disease progression prior to ZUMA-5 and initiation of lymphodepleting chemotherapy.

Table 18. Duration of response in patients with relapsed or refractory FL in ZUMA-5.

	From N = 81
Number of responders	74
DOR (Months)[a] Median[b] (95% CI) Range[c]	 NE (20.8, NE) 0.0, 25.0+
Rate of continued remission[a, b, d]	
At 12 months (95% CI), % At 18 months (95% CI), %	76.2 (63.9, 84.7) 74.2 (61.5, 83.2)
Median follow-up for DOR (months) [a,b]	14.5

CR, complete remission; DOR, duration of response; NE, not estimable; PR, partial remission.

[a]Among all responders in the primary efficacy population. DOR is measured from the date of first objective response to the date of progression or death from any cause.
[b]Kaplan-Meier estimate.

[c]A "+" sign indicates a censored value.

[d]Measured from the date of first objective response to the date of progression or death.

[Author's comments: this is a single armed study. However, in this heavily pre-treated population, the complete response rate was 60%, the median duration of response was not reached with a range of 0.0 to 25.0+ months while the duration of remission was 76% at 12 months and 74% at 18 months. These are impressive results].

10.3. BREXUCABTAGENE/TECARTUS

[Author's comment:

Current similarities between tisangelecleucel/Kymriah, axicabtagene ciloleucel/Yescarta and brexucabtagene/Tecartus are that

1. All three target CD19.

2. All three are FDA-approved for adults with relapsed or refractory (r/r) diffuse B cell non-Hodgkin lymphomas.

Current differences between the three are that

1. *Kymriah is approved for children and young adults with r/r B cell ALL, whereas Yescarta is not. Tescartus is approved for adults with r/r B cell ALL*
2. *Yescarta is approved for r/r follicular lymphoma, whereas Kymriah and Tecartus are not.*
3. *Tecartus is approved for adults with r/r mantle cell lymphoma, whereas Kymriah and Yescarta are not.*
4. *The co-stimulatory domains used in Kymriah are CD137 and CD3 zeta, whereas those used in Yescarta and Tecartus are CD28 and CD3 zeta.*

Many other aspects of the three drugs are similar – for example, the toxicities - and will not be repeated in full for Yescarta and Tecartus

Full details on Yescarta are in the FDA insert package at

https://www.fda.gov/media/108377/download].

Full details on Tecartus are in the FDA insert package at

https://www.fda.gov/media/140409/download].

WARNING: CYTOKINE RELEASE SYNDROME and NEUROLOGIC TOXICITIES

• Cytokine release syndrome (CRS), including life-threatening reactions, occurred in patients receiving TECARTUS. Do not administer TECARTUS to patients with active infection or inflammatory disorders. Treat severe or life-threatening CRS with tocilizumab or tocilizumab and corticosteroids

• Neurologic toxicities, including life-threatening reactions, occurred in patients receiving TECARTUS, including concurrently with CRS or after CRS resolution. Monitor for neurologic toxicities after treatment with TECARTUS. Provide supportive care and/or corticosteroids, as needed.

• TECARTUS is available only through a restricted program under a Risk Evaluation and Mitigation Strategy (REMS) called the YESCARTA and TECARTUS REMS Program.

DESCRIPTION

TECARTUS (brexucabtagene autoleucel) is a CD19-directed genetically modified autologous T cell immunotherapy. To prepare TECARTUS, a patient's own T cells are harvested and genetically modified ex vivo by retroviral transduction to express a chimeric antigen receptor (CAR) comprising a murine **anti-CD19** single-chain variable fragment (scFv) linked to **CD28 and CD3 zeta** co-stimulatory domains. The anti-CD19 CAR T cells are expanded and infused back into the patient, where they can recognize and eliminate CD19- expressing target cells. TECARTUS is prepared from the patient's peripheral blood mononuclear cells, which are obtained via a standard leukapheresis procedure. The mononuclear cells are enriched for T cells and activated with anti-CD3 and anti-CD28 antibodies in the presence of IL-2, then transduced with a replication-incompetent retroviral vector containing the anti-CD19 CAR transgene. The transduced T cells are expanded in cell culture, washed, formulated into a suspension, and cryopreserved. The manufacture of TECARTUS includes a T cell enrichment step that may reduce the likelihood of circulating CD19-expressing tumor cells in patients' leukapheresis material driving the activation, expansion, and exhaustion of the anti-CD19 CAR T cells during the ex vivo manufacturing process. The product must pass a sterility test before release for shipping as a frozen suspension in a patient-specific infusion bag. The product is thawed prior to infusion. In addition to T cells, TECARTUS may contain natural killer (NK) cells. The formulation contains CryoStor (dimethyl sulfoxide [DMSO], final concentration, 5%), sodium chloride (NaCl), and Human Serum Albumin (HSA).

Mechanism of action

TECARTUS, a CD19-directed genetically modified autologous T cell immunotherapy, binds to CD19-expressing cancer cells and normal B cells. Studies demonstrated that following anti-CD19 CAR T cell engagement with CD19-expressing target cells, the CD28 and CD3 zeta co-stimulatory domains activate downstream signaling cascades that lead to T cell activation, proliferation, acquisition of effector functions, and secretion of inflammatory cytokines and chemokines. This sequence of events leads to killing of CD19- expressing cells.

INDICATIONS AND USAGE

TECARTUS is a CD19-directed genetically modified autologous T cell immunotherapy indicated for the treatment of

1. **Mantle Cell Lymphoma**

Adult patients with relapsed or refractory mantle cell lymphoma (MCL). This indication is approved under accelerated approval based on overall response rate and durability of response. Continued approval for this indication may be contingent upon verification and description of clinical benefit in a confirmatory trial.

[Mantle cell lymphoma

Mantle cell lymphoma (MCL) is a type of non-Hodgkin's lymphoma (NHL), comprising about 6% of NHL cases. It is named for the mantle zone of the lymph nodes.

MCL is a subtype of B cell lymphoma, due to CD5 positive antigen-naive pregerminal center B cell within the mantle zone that surrounds normal germinal center follicles. MCL cells generally over-express cyclin D1 due to a t(11:14)[3] chromosomal translocation in the DNA. Specifically, the translocation is at t(11;14)(q13;q32).

At diagnosis, patients typically are in their 60s and present to their physician with advanced disease. About half have B symptoms such as fever, night sweats, or unexplained weight loss (over 10% of body weight). Enlarged lymph nodes or enlargement of the spleen are usually present. Bone marrow, liver and gastrointestinal tract involvement occurs relatively early in the course of the disease. Mantle cell lymphoma has been reported in rare cases to be associated with severe allergic reactions to mosquito bites.

MCL, like most cancers, results from the acquisition of a combination of (non-inherited) genetic mutations in somatic cells. This leads to a clonal expansion of malignant B lymphocytes. The factors that initiate the genetic alterations are typically not identifiable, and usually occur in people with no particular risk factors for lymphoma development. Because it is an acquired genetic disorder, MCL is neither communicable nor inheritable.[citation needed]

A defining characteristic of MCL is mutation and overexpression of cyclin D1, a cell cycle gene that contributes to the abnormal proliferation of the malignant cells. MCL cells may also be resistant to drug-induced apoptosis, making them harder to cure with chemotherapy or radiation. Cells affected by MCL proliferate in a nodular or diffuse pattern with two main cytologic variants, typical or blastic. Typical cases are small to intermediate-sized cells with irregular nuclei. Blastic (aka blastoid) variants have intermediate to large-sized cells with finely dispersed chromatin, and are more aggressive in nature (Figures X – X).

Figure 57. Lymph node involve by with mantle cell lymphoma (low power view, H&E).

By immunohistochemistry the lymphoma cells expressed CD5, CD20 and Cyclin D1.

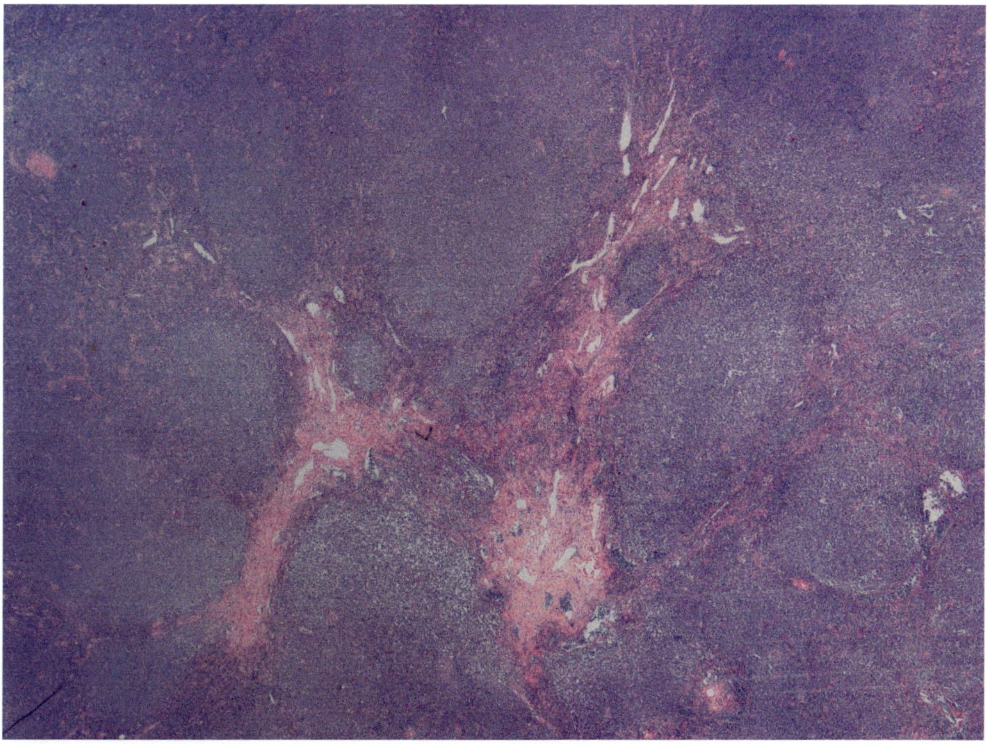

This image is by Gabriel Caponetti - Own work, CC BY-SA 3.0, https://commons.wikimedia.org/w/index.php?curid=21994668; https://en.wikipedia.org/wiki/Mantle_cell_lymphoma#/media/File:Nodular_Mantle_Cell_Lymphoma_-_low_power_view_-_by_Gabriel_Caponetti.jpg. This file is licensed under the Creative Commons Attribution-Share Alike 3.0 Unported license. No changes were made to this image.

Figure 58. Mantle cell lymphoma. Note the irregular nuclear contours of the medium-sized lymphoma cells and the presence of a pink histiocyte. By immunohistochemistry the lymphoma cells expressed CD20, CD5 and Cyclin D1 (high power view, H&E).

This image is by Gabriel Caponetti - Own work, CC BY-SA 3.0, https://commons.wikimedia.org/w/index.php?curid=21994667; https://en.wikipedia.org/wiki/Mantle_cell_lymphoma#/media/File:Nodular_Mantle_Cell_Lymphoma_-_high_power_view_-_by_Gabriel_Caponetti.jpg. This file is licensed under the Creative Commons Attribution-Share Alike 3.0 Unported license. No changes were made to this image.

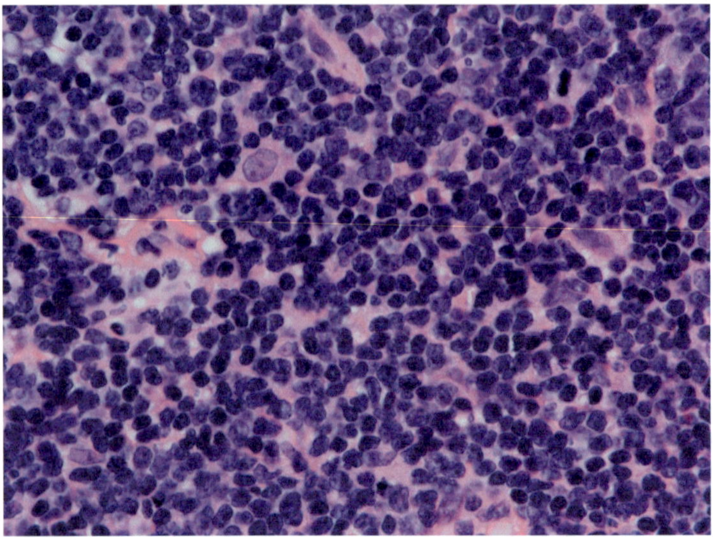

Figure 59. Micrograph of terminal ileum with mantle cell lymphoma (bottom of image). H&E stain. Note the monomorphic small lymphoid cells less than twice the size of a resting lymphocyte, abundant mitoses. sclerosed blood vessels and scattered epithelioid histiocytes.

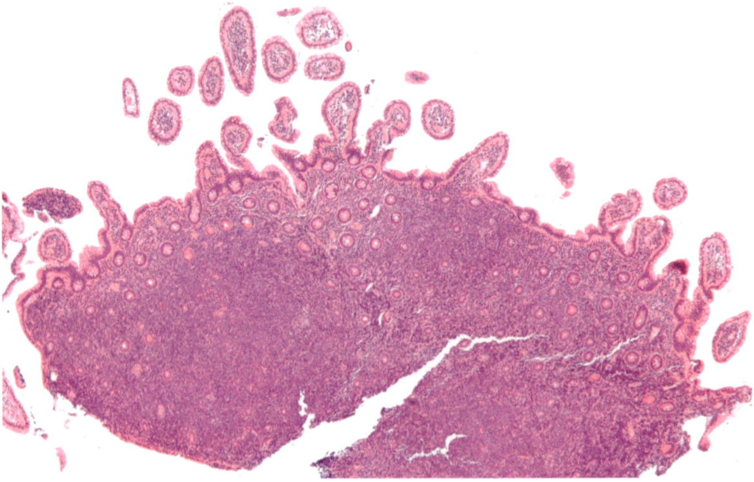

Figure 60. Micrograph of terminal ileum with mantle cell lymphoma (bottom of image - brown colour). Cyclin D1 immunostain.

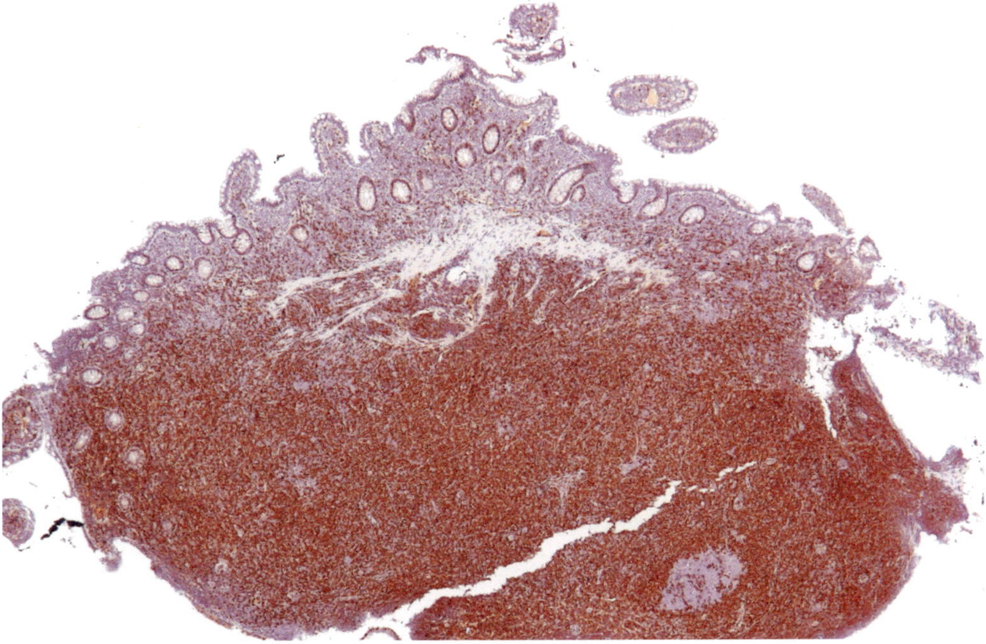

The tumor cells accumulate in the lymphoid system, including lymph nodes and the spleen, with non-useful cells eventually rendering the system dysfunctional. MCL may also replace normal cells in the bone marrow, which impairs normal blood cell production

Diagnosis generally requires stained slides of a surgically removed part of a lymph node. Other methods commonly used, including cytogenetics and fluorescence in situ hybridization (FISH). Polymerase chain reaction (PCR) and CER3 clonotypic primers are additional methods, but are less often used.

The immunophenotype profile consists of CD5+ (in about 80% of cases), CD10-/+, and it is usually CD5+ and CD10-, CD20+, CD23-/+ (though plus in rare cases). Generally, cyclin D1 is expressed. Cyclin D1-negative mantle cell lymphoma can be diagnosed by detecting the SOX11 marker. The workup for mantle cell lymphoma is similar to the workup for many indolent lymphomas and certain aggressive lymphomas. Mantle cell lymphomas also express the pan-B cell markers CD19, CD20, CD79a, CD79b and PAX-5.

Mantle cell lymphoma is a systemic disease with frequent involvement of the bone marrow and gastrointestinal tract (generally showing polyposis in the lining). There is also a not-uncommon leukemic phase, marked by its presence in the blood. For this reason, both the peripheral blood and bone marrow are evaluated for the presence of malignant cells. Chest, abdominal, and pelvic CT scans are routinely performed.

Since mantle cell lymphoma may present a lymphomatous polyposis coli and colon involvement is common, colonoscopy is considered a routine part of the evaluation. Upper endoscopy and neck CT scan may be helpful in selected cases. In some patients with the blastic variant; lumbar puncture is done to evaluate the spinal fluid for involvement.

There are no proven standards of treatment for MCL, and there is no consensus on how to treat it optimally. Many regimens are available and often have good response rates, but patients almost always have disease progression after chemotherapy. Each relapse is typically more difficult to treat, and the relapse recurrence rate is generally faster.

There are four classes of treatments in general use: chemotherapy, immunotherapy, radioimmunotherapy and biologic agents.

Chemotherapy is widely used as frontline treatment, and often is not repeated in relapse due to side-effects. Alternate chemotherapy is sometimes used at first relapse. For frontline treatment, CHOP with rituximab is the most common chemotherapy regimen, and is often given as outpatient by IV infusion. A stronger chemotherapy with greater side effects (mostly hematologic) is HyperCVAD, often given in the hospital setting, with rituximab and generally to fitter patients (some of which are over 65). HyperCVAD is becoming popular and showing promising results, especially with rituximab. It can be used on some elderly (over 65) patients, but seems only beneficial when the baseline beta-2 microglobulin blood test is normal. It is showing better complete remissions (CR) and progression-free survival (PFS) than CHOP regimens. A less intensive option is bendamustine with rituximab.

Second line treatment may include fludarabine, combined with cyclophosphamide and/or mitoxantrone, usually with rituximab. Cladribine and clofarabine are two other medications being investigated in MCL.

Another approach involves using very high doses of chemotherapy, sometimes combined with total body irradiation (TBI), in an attempt to destroy all evidence of the disease. The downside to this is the destruction of the patient's entire immune system as well, requiring rescue by transplantation of a new immune system (hematopoietic stem cell transplantation), using either autologous stem cell transplantation, or an allogeneic stem cell transplant.

Immune-based therapy is dominated by the use of the rituximab monoclonal antibody, sold under the trade name Rituxan (or as Mabthera in Europe and Australia). Rituximab may have good activity against MCL as a single agent, but it is typically given in combination with chemotherapies, which prolongs response duration.

Two Bruton tyrosine kinase inhibitors (BTKi), ibrutinib and acalabrutinib have been approved by the USA FDA for treating MCL.

Additionally, zanubrutinib (Brukinsa) was approved in the United States with an indication for the treatment of adults with mantle cell lymphoma who have received at least one prior therapy.

Cell-mediated gene therapy

Brexucabtagene autoleucel (Tecartus) was approved for medical use in the United States in July 2020, with an indication for the treatment of adults with relapsed or refractory mantle cell lymphoma. It was approved for medical use in the European Union in December 2020 (see section 8.2)].

The overall 5-year survival rate for MCL is generally 50% for advanced stage MCL to 70 for limited-stage MCL].

B cell acute lymphoblastic leukemia

Adult patients with relapsed or refractory B-cell precursor acute lymphoblastic leukemia (ALL).

Administration

TECARTUS is for autologous use only. The patient's identity must match the patient identifiers on the TECARTUS cassette and infusion bag. Do not infuse TECARTUS if the information on the patient-specific label does not match the intended patient. Preparing the patient for TECARTUS Infusion

Confirm availability of TECARTUS prior to starting the lymphodepleting chemotherapy regimen.

Pre-treatment

• MCL: administer a lymphodepleting chemotherapy regimen of cyclophosphamide 500 mg/m^2 intravenously and fludarabine 30 mg/m^2 intravenously on each of the fifth, fourth, and third day before infusion of TECARTUS.

• ALL: administer a lymphodepleting chemotherapy regimen of fludarabine 25 mg/m^2 intravenously over 30 minutes on the fourth, third, and second day and administer cyclophosphamide 900 mg/m^2 over 60 minutes on the second day before infusion of TECARTUS.

Premedication

• Premedicate with acetaminophen and diphenhydramine or another H1-antihistamine approximately 30 to 60 minutes prior to TECARTUS infusion.

• Avoid prophylactic use of systemic corticosteroids as it may interfere with the activity of TECARTUS.

Preparation of TECARTUS for infusion

Coordinate the timing of TECARTUS thaw and infusion. Confirm the infusion time in advance, and adjust the start time of TECARTUS thaw such that TECARTUS will be available for infusion when the patient is ready.

• Confirm patient identity

Prior to TECARTUS preparation, match the patient's identity with the patient identifiers on the TECARTUS cassette.

• Do not remove the TECARTUS infusion bag from the cassette if the patient information on the cassette label does not match the intended patient.

• Once patient identity is confirmed, remove the TECARTUS infusion bag from the cassette and check that the patient information on the cassette label matches the patient information on the bag label.

• Inspect the infusion bag for any breaches of container integrity such as breaks or cracks before thawing. If the bag is compromised, follow the local guidelines (or call Kite at 1-844-454-KITE).

• Place the infusion bag inside a second sterile bag per local guidelines.

• Thaw the infusion bag at approximately 37°C using either a water bath or dry-thaw method until there is no visible ice in the infusion bag.

• Gently mix the contents of the bag to disperse clumps of cellular material. If visible cell clumps remain, continue to gently mix the contents of the bag. Small clumps of cellular material should disperse with gentle manual mixing. Do not wash, spin down, and/or re-suspend TECARTUS in new media prior to infusion.

• Once thawed, TECARTUS should be administered within 30 minutes but may be stored at room temperature (20°C to 25°C) for up to three hours.

Administration

• For autologous use only.

• Ensure that tocilizumab and emergency equipment are available prior to infusion and during the recovery period.

• Do NOT use a leukodepleting filter.

• Central venous access is recommended for the administration of TECARTUS.

• Confirm that the patient's identity matches the patient identifiers on the TECARTUS infusion bag.

• Prime the tubing with normal saline prior to infusion.

• Infuse the entire contents of the TECARTUS bag within 30 minutes by either gravity or a peristaltic pump. TECARTUS is stable at room temperature for up to three hours after thaw.

• Gently agitate the TECARTUS bag during infusion to prevent cell clumping.

• After the entire contents of the TECARTUS bag are infused, rinse the tubing with normal saline at the same infusion rate to ensure all product is delivered.
TECARTUS contains human blood cells that are genetically modified with replication-incompetent retroviral vector. Follow universal precautions and local biosafety guidelines for handling and disposal of TECARTUS to avoid potential transmission of infectious diseases.

Monitoring

• Administer TECARTUS at a certified healthcare facility.

• Monitor patients at the certified healthcare facility daily for at least seven days for patients with MCL and at least 14 days for patients with ALL following infusion for signs and symptoms of Cytokine Release Syndrome (CRS) and neurologic events.

• Instruct patients to remain within proximity of the certified healthcare facility for at least four weeks following infusion.

Management of severe adverse reactions

Cytokine Release Syndrome

Identify CRS based on clinical presentation. Evaluate for and treat other causes of fever, hypoxia, and hypotension. If CRS is suspected, manage according to the recommendations in Table 13. *[This Table relates to Yescarta, but the recommendations are the same for Tescartus].* Patients who experience Grade 2 or higher CRS (e.g., hypotension, not responsive to fluids, or hypoxia requiring supplemental oxygenation) should be monitored with continuous cardiac telemetry and pulse oximetry. For patients experiencing severe CRS, consider performing an echocardiogram to assess cardiac function. For severe or life-threatening CRS, consider intensive care supportive therapy.

Neurologic Toxicity

Monitor patients for signs and symptoms of neurologic toxicities (Table 14). *[This table relates to Yescarta but the recommendations are the same for Tescartus].* Rule out other causes of neurologic symptoms. Patients who experience Grade 2 or higher neurologic toxicities should be monitored with continuous cardiac telemetry and pulse oximetry. Provide intensive care supportive therapy for severe or life-threatening neurologic toxicities. Consider non-sedating anti-seizure medicines (e.g., levetiracetam) for seizure prophylaxis for any Grade 2 or higher neurologic toxicities.

DOSAGE FORMS AND STRENGTHS

TECARTUS is available as a cell suspension for infusion.

• MCL: A single dose of TECARTUS contains 2×10^6 CAR-positive viable T cells per kg of body weight [maximum of 2×10^8 CAR-positive viable T cells (for patients 100 kg and above)] in approximately 68 mL suspension in an infusion bag.

• ALL: A single dose of TECARTUS contains 1×10^6 CAR-positive viable T cells per kg of body weight [maximum of 1×10^8 CAR-positive viable T cells (for patients 100 kg and above)] in approximately 68 mL suspension in an infusion bag.

CONTRAINDICATIONS: None

WARNINGS AND PRECAUTIONS

Cytokine Release Syndrome (CRS), including fatal or life-threatening reactions, occurred following treatment with TECARTUS. CRS occurred in 91% (75/82) of patients with MCL, including ≥ Grade 3 (Lee grading system1) CRS in 18% of patients. Among the patients with MCL who died after receiving TECARTUS, one patient had a fatal CRS event. The median time to onset of CRS was three days (range 1 to 13 days) and the median duration of CRS was ten days (range 1 to 50 days) for patients with MCL.

CRS occurred in 92% (72/78) of patients with ALL, including ≥ Grade 3 (Lee grading system1) CRS in 26% of patients. Three patients with ALL had ongoing CRS events at the time of death. The median time to onset of CRS was five days (range 1 to 12 days) and the median duration of CRS was eight days (range 2 to 63 days) for patients with ALL. The incidence of CRS (first occurrence) within the first seven days after TECARTUS infusion was 83% (68/82) in patients with MCL and 90% (70/78) in patients with ALL. In all patients combined (MCL/ALL), the incidence of first CRS (first occurrence) within the first seven days after TECARTUS infusion was 86% (138/160). Among patients with CRS, the key manifestations (>10%) were similar in MCL and ALL and included fever (93%), hypotension (62%), tachycardia (59%), chills (32%), hypoxia (31%), headache (21%), fatigue (20%), and nausea (13%). Serious events associated with CRS in MCL and ALL combined (≥ 2%) included hypotension, fever, hypoxia, tachycardia, and dyspnea. Ensure that a minimum of two doses of tocilizumab are available for each patient prior to infusion of TECARTUS. Monitor patients daily for at least seven days for patients with MCL and at least 14 days for patients with ALL at the certified healthcare facility following infusion for signs and symptoms of CRS. Monitor patients for signs or symptoms of CRS for four weeks after infusion. Counsel patients to seek immediate medical attention should signs or symptoms of CRS occur at any time.

At the first sign of CRS, institute treatment with supportive care, tocilizumab, or tocilizumab and corticosteroids as indicated.

Neurologic toxicities

Neurologic events, including those that were fatal or life-threatening, occurred following treatment with TECARTUS. Neurologic events occurred in 81% (66/82) of patients with MCL, including ≥ Grade 3 in 37% of patients. The median time to onset for neurologic events was six days (range 1 to 32 days) with a median duration of 21 days (range 2 to 454 days) in patients with MCL. Neurologic events occurred in 87% (68/78) of patients with ALL, including ≥ Grade 3 in 35% of patients. The median time to onset for neurologic events was seven days (range 1 to 51 days) with a median duration of 15 days (range 1 to 397 days) in patients with ALL. For patients with MCL, 54 (66%) patients experienced CRS before the onset of neurological events. Five (6%) patients did not experience CRS with neurologic events and eight patients (10%) developed neurological events after the resolution of CRS. Neurologic events resolved for 119 out of 134 (89%) patients treated with TECARTUS. Nine patients (three patients with MCL and six patients with ALL) had ongoing neurologic events at the time of death. For patients with ALL, neurologic events occurred before, during, and after CRS in 4 (5%), 57 (73%), and 8 (10%) of patients, respectively. Three patients (4%) had neurologic events without CRS. The onset of neurologic events can be concurrent with CRS, following resolution of CRS or in the absence of CRS. The incidence of neurologic events (first occurrence) within the first seven days after TECARTUS infusion was 56% (46/82) in patients with MCL and 55% (43/78) in patients with ALL. In all patients combined (MCL/ALL) the incidence of neurologic events (first occurrence) within the first seven days after TECARTUS infusion was 56% (89/160). Ninety-one percent of all treated patients experienced the first CRS or neurological event within the first seven days after TECARTUS infusion. The most common neurologic events (>10%) were similar in MCL and ALL and included encephalopathy (57%), headache (37%), tremor (34%), confusional state (26%), aphasia (23%), delirium (17%), dizziness (15%), anxiety (14%), and agitation (12%). Serious events (≥ 2%) including encephalopathy, aphasia, confusional state, and seizures occurred after treatment with TECARTUS. Monitor patients daily for at least seven days for patients with MCL and at least 14 days for patients with ALL at the certified healthcare facility following infusion for signs and symptoms of neurologic toxicities. Monitor patients for signs or symptoms of neurologic toxicities for four weeks after infusion and treat promptly.

YESCARTA and TECARTUS REMS Program

Because of the risk of CRS and neurologic toxicities, TECARTUS is available only through a restricted program under a Risk Evaluation and Mitigation Strategy (REMS) called the YESCARTA and TECARTUS REMS Program.

The required components of the YESCARTA and TECARTUS REMS Program are

- Healthcare facilities that dispense and administer TECARTUS must be enrolled and comply with the REMS requirements. Certified healthcare facilities must have on-site, immediate access to tocilizumab, and ensure that a minimum of two doses of tocilizumab are available for each patient for infusion within two hours after TECARTUS infusion, if needed for treatment of CRS.

- Certified healthcare facilities must ensure that healthcare providers who prescribe, dispense, or administer TECARTUS are trained in the management of CRS and neurologic toxicities. Further information is available at www.YescartaTecartus REMS.com or 1-844-454-KITE (5483).

Hemophagocytic lymphohistiocytosis/macrophage activation syndrome

[see below and also Sections 10.1, Section 10.2 and Appendix 11.4 for details of HLH and Appendix 11.5 for details of MAS],

Hemophagocytic lymphohistiocytosis/macrophage activation syndrome (HLH/MAS) including life-threatening reactions, occurred following treatment with TECARTUS. HLH/MAS occurred in 4% (3/78) of patients with ALL. Two patients experienced Grade 3 events and 1 patient experienced a Grade 4 event. The median time to onset for HLH/MAS was 8 days (range: 6 to 9 days) with a median duration of 5 days (range: 2 to 8 days). All three patients with HLH/MAS had concurrent CRS symptoms and neurologic events after TECARTUS infusion. Treatment of HLH/MAS should be administered per institutional standards.

*[**Hemophagocytic lymphohistiocytosis** (HLH), also known as haemophagocytic lymphohistiocytosis (British spelling), and hemophagocytic or haemophagocytic syndrome, is an uncommon hematologic disorder seen more often in children than in adults. It is a life-threatening disease of severe hyperinflammation caused by uncontrolled proliferation of activated lymphocytes and macrophages, characterised by proliferation of morphologically benign lymphocytes and macrophages that secrete high amounts of inflammatory cytokines. It is classified as one of the **cytokine storm syndromes.** There are inherited and non-inherited (acquired) causes of hemophagocytic lymphohistiocytosis (HLH). The onset of HLH occurs before the age of one year in approximately 70 percent of cases. Familial HLH should be suspected if siblings are diagnosed with HLH or if symptoms recur when therapy has been stopped. Familial HLH is an autosomal recessive disease, hence each sibling of a child with familial HLH has a twenty-five–percent chance of developing the disease, a fifty-percent chance of carrying the defective gene (which is very rarely associated with any risk of disease), and a twenty-five–percent chance of not being affected and not carrying the gene defect.*

Patients with HLH, especially when untreated, may need intensive therapy. Therefore, HLH should be included in the differential diagnosis of intensive care unit patients with cytopenia and hyperferritinemia. Patients in the earlier stages of HLH are frequently hospitalized at internal medicine wards.

HLH clinically manifests with fever, enlargement of the liver and spleen, enlarged lymph nodes, yellow discoloration of the skin and eyes, and a rash. Laboratory findings may include elevated triglyceride levels, low fibrinogen levels, transaminitis, and elevated ferritin levels (among others)

The underlying cause oh HLH leads to an unchecked immune response. Impaired NK-cell cytotoxicity is the hallmark of HLH. All genetic defects for familial HLH are related to granule-dependent cytotoxicity. This inability to remove infected and antigen-presenting cells and terminate the immune response leads to uncontrolled proliferation and activation of the immune system with release of excessive cytokines. These cells then infiltrate organs, releasing more cytokines, which gives the clinical picture. The fever is caused by thepro-inflammatory cytokines IL-1, IL-6 and TNF-alpha; the cytopenia is due to the suppressive effect on hematopoiesis by TNF-alpha and TNF-gamma. TNF-alpha and TNF-gamma may also lead to inhibition of lipoprotein lipase or stimulate triglyceride synthesis. Activated macrophages secrete ferritin and plasminogen activator leading to hyperfibrinolysis.

Figure 61. Colorized scanning electron micrograph of a natural killer cell from a human donor. Credit: NIAID

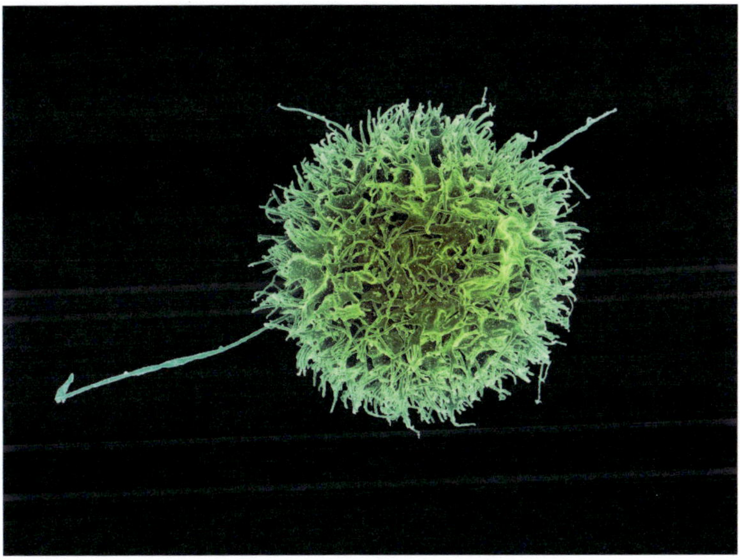

The blood count typically shows decreased numbers of blood cells - including a decreased number of circulating red blood cells, white blood cells, and platelets. The bone marrow may show hemophagocytosis. The liver function tests are usually elevated. A low level of the protein albumin in the blood is common.

The serum C reactive protein, erythrocyte sedimentation rate, and ferritin level are markedly elevated. In children, a ferritin above 10000 is very sensitive and specific for the diagnosis of HLH, however, the diagnostic utility for ferritin is less for adult HLH patients. The serum fibrinogen level is usually low and the D-dimer level is elevated. The sphingomyelinase is elevated.

Diagnostic criteria for acquired HLH are

Fulfillment of five out of the eight criteria below:

Fever (defined as a temperature >100.3 °F, >38 °C)

Enlargement of the spleen

Decreased blood cell counts affecting at least two of three lineages in the peripheral blood:

Haemoglobin <9 g/100 ml (in infants <4 weeks: haemoglobin <10 g/100 ml) (anemia)

Platelets <100×10^9/L (thrombocytopenia)

Neutrophils <1×10^9/L (neutropenia)

High blood levels of triglycerides (fasting, greater than or equal to 265 mg/100 ml) and/or decreased amounts of fibrinogen in the blood (≤ 150 mg/100 ml)

Ferritin ≥ 500 ng/ml

Haemophagocytosis in the bone marrow, spleen or lymph nodes

Low or absent natural killer cell activity

Soluble CD25 (Figure 62), (soluble IL-2 receptor) >2400 U/ml (or per local reference laboratory)

In addition, in the case of familial HLH, no evidence of malignancy should be apparent. Not all five out of eight criteria are required for diagnosis of HLH in adults, and a high index of suspicion is required for diagnosis as delay results in increased mortality. The diagnostic criteria were developed in pediatric populations and have not been validated for adult HLH patients. Attempts to improve diagnosis of HLH have included use of the HScore, which can be used to estimate an individual's risk of HLH. In adults, soluble IL-2 receptor has been found to be a very sensitive marker for HLH, demonstrating 100% sensitivity for ruling out HLH below a cutoff of 2400 U/mL and optimal cutoff for ruling in at 2515 U/mL (sensitivity, 100%; specificity, 72.5%), with 93% specificity at >10 000 U/mL.

Figure 62. Structure of the soluble interleukin-2 receptor alpha chain (CD25).

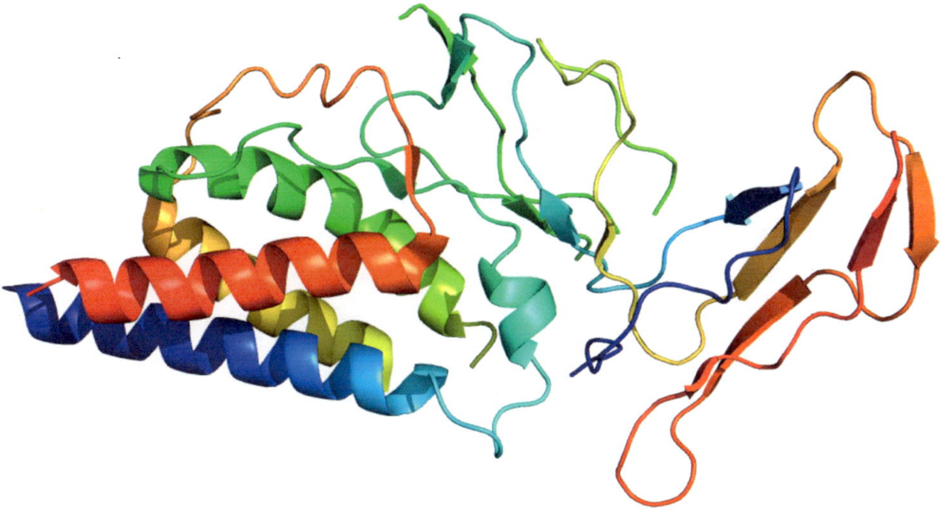

The first case report of HLH was published in 1952 by James Farquar and colleagues].

*[**Macrophage activation syndrome***

Macrophage activation syndrome is a severe, potentially life-threatening, complication of several chronic rheumatic diseases of childhood. It occurs most commonly with systemic-onset juvenile idiopathic arthritis (SoJIA). In addition, MAS has been described in association with systemic lupus erythematosus (SLE), Kawasaki disease, and adult-onset Still's disease. ***It is thought to be closely related and pathophysiologically very similar to reactive (secondary) hemophagocytic lymphohistiocytosis (HLH)*** *The incidence of MAS is unknown as there is a wide spectrum of clinical manifestations, and episodes may remain unrecognized. The hallmark clinical and laboratory features include high fever, hepatosplenomegaly, lymphadenopathy, pancytopenia, liver dysfunction, disseminated intravascular coagulation, hypofibrinogenemia, hyperferritinemia, and hypertriglyceridemia. Despite marked systemic inflammation, the erythrocyte sedimentation rate (ESR) is paradoxically depressed, caused by low fibrinogen levels. The low ESR helps to distinguish the disorder from a flare of the underlying rheumatic disorder, in which case the ESR is usually elevated. A bone marrow biopsy or aspirate usually shows hemophagocytosis. In many cases a trigger is identified, often a viral infection, or a* ***medication****. There is uncontrolled activation and proliferation of macrophages, and T lymphocytes, with a marked increase in circulating cytokines, such as IFN-gamma, and GM-CSF. The underlying causative event is unclear, and is the subject of ongoing research. In many cases of MAS, a decreased natural killer cell (NK-cell) function is found.*

Disseminated intravascular coagulation: disseminated intravascular coagulation (DIC) is a condition in which blood clots form throughout the body, blocking small blood vessels. Symptoms may include chest pain, shortness of breath, leg pain, problems speaking, or problems moving parts of the body. As clotting factors and platelets are used up, bleeding may occur. This may include blood in the urine, blood in the stool, or bleeding into the skin. Complications may include organ failure.

A febrile patient with known or suspected sJia must be considered for macrophage activation if:

Ferritin >684 ng/ml

and any 2 of the following:

Hemoglobin <90g/L (in infants <4 weeks: <100g/L)

Platelets <100 x 10^9/L

Neutrophils <1.0 x 10^9/L

Fasting triglycerides ≥3.0 mmol/L (i.e., ≥ 265 mg/dl)

Fibrinogen ≤1.5 g/L[3]

The peripheral blood smear may show fragmented red blood cells (known as schistocytes (Figure 63)) due to shear stress from thrombi. However, this finding is neither sensitive nor specific for DIC

Figure 63. Blood film showing red blood cell fragments (schistocytes)

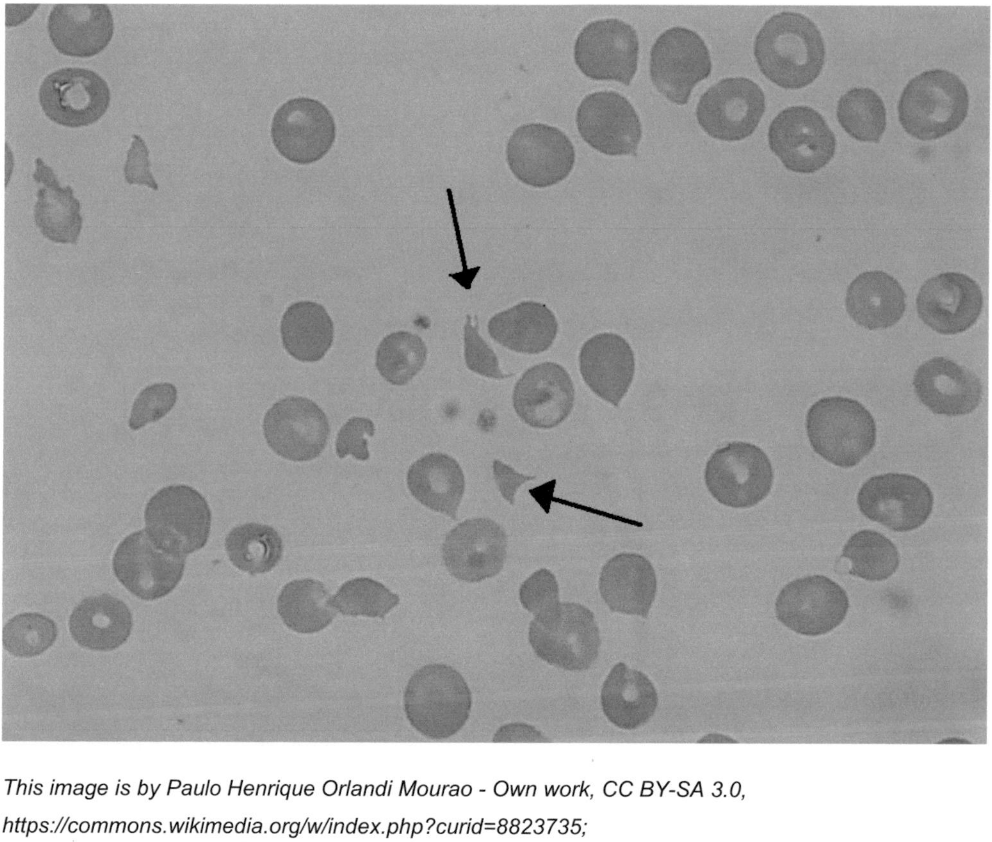

In addition, other specific markers of macrophage activation (e.g. soluble CD163), and lymphocyte activation (e.g. soluble IL-2 receptor) can be helpful. NK cell function

analysis may show depressed NK function, or, flow cytometry may show a depressed NK cell population.CD163 is the high affinity scavenger receptor for the hemoglobin-haptoglobin complex (Figure 64)

Figure 64. A model of α, β-hemoglobin/haptoglobin hexamer complex. There are 2 α, β-hemoglobin dimers depicted: one space filling model (yellow/orange), and one ribbon model (purple/blue). Each is bound by a haptoglobin molecule (both haptoglobin molecules are shown in pink, with one as a space filling model and one as a ribbon model).

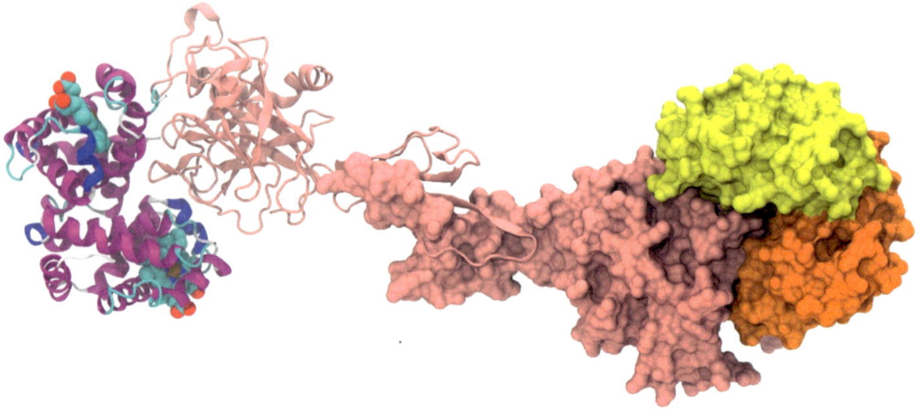

This image is by Ayacop - Own work, CC0, https://commons.wikimedia.org/w/index.php?curid=21512477; https://en.wikipedia.org/wiki/Haptoglobin#/media/File:Hem-hap_4f4o.jpg. This file is made available under the Creative Commons CC0 1.0 Universal Public Domain Dedication. No changes were made to this image].

The best treatment for MAS has not been firmly established. Most commonly used treatments include high-dose glucocorticoids, and cyclosporine. In refractory cases treatment regimens are used similar to that in HLH. Anakinra may also be effective].

Hypersensitivity reactions

Serious hypersensitivity reactions, including anaphylaxis, may occur due to dimethyl sulfoxide (DMSO) or residual gentamicin in TECARTUS.

Severe infections

Severe or life-threatening infections occurred in patients after TECARTUS infusion. Infections (all grades) occurred in 56% (46/82) of patients with MCL and 44% (34/78) of patients with ALL. Grade 3 or higher infections, including bacterial, viral, and fungal infections, occurred in 30% of patients with ALL and MCL. TECARTUS should not be administered to patients with clinically significant active systemic infections. Monitor patients for signs and symptoms of infection before and after TECARTUS infusion and treat appropriately. Administer prophylactic antimicrobials according to local guidelines. Febrile neutropenia was observed in 6% of patients with MCL and 35% of patients with ALL after TECARTUS infusion and may be concurrent with CRS. The febrile neutropenia in 27 (35%) of patients with ALL includes events of "febrile neutropenia" (11 (14%)) plus the concurrent events of "fever" and "neutropenia" (16 (21%)). In the event of febrile neutropenia, evaluate for infection and manage with broad spectrum antibiotics, fluids, and other supportive care as medically indicated. In immunosuppressed patients, life-threatening and fatal opportunistic infections have been reported. The possibility of rare infectious etiologies (e.g., fungal and viral infections such as HHV-6 and progressive multifocal leukoencephalopathy) should be considered in patients with neurologic events and appropriate diagnostic evaluations should be performed.

Hepatitis B reactivation

Hepatitis B virus (HBV) reactivation, in some cases resulting in fulminant hepatitis, hepatic failure, and death, can occur in patients treated with drugs directed against B cells. Perform screening for HBV, hepatitis C virus (HCV), and human immunodeficiency virus (HIV) in accordance with clinical guidelines before collection of cells for manufacturing.

[Figure 65. Hepatitis B viral antigens and antibodies detectable in the blood following acute infection.

This image is by User:GrahamColm - Own work, Public Domain, https://commons.wikimedia.org/w/index.php?curid=23165261; https://en.wikipedia.org/wiki/Hepatitis_B#/media/File:HBV_serum_markers.png. This work has been released into the public domain by its author, GrahamColm. No changes have been made to this image.

[Figure 65. Hepatitis B viral antigens and antibodies detectable in the blood following acute infection.

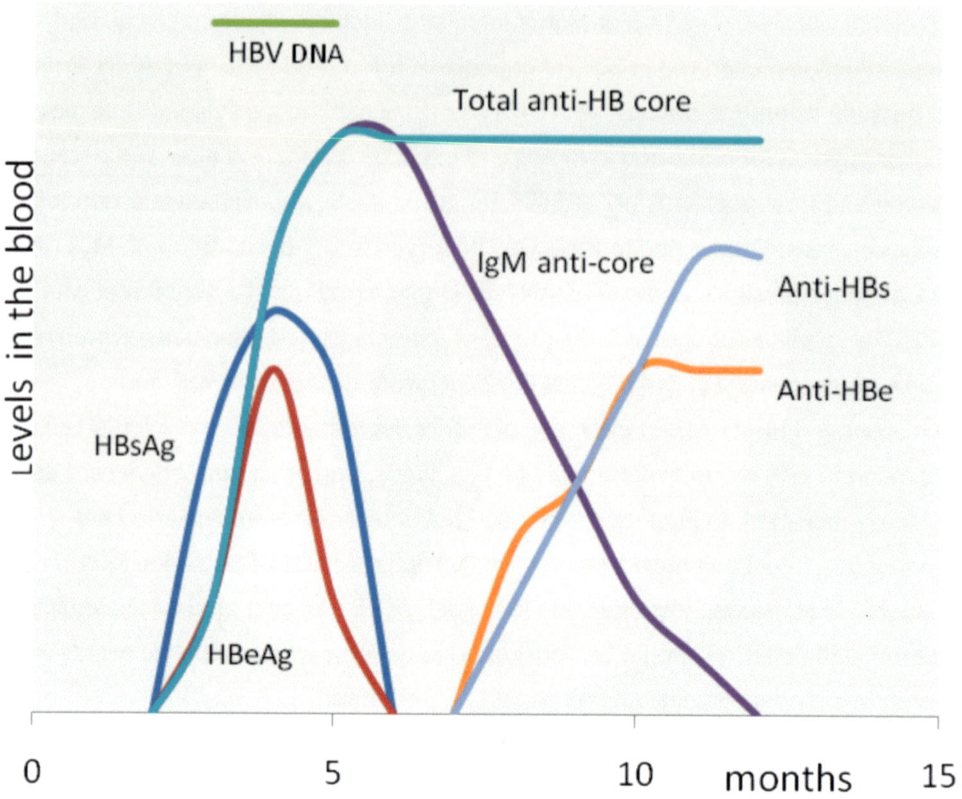

Figure 66. Serologic profile of Hepatitis C infection.

This image is by GrahamColmTalk.GrahamColm at English Wikipedia - Own work (Original text: self-made), Public Domain, https://commons.wikimedia.org/w/index.php?curid=20003582; https://en.wikipedia.org/wiki/Hepatitis_C#/media/File:Hepatitis_C_serology.png. This chart is ineligible for copyright and therefore in the public domain, because it consists entirely of information that is common property and contains no original authorship. No changes have been made to this image.

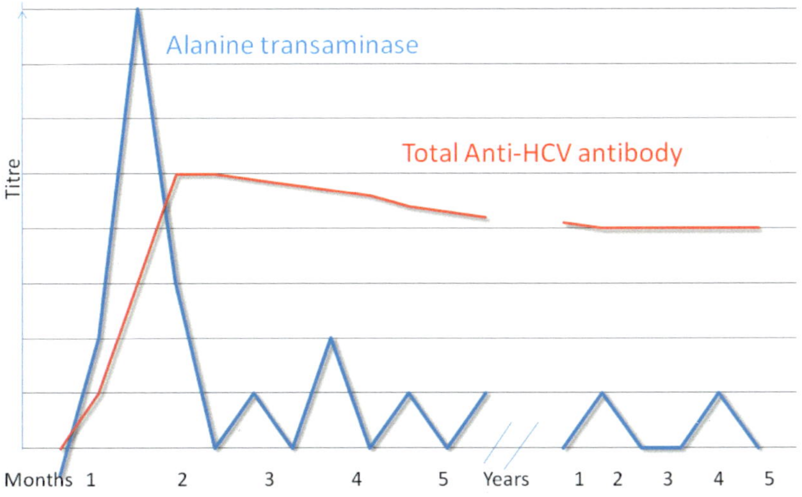

Figure 67. A generalized graph of the relationship between HIV copies (viral load) and CD4 counts over the average course of untreated HIV infection; any particular individual's disease course may vary considerably. ▯ *CD4+ T cell count (cells per μL)* ▯ *HIV RNA copies per mL of plasma.*

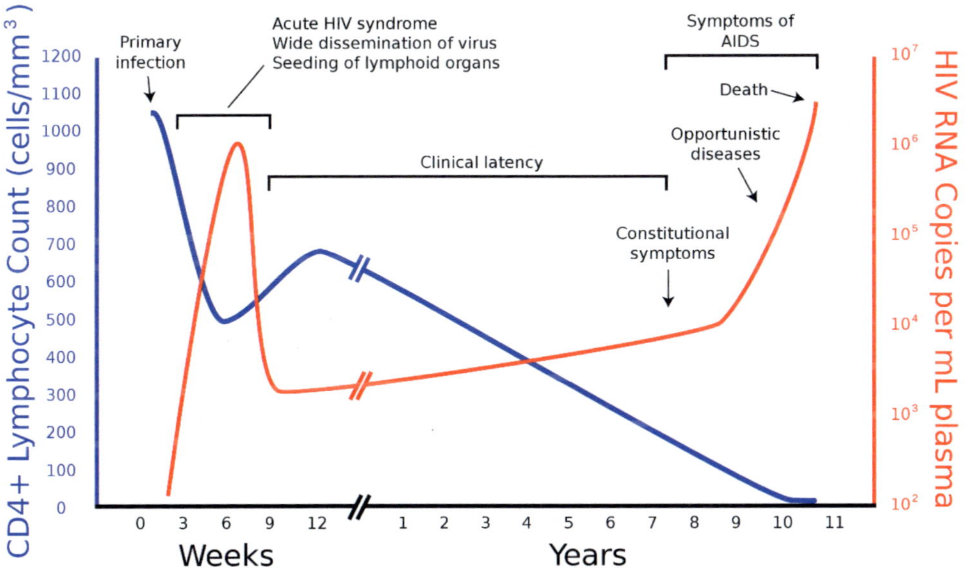

This image is by Sigve - Own work, CC0, https://commons.wikimedia.org/w/index.php?curid=15383502; https://en.wikipedia.org/wiki/HIV#/media/File:Hiv-timecourse_copy.svg. This file is made available

under the Creative Commons CC0 1.0 Universal Public Domain Dedication. No changes were made to this image].

Prolonged cytopenias

Patients may exhibit cytopenias for several weeks following lymphodepleting chemotherapy and TECARTUS infusion. In patients with MCL, Grade 3 or higher cytopenias not resolved by Day 30 following TECARTUS infusion occurred in 55% (45/82) of patients and included thrombocytopenia (38%), neutropenia (37%), and anemia (17%). In patients with ALL who were responders to TECARTUS treatment, Grade 3 or higher cytopenias not resolved by Day 30 following TECARTUS infusion occurred in 20% (7/35) of the patients and included neutropenia (12%) and thrombocytopenia (12%); Grade 3 or higher cytopenias not resolved by Day 60 following TECARTUS infusion occurred in 11% (4/35) of the patients and included neutropenia (9%) and thrombocytopenia (6%). Monitor blood counts after TECARTUS infusion.

Hypogammaglobulinemia

B cell aplasia and hypogammaglobulinemia can occur in patients receiving treatment with TECARTUS. Hypogammaglobulinemia was reported in 16% (13/82) of patients with MCL and 9% (7/78) of patients with ALL. Monitor immunoglobulin levels after treatment with TECARTUS and manage using infection precautions, antibiotic prophylaxis, and immunoglobulin replacement. The safety of immunization with live viral vaccines during or following TECARTUS treatment has not been studied. Vaccination with live virus vaccines is not recommended for at least six weeks prior to the start of lymphodepleting chemotherapy, during TECARTUS treatment, and until immune recovery following treatment with TECARTUS.

Secondary malignancies

Patients treated with TECARTUS may develop secondary malignancies. Monitor life-long for secondary malignancies. In the event that a secondary malignancy occurs, contact Kite at 1-844-454-KITE (5483) to obtain instructions on patient samples to collect for testing.

Effects on ability to drive and use machines

Due to the potential for neurologic events, including altered mental status or seizures, patients receiving TECARTUS are at risk for altered or decreased consciousness or coordination in the eight weeks following TECARTUS infusion. Advise patients to refrain from driving and engaging in hazardous occupations or activities, such as operating heavy or potentially dangerous machinery, during this initial period.

Clinical trials experience

Because clinical trials are conducted under widely varying conditions, adverse reaction rates observed in the clinical trials of a drug cannot be directly compared to rates in the clinical trials of another drug and may not reflect the rates observed in practice.

Patients with relapsed/refractory mantle cell lymphoma (MCL)

The safety of TECARTUS was evaluated in a Phase 2 single-arm clinical study (ZUMA-2) in which a total of 82 patients with relapsed/refractory MCL received a single dose of CAR-positive viable T cells (2×10^6 or 0.5×10^6 anti-CD19 CAR T cells/kg) that was weight-based. The most common adverse reactions (incidence ≥ 20%) were fever, CRS, hypotension, encephalopathy, fatigue, tachycardia, arrhythmia, infection with pathogen unspecified, chills, hypoxia, cough, tremor, musculoskeletal pain, headache, nausea, edema, motor dysfunction, constipation, diarrhea, decreased appetite, dyspnea, rash, insomnia, pleural effusion, and aphasia.

Serious adverse reactions occurred in 66% of patients. The most common serious adverse reactions (> 2%) were encephalopathy, fever, infection with pathogen unspecified, CRS, hypoxia, aphasia, renal insufficiency, pleural effusion, respiratory failure, bacterial infections, dyspnea, fatigue, arrhythmia, tachycardia, and viral infections.

The most common (≥ 10%) Grade 3 or higher reactions were anemia, neutropenia, thrombocytopenia, hypotension, hypophosphatemia, encephalopathy, leukopenia, hypoxia, fever, hyponatremia, hypertension, infection with pathogen unspecified, pneumonia, hypocalcemia, and lymphopenia.

[Details of the side-effects:

a. Coagulopathy includes coagulopathy, disseminated intravascular coagulation, international normalized ratio increased.

b. Tachycardias includes tachycardia, sinus tachycardia.

c. Bradycardias includes bradycardia, sinus bradycardia.

d. Non-ventricular arrhythmias includes atrial fibrillation, atrial flutter, cardiac flutter, palpitations, supraventricular tachycardia.

e. Abdominal pain includes abdominal pain, abdominal pain lower, abdominal pain upper, abdominal tenderness.

f. Oral pain includes oral pain, gingival pain, lip pain, oral mucosal erythema, oropharyngeal pain.

g. Vomiting includes vomiting, retching.

h. Fatigue includes fatigue, lethargy, malaise.

i. Edema includes eyelid edema, face edema, generalized edema, localised edema, edema, edema peripheral, periorbital edema, peripheral swelling, scrotal edema, swelling face.

j. Pain includes pain, allodynia, dysaesthesia, ear pain, facial pain, non-cardiac chest pain.

k. Hypogammaglobulinemia includes hypogammaglobulinemia, blood immunoglobulin G decreased.

l. Musculoskeletal pain includes musculoskeletal pain, arthralgia, back pain, bone pain, dysarthria, flank pain, groin pain, myalgia, neck pain, pain in extremity.

m. Motor dysfunction includes asthenia, intensive care acquired weakness, mobility decreased, muscle twitching, muscular weakness, myopathy.

n. Encephalopathy includes encephalopathy, altered state of consciousness, amnesia, balance disorder, cognitive disorder, confusional state, disturbance in attention, dysgraphia, dyskinesia, memory impairment, mental status changes, neurotoxicity, somnolence.

o. Headache includes headache, migraine.

p. Aphasia includes aphasia, communication disorder.

q. Dizziness includes dizziness, presyncope, syncope.

r. Neuropathy includes hyperaesthesia, neuropathy peripheral, paraesthesia, paraesthesia oral.

s. Delirium includes delirium, agitation, disorientation, hallucination, hypomania, irritability, nervousness, personality change.

t. Renal insufficiency includes acute kidney injury, blood creatinine increased.

u. Urine output decreased includes urine output decreased, urinary retention.

v. Cough includes cough, upper-airway cough syndrome.

w. Dyspnea includes dyspnea, dyspnea exertional.

x. Rash includes rash, erythema, rash erythematous, rash maculo-papular, rash pustular.

y. Hypotension includes hypotension, orthostatic hypotension.

z. Thrombosis includes thrombosis, deep vein thrombosis, embolism, pulmonary embolism.

Other clinically important adverse reactions that occurred in less than 10% of patients treated with TECARTUS include the following:

• Gastrointestinal disorders: dry mouth (7%)

• Infections and infestations disorders: fungal infections (9%)

• Metabolism and nutrition disorders: dehydration (6%)

• Nervous system disorders: ataxia (7%), seizure (5%), increased intracranial pressure (2%)

• Respiratory, thoracic and mediastinal disorders: respiratory failure (6%), pulmonary edema (4%)

• Skin and subcutaneous tissue disorders: rash (9%)

• Vascular disorders: hemorrhage (7%

Table19. Grade 3 or 4 laboratory abnormalities occurring in ≥ 10% of patients in ZUMA-2 following TECARTUS infusion (N = 82).

	Grades 3 or 4 (%)
Leukopenia	95
Neutropenia	95
Lymphopenia	86
Thrombocytopenia	63
Anemia	55
Hypophosphatemia	30
Hypocalcemia	25
Increased blood uric acid	17
Hyponatremia	16
Aspartate aminotransferase	15
Alanine aminotransferase	15
Hypokalemia	19

Patients with relapsed/refractory B-cell precursor acute lymphoblastic leukemia (ALL)

The safety of TECARTUS was evaluated in a Phase 1/2 open-label, multicenter study (ZUMA-3) in which a total of 78 patients with relapsed/refractory ALL received a single dose of CAR-positive T cells (1 x 10^6 antiCD19 CAR T cells/kg) that was weight-based. The most common non-laboratory adverse reactions (≥ 20%) were fever, cytokine release syndrome, hypotension, encephalopathy, tachycardia, nausea, chills, headache, fatigue, febrile neutropenia, diarrhea, musculoskeletal pain, hypoxia, rash, edema, tremor, infection with pathogen unspecified, constipation, decreased appetite, and vomiting.

The most common serious adverse reactions (≥ 2%) were cytokine release syndrome, febrile neutropenia, hypotension, encephalopathy, fever, infection with pathogen unspecified, hypoxia, tachycardia, bacterial infections, respiratory failure, seizure, diarrhea, dyspnea, fungal infections, viral infections, coagulopathy, delirium, fatigue, hemophagocytic lymphohistiocytosis, musculoskeletal pain, edema, and paraparesis.

The most common (≥ 10%) Grade 3 or 4 reactions were fever, febrile neutropenia, hypotension, encephalopathy, cytokine release syndrome, hypoxia, and infection with pathogen unspecified. Fatal adverse reactions occurred in 5% (4/78) of patients including cerebral edema, sepsis, and fungal pneumonia. Of the 4 patients who had fatal adverse reactions: one patient with fatal pneumonia had pre-existing pneumonia prior to study enrolment, and one patient with fatal sepsis had prolonged cytopenia and immunosuppression from prior therapies and underlying disease.

[Details of the side-effects are:]

a. Febrile neutropenia includes febrile neutropenia and fever occurring concurrently with neutropenia events.

b. Coagulopathy includes blood fibrinogen decreased, coagulopathy, disseminated intravascular coagulation, hypofibrinogenemia, international normalized ratio increased.

c. Tachycardias includes sinus tachycardia, tachycardia.

d. Arrhythmia includes arrhythmia, arrhythmia supraventricular, atrial fibrillation, atrial flutter, atrial tachycardia, bradycardia, cardiac arrest, electrocardiogram QT prolonged, electrocardiogram T wave inversion, pulseless electrical activity, sinus bradycardia, supraventricular tachycardia, ventricular tachycardia.

e. Abdominal pain includes abdominal discomfort, abdominal pain, abdominal pain upper.

f. Edema includes face edema, fluid overload, generalized edema, edema, edema peripheral, swelling face, tongue edema.

g. Fatigue includes asthenia, cancer fatigue, fatigue, malaise.

h. Infection with pathogen unspecified includes, catheter bacteremia, conjunctivitis, device related infection, mucosal infection, nasopharyngitis, parotitis, pneumonia, sepsis, septic shock, sinusitis, upper respiratory tract infection, urinary tract infection.

i. Bacterial infections includes bacteremia, bacterial disease carrier, cellulitis, cellulitis of male external genital organ, clostridial infection, clostridium difficile colitis, clostridium difficile infection, enterococcal bacteremia, enterococcal infection, escherichia bacteremia, escherichia infection, escherichia sepsis, pseudomonas infection, staphylococcal bacteremia, staphylococcal infection, wound infection staphylococcal.

j. Fungal infections includes bronchopulmonary aspergillosis, candida infection, fungal skin infection, mycotic oral candidiasis, osteomyelitis fungal, Pneumocystis jirovecii pneumonia, pneumonia fungal, sinusitis fungal.

k. Musculoskeletal pain includes arthralgia, back pain, bone pain, coccydynia, muscle strain, musculoskeletal chest pain, musculoskeletal pain, myalgia, neck pain, non-cardiac chest pain, pain in extremity.

l. Encephalopathy includes altered state of consciousness, aphasia, cognitive disorder, confusional state, depressed level of consciousness, disturbance in attention, dysarthria, dysgraphia, encephalopathy, immune effector cell-associated neurotoxicity syndrome, memory impairment, mental status changes, slow response to stimuli, slow speech, somnolence, speech disorder.

m. Dizziness includes dizziness, syncope.

n. Delirium includes agitation, delirium, delusion, disorientation, hallucination.

o. Cough includes cough, productive cough.

p. Rash includes catheter site urticaria, dermatitis bullous, drug eruption, pruritus, rash, rash macular, rash maculo-papular, rash pustular, toxic skin eruption, urticaria.

q. Hypotension includes hypotension, orthostatic hypotension.

r. Hemorrhage includes conjunctival hemorrhage, contusion, epistaxis, gastric hemorrhage, hematoma, hematoma muscle, hemorrhage intracranial, hemorrhoidal hemorrhage, menorrhagia, petechiae, pulmonary alveolar hemorrhage, retinal hemorrhage, vaginal hemorrhage, vitreous hemorrhage.

Other clinically important adverse reactions that occurred in less than 10% of patients treated with TECARTUS include the following:

• Cardiac disorder: cardiac failure (4%), palpitations (3%)

• Eye disorders: visual impairment (9%)

• Gastrointestinal disorders: dry mouth (6%), dysphagia (4%), oral pain (1%)

• Immune system disorders: hypogammaglobulinemia (9%), hemophagocytic lymphohistiocytosis (4%), drug hypersensitivity (1%)

• Infections and infestations: viral infections (6%)

• Metabolism and nutrition disorders: dehydration (5%), tumor lysis syndrome (1%)

• Musculoskeletal and connective tissue disorders: muscle spasms (4%), musculoskeletal stiffness (3%)

• Nervous system disorders: seizure (8%), ataxia (5%), peripheral neuropathy (4%), myoclonus (3%), paraparesis (3%), brain edema (1%), brain herniation (1%), cauda equina syndrome (1%), monoplegia (1%)

• Renal and urinary disorders: renal impairment (6%)

• Respiratory, thoracic and mediastinal disorders: respiratory failure (9%), pulmonary edema (6%), pleural effusion (4%), pneumonitis (4%)

• Skin and subcutaneous tissue disorders: skin lesion (4%), decubitus ulcer (3%), dry skin (3%), skin ulcer (3%), alopecia (1%), hyperhidrosis (1%), skin hyperpigmentation (1%)

• Vascular disorders: thrombosis (4%)

Grade 3 or 4 laboratory abnormalities occurring in ≥ 10% of Patients in ZUMA-3 following TECARTUS Infusion (N = 78) were similar to those listed above as occurring in patients with mantle cell lymphoma.

Immunogenicity

TECARTUS has the potential to induce anti-product antibodies, which has been evaluated using an enzyme-linked immunosorbent assay (ELISA) for the detection of binding antibodies against FMC63, the originating antibody of the anti-CD19 CAR. To date, no anti-CAR T-cell antibody immunogenicity has been observed in ZUMA-2. Based on an initial screening assay in ZUMA-2, 17 of 82 patients tested positive for antibodies at any time point; however, a confirmatory orthogonal cell-based assay demonstrated that all 17 patients were antibody negative at all time points tested. Based on an initial screening assay in ZUMA-3, 16 of 100 patients tested positive for antibodies at any time point. Among patients with evaluable samples for confirmatory testing, two patients were confirmed to be antibody-positive after treatment. One of the two patients had a confirmed positive antibody result at Month 6. The second patient had a confirmed antibody result at retreatment Day 28 and Month 3. There is no evidence that the kinetics of initial expansion and persistence of TECARTUS, or the safety or effectiveness of TECARTUS, were altered in these patients.

USE IN SPECIFIC POPULATIONS

Pregnancy

Risk summary

There are no available data with TECARTUS use in pregnant women. No animal reproductive and developmental toxicity studies have been conducted with TECARTUS to assess whether TECARTUS can cause fetal harm when administered to a pregnant woman. It is not known if TECARTUS has the potential to be transferred to the fetus. Based on the mechanism of action of TECARTUS, if the transduced cells cross the placenta, they may cause fetal toxicity, including B cell lymphocytopenia. Therefore, TECARTUS is not recommended for women who are pregnant. Pregnancy after TECARTUS infusion should be discussed with the treating physician. In the U.S. general population, the estimated background risk of major birth defects and miscarriage in clinically recognized pregnancies is 2% - 4% and 15% - 20%, respectively.

Lactation

Risk summary

There is no information regarding the presence of TECARTUS in human milk, the effect on the breastfed infant, and the effects on milk production. The developmental and health benefits of breastfeeding should be considered along with the mother's clinical need for TECARTUS and any potential adverse effects on the breastfed infant from TECARTUS or from the underlying maternal condition.

Females and males of reproductive potential

Pregnancy testing

Pregnancy status of females with reproductive potential should be verified. Sexually active females of reproductive potential should have a negative pregnancy test prior to starting treatment with TECARTUS.

Contraception

See the Prescribing Information for fludarabine and cyclophosphamide for information on the need for effective contraception in patients who receive the lymphodepleting chemotherapy. There are insufficient exposure data to provide a recommendation concerning duration of contraception following treatment with TECARTUS.

Infertility

There are no data on the effect of TECARTUS on fertility.

Pediatric use

The safety and efficacy of TECARTUS have not been established in pediatric patients.

Geriatric use

Of the 82 patients treated with TECARTUS for MCL, 42 (51%) were 65 years of age and over. Of the 78 patients treated with TECARTUS for ALL, 12 (15%) were 65 years of age and over. No overall differences in safety or effectiveness were observed between these patients and younger patients.

CLINICAL STUDIES

Relapsed or Refractory Mantle Cell Lymphoma

A single-arm, open-label, multicenter trial (ZUMA-2; NCT02601313) evaluated the efficacy and safety of a single infusion of TECARTUS in adult patients with relapsed or refractory mantle cell lymphoma (MCL) who had previously received anthracycline- or bendamustine-containing chemotherapy, an anti-CD20 antibody, and a Bruton tyrosine kinase inhibitor (BTKi; ibrutinib or acalabrutinib). Eligible patients also had disease progression after their last regimen or refractory disease to their most recent therapy. The study excluded patients with active or serious infections, prior allogeneic hematopoietic stem cell transplant (HSCT), detectable cerebrospinal fluid malignant cells or brain metastases, and any history of central nervous system (CNS) lymphoma or CNS disorders. Seventy-four patients were leukapheresed, five (7%) of whom did not begin conditioning chemotherapy or receive TECARTUS: three (4%) experienced manufacturing failure, one (1%) died of progressive disease, and one (1%) withdrew from the study. One patient (1%) received lymphodepleting chemotherapy but did not receive TECARTUS due to ongoing active atrial fibrillation. Sixty-eight of the patients who were leukapheresed received a single infusion of TECARTUS, and 60 of these patients were followed for at least six months after their first objective disease response, qualifying them as efficacy-evaluable. Among the 60 efficacy-evaluable patients, 2×10^6 CAR-positive viable T cells/kg were administered to 54 (90%). The remaining six (10%) patients received doses of 1.0, 1.6, 1.8, 1.8, 1.9, and 1.9×10^6 CAR-positive viable T cells/kg. Of the 60 efficacy-evaluable patients, the median age was 65 years (range: 38 to 79 years), 51 (85%) were male, and 56 (93%) were white. Most (50 patients; 83%) had stage IV disease. Twenty patients (33% of 60) had baseline bone marrow examinations performed per protocol; of these, ten (50%) were negative, eight (40%) were positive, and two (10%) were indeterminate. The median number of prior therapies among all 60 efficacy-evaluable patients was three (range: two to five). Twenty-six (43%) of the patients had relapsed after or were refractory to autologous HSCT. Twenty-one (35%) had relapsed after their last therapy for MCL, while 36 (60%) were refractory to their last therapy for MCL. Among the 60 efficacy-evaluable patients, 14 (23%) had blastoid MCL. Following leukapheresis and prior to administration of TECARTUS, 21 (35%) of the 60 patients received bridging therapy. Sixteen (27%) were treated with a BTKi, 9 (15%) with a corticosteroid, and 4 (7%) with both a BTKi and a corticosteroid. Among the 60 efficacy-evaluable patients, the median time from leukapheresis to product delivery was 15 days (range: 11 to 28 days), and the median time from leukapheresis to product infusion was 27 days (range: 19 to 63 days). The protocol-defined lymphodepleting chemotherapy regimen of cyclophosphamide 500 mg/m^2 intravenously and fludarabine 30 mg/m^2 intravenously, both given on each of the fifth, fourth, and third days before TECARTUS infusion, was administered to 53 (88%) of the 60 efficacy-evaluable patients. The remaining seven patients (12%) either received lymphodepletion over four or more days or received TECARTUS four or more days after completing lymphodepletion. All treated patients received TECARTUS infusion on Day 0 and were hospitalized until at least Day 7.

The median time to response was 28 days (range: 24 to 92 days) with a median follow-up time for DOR of 8.6 months.

Table 20. Efficacy results in adult patients with relapsed/refractory MCL.

	Efficacy-Evaluable Patients N = 60	All Leukapheresed Patients (ITT) N = 74
Response		
Objective Response Rate[a], n (%) [95% CI]	52 (87%) [75, 94]	59 (80%) [69, 88]
Complete Remission Rate, n (%) [95% CI]	37 (62%) [48, 74]	41 (55%) [43, 67]
Partial Remission Rate, n (%) [95% CI]	15 (25%) [15, 38]	18 (24%) [15, 36]
Duration of Response (DOR)		
Median in months [95% CI] Range[b] in months	NR [8.6, NE] 0.0+, 29.2+	NR [8.6, NE] 0.0+, 29.2+
DOR, if best response is PR, median in months [95% CI] Range[b] in months	2.2 [1.5, 5.1] 0.0+, 22.1+	22.1+ 2.2 [1.5, 5.1] 0.0+, 22.1+
Median Follow-up for DOR in months[c]	8.6 8.1	8.6 8.1

CI, confidence interval; CR, complete remission; DOR, duration of response; NE, not estimable; NR, not reached; PR, partial remission. [a]Among all responders. DOR is measured from the date of first objective response to the date of progression or death. [b]A + sign indicates a censored value. [c]At the time of primary analysis.

Relapsed or Refractory B-cell precursor Acute Lymphoblastic Leukemia

The efficacy of TECARTUS was evaluated in ZUMA-3 (NCT02614066), an open-label, single-arm, multicenter trial in adult patients with relapsed or refractory B cell precursor acute lymphoblastic leukemia (ALL). Eligible patients were adults with primary refractory ALL, first relapse following a remission lasting ≤ 12 months, relapsed or refractory ALL after second-line or higher therapy, or relapsed or refractory ALL at least 100 days after allogeneic hematopoietic stem cell transplantation (HSCT). The study excluded patients with active or serious infections, active graft-vs-host disease or taking immunosuppressive medications within 4 weeks prior to enrollment, and any history of CNS disorders, including CNS-2 disease with neurologic changes and CNS-3 disease irrespective of neurological changes. *[Author note: CNS1 = patients with white blood cell (WBC) count in CSF <5 and having no blasts in the CSF; CNS2 = patients with WBC count in CSF <5 and having blasts in the CSF; CNS3 = patients with WBC count in CSF ≥5 and having blasts in the CSF].*

Treatment consisted of lymphodepleting chemotherapy (fludarabine 25 mg/m^2 iv daily on Days -4, -3 and -2; cyclophosphamide 900 mg/m^2 iv on Day -2) followed by a single intravenous infusion of TECARTUS at a target dose of 1 × 10^6 anti-CD19 CAR T cells/kg (maximum 1 × 10^8 cells) on Day 0. All treated patients were hospitalized until at least Day 7. Seventy-one patients were enrolled and leukapheresed; six of these patients did not receive TECARTUS due to manufacturing failure, eight patients were not treated primarily due to adverse events following leukapheresis, two patients underwent leukapheresis and received lymphodepleting chemotherapy but were not treated with TECARTUS, and one patient treated with TECARTUS was inevaluable for efficacy. Among the remaining 54 efficacy-evaluable patients, the median time from leukapheresis to product delivery was 16 days (range 11 to 39 days) and the median time from leukapheresis to TECARTUS infusion was 29 days (range 20 to 60 days). Of the 54 patients who were efficacy evaluable, the median age was 40 years (range 19 to 84 years), 61% were male, and 67% were White, 6% were Asian, 2% were Black or African American, and 2% were American Indian or Alaskan Native. At enrollment, 46% had refractory relapse, 26% had primary refractory disease, 20% had untreated second or later relapse, and 7% had first untreated relapse. Among prior therapies, 43% of patients were previously treated with allogeneic HSCT, 46% with blinatumomab, and 22% with inotuzumab. Twenty-six percent of patients were Philadelphia chromosome positive (Ph+). Fifty (93%) patients had received bridging therapy between leukapheresis and lymphodepleting chemotherapy to control disease burden. The efficacy of TECARTUS was established on the basis of complete remission (CR) within 3 months after infusion and the duration of CR (DOCR). Twenty-eight (51.9%) of the 54 evaluable patients achieved CR, and with a median follow-up for responders of 7.1 months; the median DOCR was not reached (Table 21). The median time to CR was 56 days (range 25 to 86 days). All efficacy evaluable patients had potential follow-up for ≥ 10 months with a median actual follow-up time of 12.3 months (range: 0.3 to 22.1 months).

Table 21. Efficacy Results in Adult Patients with Relapsed/Refractory B-cell precursor ALL.

	Efficacy Evaluable Patients[a] N= 54	All Leukapheresed Patients N = 71
OCR rate (CR + CRi), n (%) [95% CI]	35 (64.8) [51, 77]	36 (50.7) [39, 63]
CR rate, n (%) [95% CI]	28 (51.9) [37.8, 65.7]	29 (40.9) [29.3, 53.2]
Duration of Remission, Median in months [95% CI] (Range[b] in months)	13.6 [9.4, NE] (0.03+, 16.07+)	13.6 [8.7, NE] (0.03+, 16.07+)
DOR, if best response is CR, median in months [95% CI] (Range in months)	NR [9.6, NE] (0.03+, 16.07+)	13.6 [9.4, NE] (0.03+, 16.07+)
DOR, if best response is CRi, median in months [95% CI] (Range in months)	8.7 [1.0, NE] (0.03+, 10.15+)	8.7 [1.0, NE] (0.03+, 10.15+)
Median Follow-up for CR in months	7.1 (0.03+, 16.1+)	5.0 (0.03+, 16.1+)

CI, confidence interval; CR, complete remission; CRi, complete remission with incomplete blood count recovery; DOR, duration of remission; NE, not estimable; NR, not reached, OCR, overall complete remission; NE, not estimable [a]Of the 71 patients that were enrolled (and leukapheresed), 57 patients received lymphodepleting chemotherapy, and 55 patients received TECARTUS. 54 patients were included in the efficacy evaluable population. [b]A + sign indicates a censored value.

10.4. Lisocabtagene maraleucel/BREYANZI

FULL PRESCRIBING INFORMATION WARNING: CYTOKINE RELEASE SYNDROME and NEUROLOGIC TOXICITIES

• Cytokine Release Syndrome (CRS), including fatal or life-threatening reactions, occurred in patients receiving BREYANZI. Do not administer BREYANZI to patients with active infection or inflammatory disorders. Treat severe or life-threatening CRS with tocilizumab with or without corticosteroids

• Neurologic toxicities, including fatal or life-threatening reactions, occurred in patients receiving BREYANZI, including concurrently with CRS, after CRS resolution, or in the absence of CRS. Monitor for neurologic events after treatment with BREYANZI. Provide supportive care and/or corticosteroids as needed

• BREYANZI is available only through a restricted program under a Risk Evaluation and Mitigation Strategy (REMS) called the BREYANZI REMS

INDICATIONS AND USAGE

BREYANZI is a CD19-directed genetically modified autologous T cell immunotherapy indicated for the treatment of adult patients with relapsed or refractory large B cell lymphoma after two or more lines of systemic therapy, including diffuse large B cell lymphoma (DLBCL) not otherwise specified (including DLBCL arising from indolent lymphoma), high-grade B cell lymphoma, primary mediastinal large B cell lymphoma, and follicular lymphoma grade 3B.

Limitations of use: BREYANZI is not indicated for the treatment of patients with primary central nervous system (CNS) lymphoma.

DESCRIPTION

BREYANZI (lisocabtagene maraleucel) is a **CD19**-directed genetically modified autologous T cell immunotherapy administered as a defined composition of CAR-positive viable T cells (**consisting of CD8 and CD4 components**). The CAR is comprised of the FMC63 *(anti-CD19)* monoclonal antibody-derived single-chain variable fragment (scFv), **IgG4 hinge** region, **CD28 transmembrane domain**, **4-1BB (CD137) costimulatory domain**, and **CD3 zeta activation** domain. In addition, BREYANZI includes a **nonfunctional truncated epidermal growth factor receptor** (EGFRt) that is co-expressed on the cell surface with the CD19-specific CAR. BREYANZI is a T-cell product. BREYANZI is prepared from the patient's T cells, which are obtained from the product of a standard leukapheresis procedure. The purified CD8-positive and CD4-positive T cells are separately activated and transduced with the replication-incompetent lentiviral vector containing the anti-CD19 CAR transgene. The transduced T cells are expanded in cell culture, washed, formulated into a suspension, and cryopreserved as separate CD8 and CD4 component vials that together constitute a single dose of BREYANZI. The product must pass a sterility test before release for shipping as a frozen suspension in patient-specific vials. The product is thawed prior to administration. The BREYANZI formulation contains 75% (v/v) Cryostor® CS10 [containing 7.5% dimethylsulfoxide (v/v)], 24% (v/v) Multiple Electrolytes for Injection, Type 1, 1% (v/v) of 25% albumin (human).

Mechanism of action

BREYANZI is a CD19-directed genetically modified autologous cell immunotherapy administered as a defined composition to reduce variability in CD8-positive and CD4-positive T cell dose. The CAR is comprised of an FMC63 monoclonal antibody-derived single chain variable fragment (scFv), IgG4 hinge region, CD28 transmembrane domain, 4-1BB (CD137) costimulatory domain, and CD3 zeta activation domain. CD3 zeta signaling is critical for initiating activation and antitumor activity, while 4-1BB (CD137) signaling enhances the expansion T cell and persistence of BREYANZI.

DOSAGE AND ADMINISTRATION

For autologous use only. For intravenous use only.

Dose

A single dose of BREYANZI contains 50 to 110 × 10^6 CAR-positive viable T cells (consisting of 1:1 CAR-positive viable T cells of the CD8 and CD4 components), with each component supplied separately in one to four single-dose vials.

Administration BREYANZI is for autologous use only. The patient's identity must match the patient identifiers on the BREYANZI cartons, vials and syringe labels. Do not infuse BREYANZI if the information on the patient-specific labels does not match the intended patient.

Preparing the Patient for BREYANZI

Confirm the availability of BREYANZI before starting lymphodepleting chemotherapy.
Pretreatment

Administer the lymphodepleting chemotherapy regimen before infusion of BREYANZI: fludarabine 30 mg/m^2 /day intravenously (IV), and cyclophosphamide 300 mg/m^2 /day IV for 3 days. See the prescribing information for fludarabine and cyclophosphamide for information on dose adjustment in renal impairment. Infuse BREYANZI 2 to 7 days after completion of lymphodepleting chemotherapy. Delay the infusion of BREYANZI if the patient has unresolved serious adverse events from preceding chemotherapies, active uncontrolled infection, or active graft-versus-host disease (GVHD).

Premedication

To minimize the risk of infusion reactions, premedicate the patient with acetaminophen (650 mg orally) and diphenhydramine (25-50 mg, IV or orally), or another H1-antihistamine, 30 to 60 minutes prior to treatment with BREYANZI. Avoid prophylactic use of systemic corticosteroids, as they may interfere with the activity of BREYANZI.

Receipt of BREYANZI

• BREYANZI is shipped directly to the cell-associated lab or clinical pharmacy associated with the infusion center in the vapor phase of a liquid nitrogen shipper.

• Confirm the patient's identity with the patient identifiers on the shipper.

• If the patient is not expected to be ready for administration before the shipper expires and the infusion site is qualified for onsite storage, transfer BREYANZI to onsite vapor phase of liquid nitrogen storage prior to preparation.

• If the patient is not expected to be ready for administration before the shipper expires and the infusion site is not qualified for onsite storage, contact Bristol-Myers Squibb at 1-888-805-4555 to arrange for return shipment.

Dose preparation

Detailed instructionsfor thisare given on the BREYANZI product insert.

BREYANZI administration

• Do NOT use a leukodepleting filter.

• Ensure tocilizumab and emergency equipment are available prior to infusion and during the recovery period.

• Confirm the patient's identity matches the patient identifiers on the syringe label.

• Once BREYANZI has been drawn into syringes, proceed with administration as soon as possible. The total time from removal from frozen storage to patient administration should not exceed 2 hours as indicated by the time entered on the syringe label.

1. Use intravenous normal saline to flush all the infusion tubing prior to and after each CD8 or CD4 component administration.

2. Administer the entire volume of the CD8 component intravenously at an infusion rate of approximately 0.5 mL/minute, using the closest port or Y-arm. NOTE: The time for infusion will vary but will usually be less than 15 minutes for each component.

3. If more than one syringe is required for a full cell dose of the CD8 component, administer the volume in each syringe consecutively without any time between administering the contents of the syringes (unless there is a clinical reason (e.g., infusion reaction) to hold the dose).

4. After the CD8 component has been administered, flush the tubing with normal saline, using enough volume to clear the tubing and the length of the IV catheter.

5. Administer the CD4 component second, immediately after administration of the CD8 component is complete, using steps 1-4, as described for the CD8 component. Following administration of the CD4 component, flush the tubing with normal saline, using enough volume to clear the tubing and the length of the IV catheter. BREYANZI contains human blood cells that are genetically modified with replication-incompetent, self-inactivating lentiviral vector. Follow universal precautions and local biosafety guidelines applicable for the handling and disposal, to avoid potential transmission of infectious diseases.

Monitoring

• Administer BREYANZI at a REMS-certified healthcare facility.

• Monitor patients daily at a certified healthcare facility during the first week following infusion for signs and symptoms of cytokine release syndrome and neurologic toxicities.

• Instruct patients to remain within proximity of the certified healthcare facility for at least 4 weeks following infusion.

• Refrain from driving or hazardous activities for 8 weeks.

Management of Severe Adverse Reactions

Cytokine release syndrome (CRS) and neurologic toxicity are the two most severe adverse reactions of BREYANZI, as with other CAR T cells therapies. Their grading and management are described in Tables 13 and 14.

DOSAGE FORMS AND STRENGTHS

BREYANZI is a cell suspension for infusion. A single dose of BREYANZI contains of 50 to 110 × 10^6 CAR-positive viable T cells, consisting of CD8 and CD4 components, with each component supplied separately in single-dose vials. More than one vial of each of the CD8 component and/or CD4 component may be needed to achieve the dose of BREYANZI. Each vial contains between 6.9 × 10^6 and 322 x 10^6 CAR-positive viable T cells in 4.6 mL cell suspension (between 1.5 × 10^6 and 70 x 10^6 CAR-positive viable T cells/mL). The infusion volume is calculated based on the concentration of cryopreserved drug product (CAR positive viable T cells concentration). The volume may differ for each component infused.

CONTRAINDICATIONS

None.

WARNINGS AND PRECAUTIONS

Cytokine Release Syndrome

Cytokine Release Syndrome (CRS), including fatal or life-threatening reactions, occurred following treatment with BREYANZI. CRS occurred in 46% (122/268) of patients receiving BREYANZI, including ≥ Grade 3 (Lee grading system 1) CRS in 4% (11/268) of patients. One patient had fatal CRS and 2 had ongoing CRS at time of death. The median time to onset was 5 days (range 1 to 15 days). CRS resolved in 119 of 122 patients (98%) with a median duration of 5 days (range 1 to 17 days). Median duration of CRS was 5 days (range 1 to 30 days) in all patients, including those who died or had CRS ongoing at time of death. Among patients with CRS, the most common manifestations of CRS include fever (93%), hypotension (49%), tachycardia (39%), chills (28%), and hypoxia (21%). *[Further information on CRS is given in Sections10.1, 10.2 and Appendix 11.2].*

Serious events that may be associated with CRS include cardiac arrhythmias (including atrial fibrillation and ventricular tachycardia), cardiac arrest, cardiac failure, diffuse alveolar damage, renal insufficiency, capillary leak syndrome, hypotension, hypoxia, and hemophagocytic lymphohistiocytosis/macrophage activation syndrome (HLH/MAS).

*[Further information on **HLH** is given in Sections 10.1 and 10.2 and Appendix 11.4; further information on **macrophage activation syndrome** is given in Appendix 11.5].*

Ensure that 2 doses of tocilizumab are available prior to infusion of BREYANZI. Sixty-one of 268 (23%) patients received tocilizumab and/or a corticosteroid for CRS after infusion of BREYANZI. Twenty-seven (10%) patients received tocilizumab only, 25 (9%) received tocilizumab and a corticosteroid, and 9 (3%) received corticosteroids only. Monitor patients daily at a certified healthcare facility during the first week following infusion for signs and symptoms of CRS. Monitor patients for signs or symptoms of CRS for at least 4 weeks after infusion. Counsel patients to seek immediate medical attention should signs or symptoms of CRS occur at any time. At the first sign of CRS, institute treatment with supportive care, tocilizumab or tocilizumab and corticosteroids as indicated [see Dosage and Administration (2.3)]. 5.2 Neurologic Toxicities Neurologic toxicities that were fatal or life-threatening, occurred following treatment with BREYANZI. CAR T cell-associated neurologic toxicities occurred in 35% (95/268) of patients receiving BREYANZI, including ≥ Grade 3 in 12% (31/268) of patients. Three patients had fatal neurologic toxicity and 7 had ongoing neurologic toxicity at time of death. The median time to onset of the first event was 8 days (range: 1 to 46 days). The onset of all neurologic events occurred within the first 8 weeks following BREYANZI infusion. Neurologic toxicities resolved in 81 of 95 patients (85%) with a median duration of 12 days (range: 1 to 87 days). Three of four patients with ongoing neurologic toxicity at data cutoff had tremor and one subject had encephalopathy. Median duration of neurologic toxicity was 15 days (range: 1 to 785 days) in all patients, including those with ongoing neurologic events at the time of death or at data cutoff. Seventy-eight (78) of 95

(82%) patients with neurologic toxicity experienced CRS. Neurologic toxicity overlapped with CRS in 57 patients. The onset of neurologic toxicity was after onset of CRS in 30 patients, before CRS onset in 13 patients, same day as CRS onset in 7 patients, and same day as CRS resolution in 7 patients. Neurologic toxicity resolved in three patients before the onset of CRS. Eighteen patients experienced neurologic toxicity after resolution of CRS. The most common neurologic toxicities included encephalopathy (24%), tremor (14%), aphasia (9%), delirium (7%), headache (7%), ataxia (6%), and dizziness (6%). Serious events including cerebral edema and seizures occurred with BREYANZI. Fatal and serious cases of leukoencephalopathy, some attributable to fludarabine, have occurred in patients treated with BREYANZI. Monitor patients daily at a certified healthcare facility during the first week following infusion for signs and symptoms of neurologic toxicities. Monitor patients for signs or symptoms of neurologic toxicities for at least 4 weeks after infusion; evaluate and treat promptly Counsel patients to seek immediate medical attention should signs or symptoms of neurologic toxicity occur at any time.

BREYANZI REMS

Because of the risk of CRS and neurologic toxicities, BREYANZI is available only through a restricted program under a Risk Evaluation and Mitigation Strategy (REMS) called the BREYANZI REMS.

The required components of the BREYANZI REMS are:

• Healthcare facilities that dispense and administer BREYANZI must be enrolled and comply with the REMS requirements.

• Certified healthcare facilities must have on-site, immediate access to tocilizumab.

• Ensure that a minimum of 2 doses of tocilizumab are available for each patient for infusion within 2 hours after BREYANZI infusion, if needed for treatment of CRS.

• Certified healthcare facilities must ensure that healthcare providers who prescribe, dispense, or administer BREYANZI are trained on the management of CRS and neurologic toxicities. Further information is available at www.BreyanziREMS.com, or contact Bristol-Myers Squibb at 1- 888-423-5436.

Hypersensitivity reactions

Allergic reactions may occur with the infusion of BREYANZI. Serious hypersensitivity reactions, including anaphylaxis, may be due to dimethyl sulfoxide (DMSO).

Serious Infections

Severe infections, including life-threatening or fatal infections, have occurred in patients after BREYANZI infusion. Infections (all grades) occurred in 45% (121/268) of patients. Grade 3 or higher infections occurred in 19% of patients. Grade 3 or higher infections with an unspecified pathogen occurred in 16% of patients, bacterial infections occurred in 5%, and viral and fungal infections occurred in 1.5% and 0.4% of patients, respectively. Monitor patients for signs and symptoms of infection before and after BREYANZI administration and treat appropriately. Administer prophylactic antimicrobials according to standard institutional guidelines.

Febrile neutropenia has been observed in 9% (24/268) of patients after BREYANZI infusion and may be concurrent with CRS. In the event of febrile neutropenia, evaluate for infection and manage with broad-spectrum antibiotics, fluids, and other supportive care as medically indicated. Avoid administration of BREYANZI in patients with clinically significant active systemic infections.

Viral reactivation

Hepatitis B virus (HBV) reactivation, in some cases resulting in fulminant hepatitis, hepatic failure, and death, can occur in patients treated with drugs directed against B cells. Ten of the 11 patients in the TRANSCEND study with a prior history of HBV were treated with concurrent antiviral suppressive therapy to prevent HBV reactivation during and after treatment with BREYANZI. Perform screening for HBV, HCV, and HIV in accordance with clinical guidelines before collection of cells for manufacturing. *[Further information on viral reactivation isgiven in Section 9.2].*

Prolonged cytopenias

Patients may exhibit cytopenias not resolved for several weeks following lymphodepleting chemotherapy and BREYANZI infusion. Grade 3 or higher cytopenias persisted at Day 29 following BREYANZI infusion in 31% (84/268) of patients, and included thrombocytopenia (26%), neutropenia (14%), and anemia (3.0%). Monitor complete blood counts prior to and after BREYANZI administration.

Hypogammaglobulinemia

B cell aplasia and hypogammaglobulinemia can occur in patients receiving treatment with BREYANZI. The adverse event of hypogammaglobulinemia was reported as an adverse reaction in 14% (37/268) of patients; laboratory IgG levels fell below 500 mg/dL after infusion in 21% (56/268) of patients. Hypogammaglobulinemia, either as an adverse reaction or laboratory IgG level below 500 mg/dL after infusion, was reported in 32% (85/268) of patients. Monitor immunoglobulin levels after treatment with BREYANZI and manage using infection precautions, antibiotic prophylaxis, and immunoglobulin replacement as clinically indicated. *[Further information on hypogammaglobulinemia isgiven in Section 9.1].*

Live vaccines

The safety of immunization with live viral vaccines during or following BREYANZI treatment has not been studied. Vaccination with live virus vaccines is not recommended for at least 6 weeks prior to the start of lymphodepleting chemotherapy, during BREYANZI treatment, and until immune recovery following treatment with BREYANZI.

Secondary malignancies

Patients treated with BREYANZI may develop secondary malignancies. Monitor lifelong for secondary malignancies. In the event that a secondary malignancy occurs, contact Bristol-Myers Squibb at 1-888-805-4555 for reporting and to obtain instructions on collection of patient samples for testing.

Effects on ability to drive and use machines

Due to the potential for neurologic events, including altered mental status or seizures, patients receiving BREYANZI are at risk for altered or decreased consciousness or impaired coordination in the 8 weeks following BREYANZI administration. Advise patients to refrain from driving and engaging in hazardous occupations or activities, such as operating heavy or potentially dangerous machinery, during this initial period.

Summary of Adverse Reactions Observed in at Least 10% of the Patients Treated with BREYANZI in the TRANSCEND Study (N=268).

Tachycardia including heart rate increased, sinus tachycardia, tachycardia.

Abdominal pain including abdominal dominal discomfort, abdominal pain, abdominal pain lower, abdominal pain upper, abdominal tenderness.

Fatigue including asthenia, fatigue, malaise.

Edema including edema, edema peripheral, fluid overload, fluid retention, generalized edema, hypervolemia, peripheral swelling, pulmonary congestion, pulmonary edema, swelling.

Hypogammaglobulinemia including subjects with adverse events of hypogammaglobulinemia (14%) and/or laboratory IgG levels that fell below 500 mg/dL after infusion (21%).

Infections and infestations are grouped by pathogen type and selected clinical syndromes.

Infections – pathogen unspecified contains febrile neutropenia (9%).

Bacterial infection including infections by pathogen type plus appendicitis, diverticulitis, peritonitis, skin infection, tooth infection.

Upper respiratory tract infections including nasopharyngitis, pharyngitis, rhinitis, rhinovirus infection, sinusitis, upper respiratory tract congestion, upper respiratory tract infection.

Musculoskeletal pain including arthralgia, back pain, bone pain, musculoskeletal chest pain, musculoskeletal discomfort, musculoskeletal pain, musculoskeletal stiffness, myalgia, neck pain, pain in extremity, spinal pain.

Motor dysfunction including eyelid ptosis, motor dysfunction, muscle rigidity, muscle spasms, muscle spasticity, muscle tightness, muscle twitching, muscular weakness, myoclonus, myopathy.

Headache including headache, head discomfort, migraine, sinus headache.

Encephalopathy including amnesia, bradyphrenia, cognitive disorder, confusional state, depersonalization/derealization disorder, depressed level of consciousness, disturbance in attention, encephalopathy, flat affect, hypersomnia, incoherent, lethargy, leukoencephalopathy, loss of consciousness, memory impairment, mental impairment, mental status changes, somnolence.

Dizziness including dizziness, presyncope, syncope, vertigo.

Tremor including essential tremor, resting tremor, tremor.

Peripheral neuropathy includes hyperesthesia, hypoesthesia, meralgia paresthetica, neuralgia, neuropathy peripheral, paresthesia, peripheral sensory neuropathy, sciatica, sensory loss.

Aphasia includes aphasia, disorganized speech, dysarthria, dysphemia, dysphonia, slow speech, speech disorder.

Insomnia includes insomnia, somnambulism.

Anxiety includes anxiety, panic attack.

Delirium includes agitation, delirium, delusion, disorientation, hallucination, 'hallucination, visual', irritability, restlessness.

Renal failure includes acute kidney injury, blood creatinine increased, chronic kidney disease, renal failure, renal injury.

Cough including cough, productive cough, upper airway cough syndrome.

Dyspnea including acute respiratory failure, dyspnea, dyspnea exertional, respiratory failure.

Rash including erythema, dermatitis acneiform, perineal rash, rash, rash erythematous, rash macular, rash maculopapular, rash morbilliform, rash papular, rash pruritic, rash pustular.

Hypotension including hypotension, orthostatic hypotension.

Hemorrhage including catheter site hemorrhage, conjunctival hemorrhage, epistaxis, hematoma, hematuria, hemorrhage, hemorrhage intracranial, pulmonary hemorrhage, retinal hemorrhage, vaginal hemorrhage.

Immunogenicity

BREYANZI has the potential to induce anti-product antibodies. The immunogenicity of BREYANZI has been evaluated using an electrochemiluminescence (ECL) immunoassay for the detection of binding antibodies against the extracellular CD19-binding domain of BREYANZI. Preexisting anti-product antibodies were detected in

11% (28/261) of patients. Treatment-induced or treatment-boosted anti-product antibodies were detected in 11% (27/257) of patients. Due to the small number of patients who had anti-product antibodies, the relationship between anti-product antibody status and efficacy, safety, or pharmacokinetics was not conclusive.

DRUG INTERACTIONS

Drug-laboratory test interactions

The HIV and the lentivirus used to make BREYANZI have limited, short spans of identical genetic material (RNA). Therefore, some commercial HIV nucleic acid tests may yield false-positive results in patients who have received BREYANZI.

USE IN SPECIFIC POPULATIONS

Pregnancy

Risk Summary

There are no available data with BREYANZI use in pregnant women. No animal reproductive and developmental toxicity studies have been conducted with BREYANZI to assess whether it can cause fetal harm when administered to a pregnant woman. It is not known if BREYANZI has the potential to be transferred to the fetus. Based on the mechanism of action, if the transduced cells cross the placenta, they may cause fetal toxicity, including B-cell lymphocytopenia and hypogammaglobulinemia. Therefore, BREYANZI is not recommended for women who are pregnant, and pregnancy after BREYANZI infusion should be discussed with the treating physician. In the U.S. general population, the estimated background risk of major birth defects and miscarriage in clinically recognized pregnancies is 2% to 4% and 15% to 20%, respectively.

Lactation risk summary

There is no information regarding the presence of BREYANZI in human milk, the effect on the breastfed infant, and the effects on milk production. The developmental and health benefits of breastfeeding should be considered along with the mother's clinical need for BREYANZI and any potential adverse effects on the breastfed infant from BREYANZI or from the underlying maternal condition.

Females and males of reproductive potential

Pregnancy testing

Pregnancy status of females with reproductive potential should be verified. Sexually active females of reproductive potential should have a pregnancy test prior to starting treatment with BREYANZI.

Contraception

See the prescribing information for fludarabine and cyclophosphamide for information on the need for effective contraception in patients who receive lymphodepleting chemotherapy. There are insufficient exposure data to provide a recommendation concerning duration of contraception following treatment with BREYANZI.

Infertility

There are no data on the effects of BREYANZI on fertility.

Pediatric use

The safety and efficacy of BREYANZI have not been established in pediatric patients.

Geriatric use

In clinical trials of BREYANZI, 111 (41%) of the 268 patients in TRANSCEND were 65 years of age or older, and 27 (10%) were 75 years of age or older. No clinically important differences in safety or effectiveness of BREYANZI were observed between these patients and younger patients.

10.5. Idecabtagene vicleucil/Abcema

FULL PRESCRIBING INFORMATION WARNING:

CYTOKINE RELEASE SYNDROME, NEUROLOGIC TOXICITIES, HLH/MAS, AND PROLONGED CYTOPENIA

• Cytokine Release Syndrome (CRS), including fatal or life-threatening reactions, occurred in patients following treatment with ABECMA. Do not administer ABECMA to patients with active infection or inflammatory disorders. Treat severe or life-threatening CRS with tocilizumab or tocilizumab and corticosteroids

• Neurologic toxicities, which may be severe or life-threatening, occurred following treatment with ABECMA, including concurrently with CRS, after CRS resolution, or in the absence of CRS. Monitor for neurologic events after treatment with ABECMA. Provide supportive care and/or corticosteroids as needed

• Hemophagocytic Lymphohistiocytosis/Macrophage Activation Syndrome (HLH/MAS) including fatal and life-threatening reactions, occurred in patients following treatment with ABECMA. HLH/MAS can occur with CRS or neurologic toxicities

• Prolonged cytopenia with bleeding and infection, including fatal outcomes following stem cell transplantation for hematopoietic recovery, occurred following treatment with ABECMA.

• ABECMA is available only through a restricted program under a Risk Evaluation and Mitigation Strategy (REMS) called the ABECMA REMS

INDICATIONS AND USAGE

ABECMA is a **B cell maturation antigen** (BCMA)-directed genetically modified autologous T cell immunotherapy indicated for the treatment of adult patients with relapsed or refractory **multiple myeloma** after four or more prior lines of therapy, including an immunomodulatory agent, a proteasome inhibitor, and an antiCD38 monoclonal antibody.

DESCRIPTION

ABECMA is a BCMA-directed genetically modified autologous T cell immunotherapy product consisting of a patient's own T cells that are harvested and genetically modified ex vivo through transduction with an anti-BCMA02 chimeric antigen receptor (CAR) lentiviral vector (LVV). Autologous T cells transduced with the anti-BCMA02 CAR LVV express the anti-BCMA CAR on the T cell surface. The CAR is comprised of a murine extracellular single-chain variable fragment (scFv) specific for recognizing B cell maturation antigen (BCMA) followed by a human **CD8α hinge** and transmembrane domain fused to the **T cell cytoplasmic signaling domains of CD137 (4-1BB) and CD3ζ** *[CD3 zeta]* **chain, in tandem**. Binding of ABECMA to

BCMA-expressing target cells leads to signaling initiated by CD3ζ and 4-1BB domains, and subsequent CAR-positive T cell activation. Antigen-specific activation of ABECMA results in CAR-positive T cell proliferation, cytokine secretion, and subsequent cytolytic killing of BCMA-expressing cells. ABECMA is prepared from the patient's peripheral blood mononuclear cells (PBMCs), which are obtained via a standard leukapheresis procedure. The mononuclear cells are enriched for T cells, through activation with anti-CD3 and anti-CD28 antibodies in the presence of IL-2, which are then transduced with the replication-incompetent lentiviral vector containing the anti-BCMA CAR transgene. The transduced T cells are expanded in cell culture, washed, formulated into a suspension, and cryopreserved. The product must pass a sterility test before release for shipping as a frozen suspension in one or more patient-specific infusion bag(s). The product is thawed prior to infusion back into the patient. The ABECMA formulation contains 50% Plasma-Lyte A and 50% CryoStor® CS10, resulting in a final DMSO concentration of 5%.

Mechanism of action

ABECMA is a chimeric antigen receptor (CAR)-positive T cell therapy targeting B-cell maturation antigen (BCMA), which is expressed on the surface of normal and malignant plasma cells. The CAR construct includes an anti-BCMA scFv-targeting domain for antigen specificity, a transmembrane domain, a CD3 zeta T cell activation domain, and a 4-1BB costimulatory domain. Antigen-specific activation of ABECMA results in CAR-positive T cell proliferation, cytokine secretion, and subsequent cytolytic killing of BCMA-expressing cells.

DOSAGE AND ADMINISTRATION

For autologous use only. For intravenous use only.

Dose

ABECMA is provided as a single dose for infusion containing a suspension of chimeric antigen receptor (CAR)-positive T cells in one or more infusion bags. The recommended dose range is 300 to 460 x 10^6 CAR-positive T cells.

Administration

ABECMA is for autologous use only. The patient's identity must match the patient identifiers on the ABECMA cassette(s) and infusion bag(s). Do not infuse ABECMA if the information on the patient-specific label(s) does not match the intended patient.

Preparing the patient for ABECMA infusion

Confirm the availability of ABECMA prior to starting the lymphodepleting chemotherapy regimen. Pretreatment: administer the lymphodepleting chemotherapy regimen: cyclophosphamide 300 mg/m^2 intravenously (IV) and fludarabine 30 mg/m^2 IV for 3 days. See the prescribing information of cyclophosphamide and fludarabine for information on dose adjustment in renal impairment. Administer ABECMA 2 days after completion of lymphodepleting chemotherapy.

Delay the infusion of ABECMA up to 7 days if a patient has any of the following conditions:

•unresolved serious adverse events (especially pulmonary events, cardiac events, or hypotension), including those after preceding chemotherapies

•active infections or inflammatory disorders

Premedication

Administer acetaminophen (650 mg orally) and diphenhydramine (12.5 mg IV or 25 to 50 mg orally, or another H1-antihistamine) approximately 30 to 60 minutes before infusion of ABECMA. Avoid prophylactic use of dexamethasone or other systemic corticosteroids, as the use may interfere with the activity of ABECMA.

Receipt of ABECMA

• ABECMA is shipped directly to the cell laboratory or clinical pharmacy associated with the infusion center in the vapor phase of a liquid nitrogen shipper.

• Confirm the patient's identity with the patient identifiers on the shipper.

• If the patient is not expected to be ready for same-day administration before the shipper expires and the infusion site is qualified for onsite storage, transfer ABECMA to onsite vapor phase of liquid nitrogen storage.

• If the patient is not expected to be ready for same day administration before the shipper expires and the infusion site is not qualified for onsite storage, contact Bristol-Myers Squibb at 1-888-805-4555 to arrange for return shipment.

Preparation of ABECMA for infusion

1. Coordinate the timing of ABECMA thaw and infusion. Confirm the infusion time in advance and adjust the start time of the thaw of ABECMA so that it will be available for infusion when the patient is ready.

2. Prior to thawing the product, confirm that tocilizumab and emergency equipment are available prior to the infusion and during the recovery period.

3. An ABECMA dose may be contained in one or more patient-specific infusion bag(s). Verify the number of bags received for the indicated dose of ABECMA prior to preparation of ABECMA for infusion.

4. Confirm patient identity: Prior to preparation of ABECMA, match the patient's identity with the patient identifiers on the ABECMA cassette(s), infusion bag(s), and the RFI Certificate. Note: The patient identifier number may be preceded by the letters DIN or Aph ID.

5. Do not remove the ABECMA infusion bag(s) from the cassette(s) if the information on the patientspecific cassette label(s) does not match the intended patient. Contact Bristol-Myers Squibb at 1-888-805- 4555 if there are any discrepancies between the labels and the patient identifiers.

6. Once patient identity is confirmed, remove the ABECMA infusion bag(s) from the cassette(s) and check that the patient information on the cassette label(s) matches the patient information on the bag label(s).

Figure 1: ABECMA Bag Label(s)

7. Inspect the infusion bag(s) for any breaches of container integrity such as breaks or cracks before thawing. If the bag(s) is compromised, contact Bristol-Myers Squibb at 1-888-805-4555. 8. If more than one infusion bag has been received to achieve the treatment dose, thaw each infusion bag one at a time. Do not initiate thaw of the next bag until infusion of the previous bag is complete.

Figure 1: ABECMA Bag Label(s)

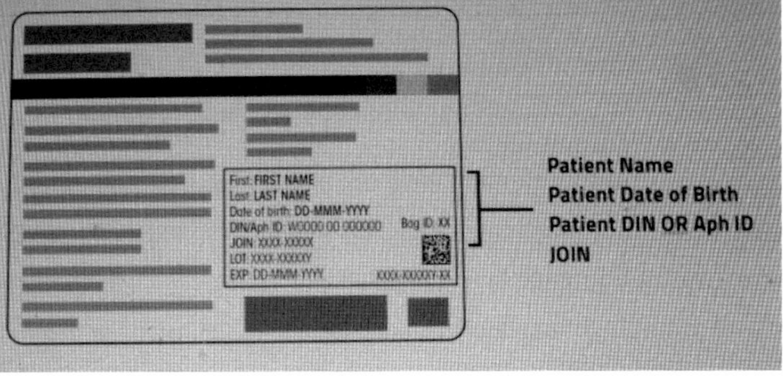

9. Place the infusion bag(s) inside a second sterile bag per local guidelines.

10. Thaw ABECMA infusion bag(s) at approximately 37°C using an approved thaw device or water bath until there is no visible ice in the infusion bag. Gently mix the contents of the bag to disperse clumps of cellular material. If visible cell clumps remain, continue to gently mix the contents of the bag. Small clumps of cellular material should disperse with gentle manual mixing. Do not wash, spin down, and/or resuspend ABECMA in new media prior to infusion.

11. ABECMA should be administered within 1 hour of the start of thaw. ABECMA is stable for 2 hours at room temperature once thawed.

ABECMA Administration

• For autologous use only.

• Do NOT use a leukodepleting filter.

• Ensure that a minimum of 2 doses of tocilizumab and emergency equipment are available prior to infusion and during the recovery period.

• Central venous access may be utilized for the infusion of ABECMA and is encouraged in patients with poor peripheral access.

1. Confirm that the patient's identity matches the patient identifiers on the ABECMA infusion bag(s).

2. Prime the tubing of the infusion set with normal saline prior to infusion.

3. Infuse the entire contents of the ABECMA infusion bag within 1 hour after start of thaw by gravity flow.

4. After the entire content of the infusion bag is infused, rinse the tubing with 30 to 60 mL of normal saline at the same infusion rate to ensure all product is delivered.

5. If more than one infusion bag has been received, administer all bags as directed, following steps 1-4 for all subsequent infusion bags. Do not initiate thaw of the next bag until infusion of the previous bag is complete. ABECMA contains human blood cells that are genetically modified with replication-incompetent, self-inactivating lentiviral vector. Follow universal precautions and local biosafety guidelines for handling and disposal of ABECMA to avoid potential transmission of infectious diseases.

Monitoring

- Administer ABECMA at a REMS-certified healthcare facility.

- Monitor patients at least daily for 7 days following ABECMA infusion at the certified healthcare facility for signs and symptoms of CRS and neurologic toxicities

- Instruct patients to remain within proximity of the certified healthcare facility for at least 4 weeks following infusion.

- Instruct patients to refrain from driving or hazardous activities for at least 8 weeks following infusion.

Management of severe adverse reactions

The management of cytokine release syndrome and nurologic toxicity are described in Sections 9.1 and 9.2. Hemophagocytic lymphohistiocytosis/macrophage activation syndrome (HLH/MAS) is described in Section 9.1. Prolonged cytopenias and hypogammaglobulinemia are also described in Section 9.1.

DOSAGE FORMS AND STRENGTHS

ABECMA is a cell suspension for intravenous infusion. A single dose of ABECMA contains a cell suspension of 300 to 460 x 10^6 chimeric antigen receptor (CAR)-positive T cells in one or more infusion bags.

CONTRAINDICATIONS

None.

ABECMA REMS

Because of the risk of CRS and neurologic toxicities, ABECMA is available only through a restricted program under a Risk Evaluation and Mitigation Strategy (REMS) called the ABECMA REMS. The required components of the ABECMA REMS are:

- Healthcare facilities that dispense and administer ABECMA must be enrolled and comply with the REMS requirements.
- Certified healthcare facilities must have on-site, immediate access to tocilizumab.
- Ensure that a minimum of 2 doses of tocilizumab are available for each patient for infusion within 2 hours after ABECMA infusion, if needed for treatment of CRS.
- Certified healthcare facilities must ensure that healthcare providers who prescribe, dispense, or administer ABECMA are trained in the management of CRS and neurologic toxicities.
- Further information is available at www.AbecmaREMS.com or contact Bristol-Myers Squibb at 1-888-423-5436.

Hypersensitivity reactions

Allergic reactions may occur with the infusion of ABECMA. Serious hypersensitivity reactions, including anaphylaxis, may be due to dimethyl sulfoxide (DMSO) in ABECMA.

Infections

ABECMA should not be administered to patients with active infections or inflammatory disorders. Severe, life-threatening, or fatal infections occurred in patients after ABECMA infusion. Infections (all grades) occurred in 70% of patients. Grade 3 or 4 infections occurred in 23% of patients. Grade 3 or 4 infections with an unspecified pathogen occurred in 15%, viral infections in 9%, bacterial infections in 3.9%, and fungal infections in 0.8% of patients. Overall, four patients had Grade 5 infections (3%); two patients (1.6%) had Grade 5 events of pneumonia, 1 patient

(0.8%) had Grade 5 bronchopulmonary aspergillosis, and 1 patient (0.8%) had cytomegalovirus (CMV) pneumonia associated with Pneumocystis jirovecii. Monitor patients for signs and symptoms of infection before and after ABECMA infusion and treat appropriately. Administer prophylactic, pre-emptive, and/or therapeutic antimicrobials according to standard institutional guidelines.

Febrile neutropenia (was observed in 16% (20/127) of patients after ABECMA infusion and may be concurrent with CRS. In the event of febrile neutropenia, evaluate for infection and manage with broad-spectrum antibiotics, fluids, and other supportive care as medically indicated.

Viral reactivation

Cytomegalovirus (CMV) infection resulting in pneumonia and death has occurred following ABECMA administration. Monitor and treat for CMV reactivation in accordance with clinical guidelines.

Hepatitis B virus (HBV) reactivation, in some cases resulting in fulminant hepatitis, hepatic failure, and death, can occur in patients treated with drugs directed against plasma cells. Perform screening for CMV, HBV, hepatitis C virus (HCV), and human immunodeficiency virus (HIV) in accordance with clinical guidelines before collection of cells for manufacturing. Consider antiviral therapy to prevent viral reactivation per local institutional guidelines/clinical practice.

Prolonged cytopenias

Patients may exhibit prolonged cytopenias following lymphodepleting chemotherapy and ABECMA infusion. In the KarMMa study, 41% of patients (52/127) experienced prolonged Grade 3 or 4 neutropenia and 49% (62/127) experienced prolonged Grade 3 or 4 thrombocytopenia that had not resolved by Month 1 following ABECMA infusion. Rate of prolonged neutropenia was 49% in the 450 x 106 CAR-positive T cells dose cohort and 34% in the 300 x 106 CAR-positive T cells dose cohort. In 83% (43/52) of patients who recovered from Grade 3 or 4 neutropenia after Month 1, the median time to recovery from ABECMA infusion was 1.9 months. In 65% (40/62) of patients who recovered from Grade 3 or 4 thrombocytopenia, the median time to recovery was 2.1 months. Median time to cytopenia recovery was similar across the 300 and 450 x 106 CAR-positive T cells dose cohort. Three patients underwent hematopoietic stem cell transplantation (2 patients with autologous and 1 with allogeneic cells) for hematopoietic reconstitution due to prolonged cytopenia. Two of the three patients died from complications of prolonged cytopenia, which occurred in the setting of ongoing or prior severe CRS or HLH/MAS. Cause of death included lower gastrointestinal bleeding in the setting of prolonged thrombocytopenia in one patient and bronchopulmonary aspergillosis in the setting of prolonged neutropenia in another patient. The third patient recovered from neutropenia after autologous hematopoietic stem cell transplantation. Monitor blood counts prior to and after ABECMA infusion. Manage cytopenia with myeloid growth factor and blood product transfusion support according to local institutional guidelines.

Hypogammaglobulinemia

Plasma cell aplasia and hypogammaglobulinemia can occur in patients receiving treatment with ABECMA. Hypogammaglobulinemia was reported as an adverse event in 21% (27/127) of patients; laboratory IgG levels fell below 500 mg/dL after infusion in 25% (32/127) of patients treated with ABECMA. Hypogammaglobulinemia either as an adverse reaction or laboratory IgG level below 500 mg/dL after infusion occurred in 41% (52/127) of patients treated with ABECMA. Sixty-one percent of patients received intravenous immunoglobulin (IVIG) post-ABECMA for serum IgG.

Use of live vaccines

The safety of immunization with live viral vaccines during or following ABECMA treatment has not been studied. Vaccination with live virus vaccines is not recommended for at least 6 weeks prior to the start of lymphodepleting chemotherapy, during ABECMA treatment, and until immune recovery following treatment with ABECMA.

Secondary malignancies

Patients treated with ABECMA may develop secondary malignancies. Monitor life-long for secondary malignancies. In the event that a secondary malignancy occurs, contact Bristol-Myers Squibb at 1-888-805-4555 for reporting and to obtain instructions on collection of patient samples for testing of secondary malignancy of T cell origin.

Effects on ability to drive and use machines

Due to the potential for neurologic events, including altered mental status or seizures, patients receiving ABECMA are at risk for altered or decreased consciousness or coordination in the 8 weeks following ABECMA infusion. Advise patients to refrain from driving and engaging in hazardous occupations or activities, such as operating heavy or potentially dangerous machinery, during this initial period.

Adverse reactions observed in at least 10% of patients treated with ABECMA in the KarMMa Study

Tachycardia including sinus tachycardia, tachycardia.

Oral pain including oral pain, oropharyngeal pain, toothache.

Fatigue including asthenia, fatigue, malaise.

Edema including edema, face edema, fluid overload, fluid retention, generalized edema, peripheral edema, peripheral swelling, scrotal swelling, swelling.

Hypogammaglobulinemia including patients with adverse events (21%) of blood immunoglobulin G decreased, hypogammaglobulinemia, hypoglobulinemia; and/or patients with laboratory IgG levels below 500 mg/dL following ABECMA infusion (25%).

Infections and infestations

Pneumonia including bronchopulmonary aspergillosis, lung infection, pneumonia, pneumonia aspiration, pneumonia cytomegaloviral, pneumonia pneumococcal, pneumonia pseudomonal.

Upper respiratory tract infection including laryngitis, nasopharyngitis, pharyngeal erythema, pharyngitis, respiratory tract congestion, respiratory tract infection, rhinitis, rhinovirus infection, sinusitis, upper respiratory tract infection, upper respiratory tract infection bacterial.

Decreased appetite including decreased appetite, hypophagia.

Musculoskeletal pain including arthralgia, back pain, bone pain, musculoskeletal chest pain, musculoskeletal discomfort, musculoskeletal pain, musculoskeletal stiffness, myalgia, neck pain, spinal pain.

Motor dysfunction including dysphonia, eyelid ptosis, hypotonia, motor dysfunction, muscle spasms, muscular weakness, restless legs syndrome.

Encephalopathy including amnesia, bradyphrenia, cognitive disorder, confusional state, depressed level of consciousness, disturbance in attention, dyscalculia, dysgraphia, encephalopathy, lethargy, memory impairment, mental status changes, metabolic encephalopathy, somnolence, toxic encephalopathy.

Headache including headache, head discomfort, sinus headache.

Dizziness including dizziness, presyncope, syncope, vertigo.

Neuropathy peripheral including carpal tunnel syndrome, hypoesthesia, hypoesthesia oral, neuralgia, neuropathy peripheral, paresthesia, peripheral sensorimotor neuropathy, peripheral sensory neuropathy, sciatica.

Tremor including asterixis, tremor.

Insomnia including insomnia, sleep deficit, sleep disorder.

Anxiety including anxiety, feeling jittery, nervousness.

Other clinically important adverse reactions that occurred in less than 10% of patients treated with ABECMA include the following:

Coagulopathy including activated partial thromboplastin time prolonged, anticoagulation drug level above therapeutic, disseminated intravascular coagulation, international normalized ratio increased.

Cardiomyopathy including stress cardiomyopathy, ventricular hypertrophy.

Gastrointestinal hemorrhage including gastrointestinal hemorrhage, hemorrhoidal hemorrhage, melena.

Sepsis including bacteremia, enterococcal bacteremia, Escherichia bacteremia, sepsis, septic shock, Serratia bacteremia, streptococcal bacteremia.

Aphasia including aphasia, dysarthria.

Ataxia including ataxia, gait disturbance, Romberg test positive.

Paresis including cranial nerve disorder, hemiparesis.

Delirium including delirium, disorientation, hallucination.

Thrombosis including deep vein thrombosis, jugular vein thrombosis, portal vein thrombosis, pulmonary embolism.

Table 21: Grade 3 or 4[a] laboratory abnormalities worsening from baseline in at least 10% of patients treated with ABECMA in the KarMMa study.

Laboratory Abnormality	Dose = 150 to 450 x 10^6 CAR-Positive T cells (N=127) %
	Grade3 or 4 (%)
Neutropenia	96
Leukopenia	96
Lymphopenia	93
Thrombocytopenia	63
Anemia	63
Hypophosphatemia	45
Hyponatremia	10
aPTT Increased (seconds)	10

[a]NCI CTCAE=Common Terminology Criteria for Adverse Events version 4.03. aPTT = activated partial thromboplastin time; CAR = chimeric antigen receptor; CTCAE = Common Terminology Criteria for Adverse Events; NCI = National Cancer Institute. Laboratory tests were graded according to NCI CTCAE Version 4.03. Laboratory abnormalities are sorted by decreasing frequency in the 150 to 450 $\times$ 10^6 column.

Immunogenicity

ABECMA has the potential to induce anti-product antibodies. In clinical studies, humoral immunogenicity of ABECMA was measured by determination of anti-CAR antibody in serum pre- and post-administration. In the KarMMa study, 3% of patients (4/127) tested positive for pre-infusion anti-CAR antibodies and treatment-induced anti-CAR antibodies were detected in 47% (60/127) of the patients. There is no evidence that the presence of pre-existing or post-infusion anti-CAR antibodies impact the cellular expansion, safety, or effectiveness of ABECMA.

DRUG INTERACTIONS

Drug/laboratory test interactions

HIV and the lentivirus used to make ABECMA have limited, short spans of identical genetic material (RNA). Therefore, some commercial HIV nucleic acid tests may yield false-positive results in patients who have received ABECMA.

USE IN SPECIFIC POPULATIONS

Pregnancy

Risk summary

There are no available data with ABECMA use in pregnant women. No animal reproductive and developmental toxicity studies have been conducted with ABECMA to assess whether it can cause fetal harm when administered to a pregnant woman. It is not known if ABECMA has the potential to be transferred to the fetus. Based on the mechanism of action, if the transduced cells cross the placenta, they may cause fetal toxicity, including plasma cell aplasia or hypogammaglobulinemia. Therefore, ABECMA is not recommended for women who are pregnant, and pregnancy after ABECMA infusion should be discussed with the treating physician. Assess immunoglobulin levels in newborns of mothers treated with ABECMA.

The estimated background risk of major birth defects and miscarriage for the indicated population is unknown. The estimated background risk in the U.S. general population of major birth defects is 2% to 4% and of miscarriage is 15% to 20% of clinically recognized pregnancies.

Lactation

Risk summary

There is no information regarding the presence of ABECMA in human milk, the effect on the breastfed infant, and the effects on milk production. The developmental and health benefits of breastfeeding should be considered along with the mother's clinical need for ABECMA and any potential adverse effects on the breastfed infant from ABECMA or from the underlying maternal condition.

Females and males of reproductive potential

Pregnancy testing

Pregnancy status of sexually-active females with reproductive potential should be verified via pregnancy testing prior to starting treatment with ABECMA.

Contraception

See the prescribing information for fludarabine and cyclophosphamide for information on the need for effective contraception in patients who receive the lymphodepleting chemotherapy. There are insufficient exposure data to provide a recommendation concerning duration of contraception following treatment with ABECMA.

Infertility

There are no data on the effect of ABECMA on fertility.

Pediatric use

The safety and efficacy of ABECMA in patients under 18 years of age have not been established.

Geriatric use

In the clinical trial of ABECMA, 45 (35%) of the 127 patients in the KarMMa study were 65 years of age or older and 4/127 (3%) patients were 75 years of age or older. All five cases of Grade 3 neurotoxicity occurred in patients ≥65 years of age (66 to 74 years). No clinically important differences in effectiveness of ABECMA were observed between these patients and patients younger than 65 years of age.

10.6. Ciltacabtagene autoleucel/Carvikti

FULL PRESCRIBING INFORMATION WARNING:

CYTOKINE RELEASE SYNDROME, NEUROLOGIC TOXICITIES, HLH/MAS and PROLONGED and RECURRENT CYTOPENIA

Cytokine Release Syndrome (CRS), including fatal or life-threatening reactions, occurred in patients following treatment with CARVYKTI. Do not administer CARVYKTI to patients with active infection or inflammatory disorders. Treat severe or life-threatening CRS with tocilizumab or tocilizumab and corticosteroids.

Warnings and Precautions

Immune effector cell-associated neurotoxicity syndrome (ICANS), which may be fatal or life-threatening, occurred following treatment with CARVYKTI, including before CRS onset, concurrently with CRS, after CRS resolution, or in the absence of CRS. Monitor for neurologic events after treatment with CARVYKTI. Provide supportive care and/or corticosteroids as needed.

Parkinsonism and Guillain-Barré syndrome and their associated complications resulting in fatal or life-threatening reactions have occurred following treatment with CARVYKTI.

Hemophagocytic Lymphohistiocytosis/Macrophage Activation Syndrome (HLH/MAS), including fatal and life-threatening reactions, occurred in patients following treatment with CARVYKTI. HLH/MAS can occur with CRS or neurologic toxicities. *[Further information on HLH is given in Sections10.1, 10.2 and Appendix11.4].*

Prolonged and/or recurrent cytopenias with bleeding and infection and requirement for hematopoietic stem cell transplantation for hematopoietic recovery occurred following treatment with CARVYKTI

CARVYKTI is available only through a restricted program under a Risk Evaluation and Mitigation Strategy (REMS) called the CARVYKTI REMS Program.

INDICATIONS AND USAGE

CARVYKTI is a B cell maturation antigen (BCMA)-directed genetically modified autologous T cell immunotherapy indicated for the treatment of adult patients with relapsed or refractory multiple myeloma, after four or more prior lines of therapy, including a proteasome inhibitor, an immunomodulatory agent, and an anti-CD38 monoclonal antibody.

DESCRIPTION

CARVYKTI (ciltacabtagene autoleucel) is a BCMA-directed genetically modified autologous T cell immunotherapy. CARVYKTI is prepared from the patient's peripheral blood mononuclear cells, which are obtained via a standard leukapheresis procedure. The mononuclear cells are enriched for T cells and genetically modified ex vivo by transduction with a replication-incompetent lentiviral vector to express a chimeric antigen receptor (CAR) comprising an anti-BCMA targeting domain, which consists of two single-domain antibodies linked to a **4-1BB costimulatory domain** and a **CD3 zeta signaling domain**. The transduced anti-BCMA CAR T cells are expanded in cell culture, washed, formulated into a suspension and cryopreserved. The product must pass a sterility test before release for shipping as a frozen suspension in a patient-specific infusion bag. The product is thawed and then infused back into the patient, where the anti-BCMA CAR T cells can recognize and eliminate BCMA-expressing target cells.

In addition to T cells, CARVYKTI may contain Natural Killer (NK) cells. The formulation contains 5% dimethyl sulfoxide (DMSO).

Mechanism of Action

CARVYKTI is a BCMA-directed, genetically modified autologous T cell immunotherapy, which involves reprogramming a patient's own T cells with a transgene encoding a chimeric antigen receptor (CAR) that identifies and eliminates cells that express BCMA. The CARVYKTI CAR protein features two BCMA-targeting single-domain antibodies designed to confer high avidity against human BCMA, a 4-1BB co-stimulatory domain and a CD3 zeta (CD3ζ) signaling cytoplasmic domain. Upon binding to BCMA-expressing cells, the CAR promotes T cell activation, expansion, and elimination of target cells.

DOSAGE AND ADMINISTRATION

For autologous use only. For intravenous use only.

Dose

CARVYKTI is provided as a single dose for infusion containing a suspension of chimeric antigen receptor (CAR)-positive viable T cells in one infusion bag. The recommended dose range is $0.5\text{-}1.0 \times 10^6$ CAR-positive viable T cells per kg of body weight, with a maximum dose of 1×10^8 CAR-positive viable T cells per single infusion.

Administration

CARVYKTI is for autologous use only. The patient's identity must match the patient identifiers on the CARVYKTI cassette and infusion bag. Do not infuse CARVYKTI if the information on the patient-specific labels does not match the intended patient.

Preparing the Patient for CARVYKTI Infusion

Confirm availability of CARVYKTI prior to starting the lymphodepleting chemotherapy regimen. Pretreatment Administer the lymphodepleting chemotherapy regimen: cyclophosphamide 300 mg/m^2 intravenously (IV) and fludarabine 30 mg/m^2 IV daily for 3 days. See the prescribing information of cyclophosphamide and fludarabine for information on dose adjustment in renal impairment. Lymphodepleting regimen must be delayed if a patient has serious adverse reactions from preceding bridging therapies (including clinically significant active infection, cardiac toxicity, and pulmonary toxicity) or active-graft-versus host disease in patients with prior allogeneic hematopoietic stem cell transplantation. Consider repeating the lymphodepleting regimen if CARVYKTI dosing is delayed by more than 14 days and the patient has recovered from toxicity of the first lymphodepleting regimen.

Administer CARVYKTI infusion 2 to 4 days after the completion of the lymphodepleting chemotherapy regimen. CARVYKTI infusion should be delayed if a patient has any of the following conditions:

• clinically significant active infection or inflammatory disorders.

• grade ≥3 non-hematologic toxicities of cyclophosphamide and fludarabine conditioning, except for Grade 3 nausea, vomiting, diarrhea, or constipation. CARVYKTI infusion should be delayed until resolution of these events to Grade ≤1.

Premedication

Administer the following pre-infusion medications to all patients 30 - 60 minutes prior to CARVYKTI infusion:

• Antipyretics (oral or intravenous acetaminophen 650 to 1000 mg).

• Antihistamine (oral or intravenous diphenhydramine 25 to 50 mg or equivalent). Avoid prophylactic use of systemic corticosteroids, because their use may interfere with the activity of CARVYKTI.

Receipt of CARVYKTI

• All sites approved for infusion will support required storage conditions for vapor phase of liquid nitrogen.

• CARVYKTI is shipped directly to the cell laboratory or clinical pharmacy associated with the infusion center in the vapor phase of a liquid nitrogen shipper.

• Confirm the patient's identity with the patient identifiers on the shipper.

• If the patient is not expected to be ready for same-day administration, before the shipper expires, transfer CARVYKTI to onsite vapor phase of liquid nitrogen storage.

Preparation of CARVYKTI for infusion

Do not thaw the product until it is ready to be used. Coordinate the timing of CARVYKTI thaw and infusion. Confirm the infusion time in advance and adjust the start time for thaw so that CARVYKTI is available for infusion when the patient is ready. Once thawed, the CARVYKTI infusion must be completed within 2.5 hours at room/ambient temperature (20°C to 25°C). Prior to thawing the product, confirm that tocilizumab and emergency equipment are available prior to the infusion and during the recovery period.

1. Confirm patient identity: Prior to CARVYKTI preparation, match the patient's identity with the patient identifiers on the CARVYKTI cassette. Do not remove the CARVYKTI infusion bag from the cassette if the information on the patient-specific label does not match the intended patient. Contact Janssen Biotech, Inc. at 1-800-526-7736 if there are any discrepancies between the labels and the patient identifiers.

2. Once patient identification is confirmed, remove the CARVYKTI product bag from the cassette and check that the patient information on the cassette label matches the patient information on the bag label.

3. Inspect the product bag for any breaches of container integrity, such as breaks or cracks before thawing. Do not administer if the bag is compromised, and contact Janssen Biotech, Inc. at 1-800-526-7736.

4. Place the infusion bag inside a sealable plastic bag (preferably sterile) prior to thawing.

5. Thaw CARVYKTI at 37°C±2°C using either a water bath or dry thaw method until there is no visible ice in the infusion bag. Total time from start of thaw until completion of thawing should be no more than 15 minutes.

6. Remove the infusion bag from the sealable plastic bag and wipe dry. Gently mix the contents of the bag to disperse clumps of cellular material. If visible cell clumps remain, continue to gently mix the contents of the bag. Small clumps of cellular material should disperse with gentle manual mixing. Do not pre-filter into a different container, wash, spin down, or resuspend CARVYKTI in new media prior to infusion.

7. Do not re-freeze or refrigerate thawed product.

Administration

- For autologous infusion only.

- Do NOT use a leukocyte-depleting filter.

- Ensure that a minimum of two doses of tocilizumab and emergency equipment are available prior to infusion and during the recovery period.

- Central venous access may be utilized for the infusion of CARVYKTI and is encouraged in patients with poor peripheral access.

1. Confirm the patient's identity with the patient identifiers on the infusion bag. Do not infuse CARVYKTI if the information on the patient-specific label does not match the intended patient.

2. Prime the tubing of the infusion set with normal saline prior to infusion.

3. Once thawed, administer the entire contents of the CARVYKTI bag by intravenous infusion within 2.5 hours using infusion sets fitted with an in-line filter.

4. Gently mix the contents of the bag during CARVYKTI infusion to disperse cell clumps.

5. After the entire content of the product bag is infused, flush the administration line, inclusive of the in-line filter, with normal saline with a volume equal or greater to the total hold up volume of the primary administration set used inclusive of the drip tube, to ensure that all product is delivered.

CARVYKTI contains human blood cells that are genetically modified with replicationincompetent, self-inactivating, lentiviral vector. Follow universal precautions and local biosafety guidelines for handling and disposal of CARVYKTI to avoid potential transmission of infectious diseases.

Monitoring after infusion

Administer CARVYKTI at a REMS-certified healthcare facility. Monitor patients at least daily for 10 days following CARVYKTI infusion at a certified healthcare facility for signs and symptoms of cytokine release syndrome (CRS) and neurologic toxicities. Monitor periodically for 4 weeks for signs and symptoms of delayed neurologic toxicity. Instruct patients to remain within proximity of a certified healthcare facility for at least 4 weeks following infusion. Instruct patients to refrain from driving or hazardous activities for at least 8 weeks following infusion.

Management of severe adverse reactions

Cytokine Release Syndrome (CRS)

[Please see Sections10.1 and 10.2 and Appendix 11.2 for further information on CRS].

Neurologic Toxicities

[Please also see Section 10.2 for further information on ICANS and other neurologic toxicities]

Immune effector cell-associated neurotoxicity syndrome (ICANS)

Patients receiving CARVYKTI may experience fatal or life-threatening ICANS following treatment with CARVYKTI, including before CRS onset, concurrently with CRS, after CRS resolution, or in the absence of CRS. ICANS occurred in 23% (22/97) of patients receiving ciltacabtagene autoleucel including Grade 3 or 4 events in 3% (3/97) and Grade 5 (fatal) events in 2% (2/97). Two patients had ongoing Grade 3 and Grade 1 ICANS at last known alive date and one patient had Grade 1 ICANS ongoing at time of death from neurologic toxicity with parkinsonian features. The median time to onset of ICANS was 8 days (range: 1 to 28 days). ICANS resolved in 17 of 22 patients (77%), and the median time to resolution was 6 days (range: 2 to 143 days). Median duration of ICANS in all patients, including those with fatal ICANS, ICANS ongoing at time of death from other causes or ongoing at last known alive date, was 7.5 days (range: 2 to 927 days). All 22 patients with ICANS had CRS. The onset of ICANS occurred during CRS in 16 patients, before the onset of CRS in 3 patients, and after the CRS event in 3 patients. The most frequent (≥5%) manifestation of ICANS included encephalopathy (23%), aphasia (8%) and headache (6%). Monitor patients at least daily for 10 days following CARVYKTI infusion at the REMS-certified healthcare facility for signs and symptoms of ICANS. Rule out other causes of ICANS symptoms. Monitor patients for signs or symptoms of ICANS for at least 4 weeks after infusion and treat promptly. Neurologic toxicity should be managed with supportive care and/or corticosteroids as needed.

Parkinsonism

Of the 25 patients in the CARTITUDE-1 study experiencing any neurotoxicity, five male patients had neurologic toxicity with several signs and symptoms of Parkinsonism, distinct from ICANS. Neurologic toxicity with Parkinsonism has been reported in other ongoing trials of ciltacabtagene autoleucel.

Patients had parkinsonian and non-parkinsonian symptoms that included tremor, bradykinesia, involuntary movements, stereotypy, loss of spontaneous movements, masked facies, apathy, flat affect, fatigue, rigidity, psychomotor retardation, micrographia, dysgraphia, apraxia, lethargy, confusion, somnolence, loss of consciousness, delayed reflexes, hyperreflexia, memory loss, difficulty swallowing, bowel incontinence, falls, stooped posture, shuffling gait, muscle weakness and wasting, motor dysfunction, motor and sensory loss, akinetic mutism and frontal lobe release signs.

[Figure 68. Front and side views of a man portrayed to be suffering from Parkinson's disease].

[This image is by William Richard Gowers (1845–1915) after St. Leger (unknown dates) - Herter, Christian Archibald (1907) [1892]. " Fig 66 — Paralysis agitans. (After St. Leger.) (Gowers)" Diagnosis of Organic Nervous Diseases (2nd ed.). New York and London: G. P. Putnam' s Sons. p. 589. Retrieved 2011-03-24., PD-US, https://en.wikipedia.org/w/index.php?curid=31434429; https://en.wikipedia.org/wiki/Parkinson%27s_disease#/media/File:Paralysis_agitans_(1907,_after_St._Leger).png. This image is in the public domain in the United States because it was first published outside the United States prior to January 1, 1927 No changes were made to this image].

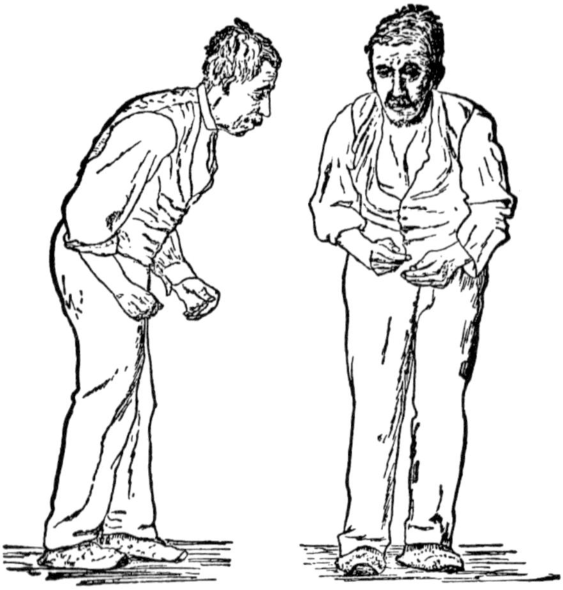

[Figure 69. Example of writing by a patient with Parkinson's disease; possibly showing micrographia in addition to other abnormal characteristics.

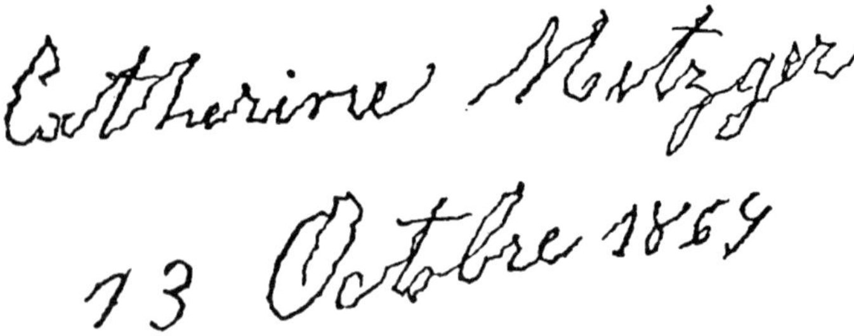

[This image is by Jean-Martin Charcot - Lectures on the diseases of the nervous system. Published 1879. Second edition by H. C. Lea in Philadelphia. Lecture V: On paralysis agitans. (p. 112), Public Domain, https://commons.wikimedia.org/w/index.php?curid=14869916; https://en.wikipedia.org/wiki/Parkinson%27s_disease#/media/File:Writing_by_a_Parkinson's_disease_patient.png. This work is in the public domain in its country of origin and other countries and areas where the copyright term is the author's life plus 100 years or fewer. PD 1925. No changes were made to this image].

Symptoms did not respond to one or more of the following treatments attempted in one or more patients – systemic chemotherapy, intrathecal chemotherapy and steroids, 14 dopaminergic agents, systemic corticosteroids, plasmapheresis, and intravenous immunoglobulin and dasatinib. One patient experienced partial resolution with residual gait disturbance without treatment for Parkinsonism, immunosuppressants or chemotherapy.

The median onset of Parkinsonism in the 5 patients in CARTITUDE-1 was 43 days (range 15 to 108 days) from infusion of ciltacabtagene autoleucel. One patient died of neurologic toxicity with Parkinsonism 247 days after administration of ciltacabtagene autoleucel; two patients with ongoing Parkinsonism died of infectious causes 162 and 119 days after administration of ciltacabtagene autoleucel; in the remaining 2 patients, symptoms of Parkinsonism were ongoing up to 530 days after administration of ciltacabtagene autoleucel. Maximum toxicity grade was 2, 3, 4 and 5 in 1, 2, 1 and 1 patient respectively. All 5 patients had a history of prior CRS (n=4 Grade 2; n=1 Grade 3), while 4 of 5 patients had prior ICANS (n=3 Grade 1; n=1 Grade 2). Monitor patients for signs and symptoms of Parkinsonism that may be delayed in onset and managed with supportive care measures. There is limited efficacy information with medications used for the treatment of Parkinson's disease for the improvement or resolution of Parkinsonism symptoms following CARVYKTI treatment.

Guillain-Barré Syndrome

A fatal outcome following Guillain-Barré Syndrome (GBS) has occurred in another ongoing study of ciltacabtagene autoleucel despite treatment with intravenous immunoglobulins. Symptoms reported include those consistent with the Miller-Fisher variant of GBS, encephalopathy, motor weakness, speech disturbances, and polyradiculoneuritis.

[Figure 70. Various patterns of manifestation of Guillain–Barré syndrome.

This image is by Leonhard, S.E., Mandarakas, M.R., Gondim, F.A.A. et al. - Diagnosis and management of Guillain–Barré syndrome in ten steps. Nat Rev Neurol 15, 671–683 (2019). https://doi.org/10.1038/s41582-019-0250-9, CC BY 4.0, https://commons.wikimedia.org/w/index.php?curid=113067201; https://en.wikipedia.org/wiki/Guillain%E2%80%93Barr%C3%A9_syndrome#/media/File:Guillain_Barre_Patterns.png. This file is licensed under the Creative Commons Attribution 4.0 International license. No changes were made to this image].

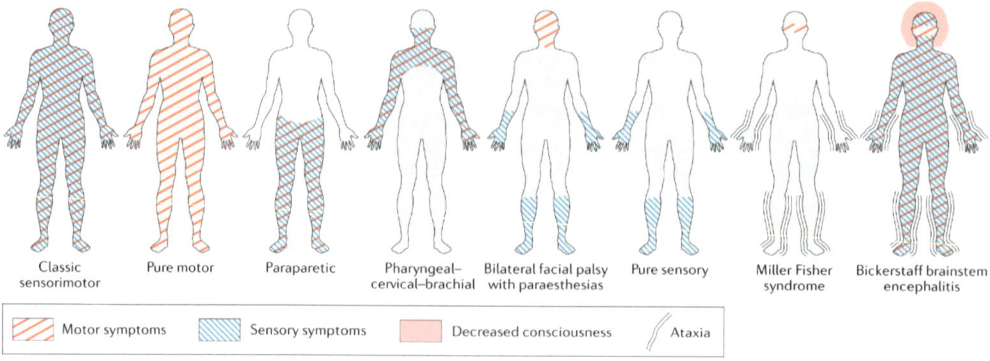

Monitor for GBS.

Evaluate patients presenting with peripheral neuropathy for GBS. Consider treatment of GBS with supportive care measures and in conjunction with immunoglobulins and plasma exchange, depending on the severity of GBS.

Peripheral Neuropathy

Six patients in CARTITUDE-1 developed peripheral neuropathy. These neuropathies presented as sensory, motor or sensorimotor neuropathies. Median time of onset of symptoms was 62 days (range 4 to 136 days), median duration of peripheral neuropathies was 256 days (range 2 to 465 days) including those with ongoing neuropathy. Of these six patients, two patients experienced Grade 3 peripheral neuropathy, and 3 had resolution of neuropathy. Treatment with corticosteroids in one patient was not associated with improvement of peripheral neuropathy. Patients who experienced peripheral neuropathy also experienced cranial nerve palsies or GBS in other ongoing trials of ciltacabtagene autoleucel.

Cranial nerve palsies

Three patients (3.1%) experienced cranial nerve palsies in CARTITUDE-1. All 3 patients had 7th cranial nerve palsy; one patient had 5th cranial nerve palsy as well. Median time to onset was 26 days (range 21 to 101 days) following infusion of ciltacabtagene autoleucel. All three patients received systemic corticosteroids and had resolution of symptoms; one patient received valacyclovir in addition to corticosteroids. Median time to resolution was 70 days (range 1 to 79 days) following onset of symptoms. Occurrence of 3rd and 6th cranial nerve palsy, bilateral 7th cranial nerve palsy, worsening of cranial nerve palsy after improvement and occurrence of peripheral neuropathy in patients with cranial nerve palsy have also been reported in ongoing trials of ciltacabtagene autoleucel. Monitor patients for signs and symptoms of cranial nerve palsies. Consider management with systemic corticosteroids, depending on the severity and progression of signs and symptoms.

[Figure 71. Palsy of the right 7th cranial nerve.

This image is by James Heilman, MD - Own work, CC BY-SA 3.0, https://commons.wikimedia.org/w/index.php?curid=11520707; https://en.wikipedia.org/wiki/Bell%27s_palsy#/media/File:Bellspalsy.JPG. This file is licensed under the Creative Commons Attribution-Share Alike 3.0 Unported license. The uploader asserts the following regarding consent of identifiable persons: I personally created this media. All identifiable persons shown specifically consented to publication of this photograph or video. No changes were made to this image].

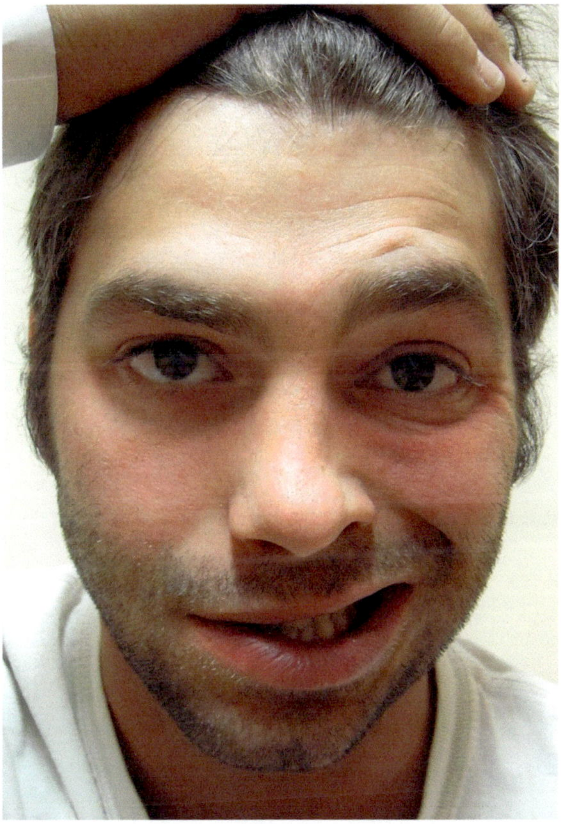

Hemophagocytic Lymphohistiocytosis (HLH)/Macrophage Activation Syndrome (MAS)

Fatal HLH occurred in one patient (1%), 99 days after ciltacabtagene autoleucel infusion. The HLH event was preceded by prolonged CRS lasting 97 days. The manifestations of HLH/MAS include hypotension, hypoxia with diffuse alveolar damage, coagulopathy, cytopenia and multi-organ dysfunction, including renal dysfunction. HLH is a life-threatening condition with a high mortality rate if not recognized and treated early. Treatment of HLH/MAS should be administered per institutional standards. *[Further information on HLH is given in Sections 10.1, 10.2 and Appendix 11.4].*

CARVYKTI REMS

Because of the risk of CRS and neurologic toxicities, CARVYKTI is available only through a restricted program under a Risk Evaluation and Mitigation Strategy (REMS) called the CARVYKTI REMS. The required components of the CARVYKTI REMS are:

• Healthcare facilities that dispense and administer CARVYKTI must be enrolled and comply with the REMS requirements.

• Certified healthcare facilities must have on-site, immediate access to tocilizumab.

• Ensure that a minimum of 2 doses of tocilizumab are available for each patient for infusion within 2 hours after CARVYKTI infusion, if needed for treatment of CRS.

• Certified healthcare facilities must ensure that healthcare providers who prescribe, dispense or administer CARVYKTI are trained in the management of CRS and neurologic toxicities. Further information is available at www.carvyktirems.com or 1-844-672-0067.

Prolonged and recurrent cytopenias

Patients may exhibit prolonged and recurrent cytopenias following lymphodepleting chemotherapy and CARVYKTI infusion. In Study CARTITUDE-1 (N=97), 30% (29/97) of patients experienced prolonged Grade 3 or 4 neutropenia and 41% (40/97) of patients experienced prolonged Grade 3 or 4 thrombocytopenia that had not resolved by Day 30 following ciltacabtagene autoleucel infusion. In 31% (29/95) of patients who recovered from Grade 3 or 4 neutropenia after 1 month, the median time to recovery from ciltacabtagene autoleucel infusion was 1.8 months (range 1.0 to 3.7 months). In 52% (32/61) of patients who recovered from Grade 3 or 4 thrombocytopenia after 1 month, the median time to recovery from ciltacabtagene autoleucel infusion was 1.9 months (range 1.1 to 8.5 months). One patient underwent autologous stem cell transplantation for hematopoietic reconstitution due to prolonged thrombocytopenia.

Recurrent Grade 3 or 4 neutropenia, thrombocytopenia, lymphopenia, and anemia were seen in 63% (61/97), 18% (17/97), 60% (58/97), and 37% (36/97) after recovery from initial Grade 3 or 4 cytopenia following ciltacabtagene autoleucel infusion. After Day 60 following ciltacabtagene autoleucel, 31%, 12%, and 6% of patients had a recurrence of Grade 3 or higher lymphopenia, neutropenia, and thrombocytopenia, respectively, after initial recovery of their Grade 3 or 4 cytopenia.

Eighty-seven percent (84/97) of patients had one, two or three or more recurrences of Grade 3 or 4 cytopenias after initial recovery of Grade 3 or 4 cytopenia. Six and 11 patients had Grade 3 or 4 neutropenia and thrombocytopenia respectively at the time of death. Monitor blood counts prior to and after CARVYKTI infusion. Manage cytopenias with growth factors and blood product transfusion support according to local institutional guidelines.

Infections

CARVYKTI should not be administered to patients with active infection or inflammatory disorders. Severe, life-threatening, or fatal infections, occurred in patients after CARVYKTI. Infections (all grades) occurred in 57 (59%) patients. Grade 3 or 4 infections occurred in 23% (22/97) of patients; Grade 3 or 4 infections with an unspecified pathogen occurred in 17%, viral infections in 7%, bacterial infections in 1%, and fungal infections in 1% of patients. Overall, 4 patients had Grade 5 infections: lung abscess (n=1), sepsis (n=2) and pneumonia (n=1).

Monitor patients for signs and symptoms of infection before and after CARVYKTI infusion and treat patients appropriately. Administer prophylactic, pre-emptive and/or therapeutic antimicrobials according to the standard institutional guidelines. Febrile neutropenia was observed in 10% of patients after ciltacabtagene autoleucel infusion and may be concurrent with CRS. In the event of febrile neutropenia, evaluate for infection and manage with broad-spectrum antibiotics, fluids and other supportive care, as medically indicated.

Viral reactivation

Hepatitis B virus (HBV) reactivation, in some cases resulting in fulminant hepatitis, hepatic failure and death, can occur in patients with hypogammaglobulinemia. Perform screening for Cytomegalovirus (CMV), HBV, hepatitis C virus (HCV), and human immunodeficiency virus (HIV) or any other infectious agents if clinically indicated in accordance with clinical guidelines before collection of cells for manufacturing. Consider antiviral therapy to prevent viral reactivation per local institutional guidelines/clinical practice.

Hypogammaglobulinemia

Hypogammaglobulinemia can occur in patients receiving treatment with CARVYKTI. Hypogammaglobulinemia was reported as an adverse event in 12% (12/97) of patients; laboratory IgG levels fell below 500 mg/dL after infusion in 92% (89/97) of patients treated with ciltacabtagene autoleucel. Hypogammaglobulinemia either as an adverse reaction or a laboratory IgG level below 500 mg/dL, after infusion occurred in 94% (91/97) of patients treated with ciltacabtagene autoleucel. Thirty-eight percent of patients received intravenous immunoglobulin (IVIG) post ciltacabtagene autoleucel for either an adverse reaction or prophylaxis. Monitor immunoglobulin levels after treatment with CARVYKTI and administer IVIG for IgG 400 mg/dL. Manage per local institutional guidelines, including infection precautions and antibiotic or antiviral prophylaxis.

Use of live vaccines

The safety of immunization with live viral vaccines during or following CARVYKTI treatment has not been studied. Vaccination with live virus vaccines is not recommended for at least 6 weeks prior to the start of lymphodepleting chemotherapy, during CARVYKTI treatment, and until immune recovery following treatment with CARVYKTI.

Hypersensitivity reactions

Hypersensitivity reactions have occurred in 5% (5/97) of patients following ciltacabtagene autoleucel infusion. All reactions were Grade 1 and symptoms included flushing (n=4), chest discomfort (n=2), tachycardia (n=1), wheezing (n=1), tremor (n=1), and burning sensation (n=1). Serious hypersensitivity reactions, including anaphylaxis, may be due to the dimethyl sulfoxide (DMSO) in CARVYKTI. Patients should be carefully monitored for 2 hours after infusion for signs and symptoms of severe reaction. Treat promptly and manage patients appropriately according to the severity of the hypersensitivity reaction.

Secondary malignancies

Patients treated with CARVYKTI may develop secondary malignancies. Monitor life-long for secondary malignancies. In the event that a secondary malignancy occurs, contact Janssen Biotech, Inc. at 1-800-526-7736 for reporting and to obtain instructions on collection of patient samples for testing of secondary malignancy of T cell origin.

Effects on ability to drive and use machines

Due to the potential for neurologic events, including altered mental status, seizures, neurocognitive decline or neuropathy, patients receiving CARVYKTI are at risk for altered or decreased consciousness or coordination in the 8 weeks following CARVYKTI infusion. Advise patients to refrain from driving and engaging in hazardous occupations or activities, such as operating heavy or potentially dangerous machinery during this initial period, and in the event of new onset of any neurologic toxicities.

Laboratory Abnormalities Table 4 presents the most common Grade 3 or 4 laboratory abnormalities based on laboratory data, occurring in at least 10% of patients.

Table 22. Grade 3 or 4 laboratory abnormalities in at least 10% of patients treated with Carvykti.

Laboratory abnormality	**Grade 3 or 4 (%)**
Lymphopenia	99
Neutropenia	98
White blood cell count decreased	98
Anemia	72

Thrombocytopenia	63
Aspartate aminotransferase increased	21

Laboratory abnormalities graded using NCI Common Terminology Criteria for Adverse Events version 5.0. Laboratory abnormalities are sorted by decreasing frequency in the Grade column.

Other clinically important Grade 3 or 4 laboratory abnormalities (based on laboratory data) that occurred in less than 10% of patients treated with ciltacabtagene autoleucel include the following: fibrinogen decreased, hypoalbuminemia, alanine aminotransferase increased, hyponatremia, hypocalcemia, gamma glutamyl transferase increased, alkaline phosphatase increased, hypokalemia, blood bilirubin increased.

Immunogenicity

The immunogenicity of CARVYKTI has been evaluated using a validated assay for the detection of binding antibodies against the extracellular portion of the anti-BCMA CAR pre-dose, and at multiple timepoints post-infusion. In Study CARTITUDE-1, 19 of 97 (19.6%) patients were positive for anti-product antibodies. There was no clear evidence that the observed anti-product antibodies impact CARVYKTI kinetics of initial expansion and persistence, efficacy, or safety.

DRUG INTERACTIONS

HIV and the lentivirus used to make CARVYKTI have limited, short spans of identical genetic material (RNA). Therefore, some commercial HIV nucleic acid tests (NATs) may yield false-positive results in patients who have received CARVYKTI.

USE IN SPECIFIC POPULATIONS

Pregnancy

Risk summary

There are no available data on the use of CARVYKTI in pregnant women. No reproductive and developmental toxicity studies in animals have been conducted with CARVYKTI to assess whether it can cause fetal harm when administered to a pregnant woman. It is not known whether CARVYKTI has the potential to be transferred to the fetus and cause fetal toxicity. Based on the mechanism of action, if the transduced cells cross the placenta, they may cause fetal toxicity, including B-cell lymphocytopenia and hypogammaglobulinemia. Therefore, CARVYKTI is not recommended for women who are pregnant, or for women of childbearing potential not using contraception. Pregnant women should be advised that there may be risks to the fetus. Pregnancy after CARVYKTI therapy should be discussed with the treating physician. In the U.S. general population, the estimated background risk of major birth defects and miscarriage in clinically recognized pregnancies is 2%-4% and 15%-20%, respectively.

Lactation

Risk summary

There is no information regarding the presence of CARVYKTI in human milk, the effect on the breastfed infant, and the effects on milk production. The developmental and health benefits of breastfeeding should be considered along with the mother's clinical need for CARVYKTI and any potential adverse effects on the breastfed infant from CARVYKTI or from the underlying maternal condition.

Females and males of reproductive potential

Pregnancy testing

Pregnancy status for females of child-bearing age should be verified prior to starting treatment with CARVYKTI.

Contraception

There are insufficient data to provide a recommendation concerning duration of contraception following treatment with CARVYKTI. In clinical trials, female patients of childbearing potential were advised to practice a highly effective method of contraception and male patients with partners of childbearing potential or whose partners were pregnant were instructed to use a barrier method of contraception, until one year after the patient has received CARVYKTI infusion. See the prescribing information for lymphodepleting chemotherapy for information on the need for contraception in patients who receive the lymphodepleting chemotherapy.

Infertility

There are no data on the effect of CARVYKTI on fertility.

Pediatric use

Safety and effectiveness of CARVYKTI in pediatric patients have not been established.

Geriatric use

Of the 97 patients in Study CARTITUDE-1 that received ciltacabtagene autoleucel, 28% were 65 to 75 years of age, and 8% were 75 years of age or older. CARTITUDE-1 did not include sufficient numbers of patients aged 65 and older to determine whether the effectiveness differs compared with that of younger patients. In 62 patients less than 65 years of age, all grade and Grade 3 and higher neurologic toxicities occurred in 19% (12/62) and 6% (4/62) respectively. Of the 35 patients ≥65 years of age, all grade and Grade 3 and higher neurologic toxicities occurred in 37% (13/35) and 20% (7/35) respectively.

CONCLUSIONS

The first cellular therapy that entered mainstream medicine was hematopoietic stem cell transplantation in the 1970s. Other cell types have ben tried such as natural killer cells, neutrophils and mesenchymal cells but none are in standard practice with the possible exception of neutrophils in people with febrile neutropenia or severe infection due to neutropenia who are unresponsive to antimicrobial agents plus granulocyte colony-stimulating factor (G-CSF).

CAR T cells are generating intense interest with haematologists and oncologists because of their remarkable ability to induce significant responses in people with acute B cell leukemia, diffuse large B cell lymphoma, mantle cell lymphoma and multiple myeloma refractory or resistant to currently available treatment including drugs, irradiation, monoclonal antibodies and, in some cases, hematopoietic stem cell transplantation. Some are already acknowledged as being appropriate treatments for specific indications in the USA.

For example:

1. Chimeric antigen receptor T cell therapy (eg, tisagenlecleucel) is considered an acceptable alternative remission induction therapy to blinatumomab or inotuzumab

ozogamicin for patients ≤25 years old with B cell precursor ALL that is refractory or in second or later relapse.

2. Large B cell lymphoma (DLBCL) – for refractory disease or early relapse (<12 months after initial therapy), CD19-directed chimeric antigen receptor (CAR)-T cell therapy using lisocabtagene maraleucel (liso-cel) or axicabtagene ciloleucel (axi-cel), rather than autologous hematopoietic cell transplantation is recommended.

3a. Follicular cell lymphoma in early relapse: for people who are unable to achieve a complete remission (CR), options include serial novel agents (eg, lenalidomide, tazemetostat, copanlisib) with a plan for autologous hematopietic stem cell transplantation in complete remission or chimeric antigen receptor T cell therapy.

3b. Follicular lymphoma in subsequent relapse: fit patients who attain a CR may proceed with autologous HCT or CAR-T therapy in an attempt to attain long-term remission.

4. Multiple myeloma: for patients with penta-refractory disease, therapies that target BCMA or alkylator-containing regimens rather than other therapies are recommended. BCMA can be targeted using chimeric antigen receptor (CAR)-T cells or the antibody drug conjugate belantamab mafodotin. (Penta-refractory myeloma is defined as myeloma refractory to an anti-CD38 monoclonal antibody (eg, daratumumab, isatuximab), lenalidomide, pomalidomide, bortezomib and arfilzomib

It is notable that all six FDA-approved CAR T cell therapies target hematologic malignancies. Intense effort is underway to try to mirror their efficacy in solid tumors.

Of note, also, is the frequency and severity of side-effects that they produce, many of which are severe and sometimes fatal. These therapies should be administered by hospital physicians experienced in cellular therapy such as allogeneic hematopietic stem cell transplantation.

Finally, it is noteworthy that only one of the six FDA-approved CAR T cell therapies has so far been approved by the Australian Therapeutic Goods Authority for use in Australia. Australia thus currently lags significantly behind the USA in regard to CAR T cell treatments

12. APPENDICES

Appendix 1. The grading of severity of adverse clinical and laboratory events

From the U.S. DEPARTMENT OF HEALTH AND HUMAN SERVICES.

Common Terminology Criteria for Adverse Events (CTCAE) Version 5.0 Published: November 27, 2017

This quick reference extensive document (155 pages) can be found at

https://ctep.cancer.gov/protocoldevelopment/electronic_applications/docs/CTCAE_v5_Quick_Reference_5x7.pdf

SYNDROMES IN WHICH CYTOKINES ARE INVOLVED

A number of diseases or syndromes in which cytokines mediate at least some of the symptoms and signs have been described in the last 50 years and are described in Appendices 12.2 –12.13.

Appendix 12.2. Cytokine release syndrome

From the USA National Cancer Institute:

A condition that may occur after treatment with some types of immunotherapy, such as monoclonal antibodies and CAR-T cells. Cytokine release syndrome is caused by a large, rapid release of cytokines into the blood from immune cells affected by the immunotherapy. Cytokines are immune substances that have many different actions in the body. Signs and symptoms of cytokine release syndrome include fever, nausea, headache, rash, rapid heartbeat, low blood pressure, and trouble breathing. Most patients have a mild reaction, but sometimes, the reaction may be severe or life threatening.

From Wikipedia (https://en.wikipedia.org/wiki/Cytokine_release_syndrome)

Cytokine release syndrome (CRS) is a form of systemic inflammatory response syndrome (SIRS) that can be triggered by a variety of factors such as infections and certain drugs. It refers to cytokine storm syndromes (CSS) and occurs when large numbers of white blood cells are activated and release inflammatory cytokines, which in turn activate yet more white blood cells. CRS is also an adverse effect of some monoclonal antibody medications, as well as adoptive T-cell therapies. When occurring as a result of a medication, it is also known as an infusion reaction.

The term cytokine storm is often used interchangeably with CRS but, despite the fact that they have similar clinical phenotype, their characteristics are different. When occurring as a result of a therapy, CRS symptoms may be delayed until days or weeks after treatment. Immediate-onset CRS is a cytokine storm, although severe cases of CRS have also been called cytokine storm

Symptoms include fever, fatigue, loss of appetite, muscle and joint pain, nausea, vomiting, diarrhea, rashes, fast breathing, rapid heartbeat, low blood pressure, seizures, headache, confusion, delirium, hallucinations, tremor, and loss of coordination.

Laboratory tests and clinical monitoring show low blood oxygen, widened pulse pressure, increased cardiac output (early), potentially diminished cardiac output (late), high levels of nitrogen compounds in the blood, elevated D-dimer, elevated transaminases, factor I deficiency and excessive bleeding, higher-than-normal level of bilirubin.

CRS occurs when large numbers of white blood cells, including B cells, T cells, natural killer cells, macrophages, dendritic cells, and monocytes are activated and release inflammatory cytokines, which activate more white blood cells in a positive feedback loop of pathogenic inflammation. Immune cells are activated by stressed or infected cells through receptor-ligand interactions.

This can occur when the immune system is fighting pathogens, as cytokines produced by immune cells recruit more effector immune cells such as T-cells and inflammatory monocytes (which differentiate into macrophages) to the site of inflammation or infection. In addition, pro-inflammatory cytokines binding their cognate receptor on immune cells results in activation and stimulation of further cytokine production. This process, when dysregulated, can be life-threatening due to systemic hyper-inflammation, hypotensive shock, and multi-organ failure.

Adoptive cell transfer of autologous T-cells modified with chimeric antigen receptors (CAR-T cell therapy) also causes CRS. Serum samples of patients with CAR-T associated CRS have elevated levels of IL-6, IFN-γ, IL-8 (CXCL8), IL-10,

GM-CSF, MIP-1α/β, MCP-1 (CCL2), CXCL9, and CXCL10 (IP-10). The most predictive biomarkers 36h after CAR-T infusion of CRS are a fever ≥38.9 °C (102 °F) and elevated levels of MCP-1 in serum. Many of the cytokines elevated in CRS are not produced by CAR-T cells, but by myeloid cells that are pathogenically licensed through T-cell-mediated activating mechanisms. For example, in vitro co-culture experiments have demonstrated IL-6, MCP-1, and MIP-1 are not produced by CAR-T cells, but rather by inflammatory myeloid lineage cells. In vivo models have demonstrated NSG (NOD/SCID/γ-chain deficient mice) with defects of both lymphocyte and myeloid lineage compartments do not develop CRS after CAR-T cell infusion.

In addition to adoptive T-cell therapies, severe CRS or cytokine reactions can occur in a number of infectious and non-infectious diseases including graft-versus-host disease (GVHD), coronavirus disease 2019 (COVID-19), acute respiratory distress syndrome (ARDS), sepsis, Ebola, avian influenza, smallpox, and systemic inflammatory response syndrome (SIRS).

Although severe acute respiratory syndrome coronavirus 2 (SARS-CoV-2) is sufficiently cleared by the early acute phase anti-viral response in most individuals, some progress to a hyperinflammatory condition, often with life-threatening pulmonary involvement. This systemic hyperinflammation results in inflammatory lymphocytic and monocytic infiltration of the lung and the heart, causing ARDS and cardiac failure. Patients with fulminant COVID-19 and ARDS have classical serum biomarkers of CRS including elevated CRP, LDH, IL-6, and ferritin.

Hemophagocytic lymphohistiocytosis and Epstein-Barr virus-related hemophagocytic lymphohistiocytosis are caused by extreme elevations in cytokines and can be regarded as one form of severe cytokine release syndrome.

Cytokine reaction syndrome may also be induced by certain medications, such as the CD20 antibody rituximab and the CD19 CAR T cell tisagenlecleucel. The experimental drug TGN1412 - also known as theralizumab - caused extremely serious symptoms when given to six participants in a Phase I trial. A controlled and limited CRS is triggered by active fever therapy with mixed bacterial vaccines (MBV) according to Coley; it is used for oncological and certain chronic diseases. CRS has also arisen with biotherapeutics intended to suppress or activate the immune system through receptors on white blood cells. Muromonab-CD3, an anti-CD3 monoclonal antibody intended to suppress the immune system to prevent rejection of organ transplants; alemtuzumab, which is anti-CD52 and used to treat blood cancers as well as multiple sclerosis and in organ transplants; and rituximab, which is anti-CD20 and used to treat blood cancers and auto-immune disorders, all cause CRS.

CRS needs to be distinguished from symptoms of the disease itself and, in the case of drugs, from other adverse effects—for example tumor lysis syndrome requires different interventions. As of 2015, differential diagnoses depended on the judgement of doctor as there were no objective tests.

CRS is a form of systemic inflammatory response syndrome and is an adverse effect of some drugs.

Appendix 12.3. Cytokine storm

From Wikipedia (https://en.wikipedia.org/wiki/Cytokine_storm)

A cytokine storm, also called hypercytokinemia, is a physiological reaction in humans and other animals in which the innate immune system causes an uncontrolled and excessive release of pro-inflammatory signaling molecules called cytokines. Normally, cytokines are part of the body's immune response to infection, but their sudden release in large quantities can cause multisystem organ failure and death.

Cytokine storms can be caused by a number of infectious and non-infectious etiologies, especially viral respiratory infections such as H1N1 influenza, H5N1 influenza, SARS-CoV-1, and SARS-CoV-2, Influenza B, Parainfluenza virus, and Ebola. Other causative agents include the Epstein-Barr virus, cytomegalovirus, group A streptococcus, and non-infectious conditions such as graft-versus-host disease. The viruses can invade lung epithelial cells and alveolar macrophages to produce viral nucleic acid, which stimulates the infected cells to release cytokines and chemokines, activating macrophages, dendritic cells, and others.

Cytokine storm syndrome is a diverse set of conditions that can result in a cytokine storm. Cytokine storm syndromes include familial hemophagocytic lymphohistiocytosis, Epstein-Barr virus–associated hemophagocytic lymphohistiocytosis, systemic or non-systemic juvenile idiopathic arthritis–

associated macrophage activation syndrome, NLRC4 macrophage activation syndrome, cytokine release syndrome and sepsis.

Cytokine storms versus cytokine release syndrome

The term "cytokine storm" is often loosely used interchangeably with cytokine release syndrome (CRS) but is more precisely a differentiable syndrome that may represent a severe episode of cytokine release syndrome or a component of another disease entity, such as macrophage activation syndrome. When occurring as a result of a therapy, CRS symptoms may be delayed until days or weeks after treatment. Immediate-onset (fulminant) CRS appears to be a cytokine storm.

Appendix 12.4. Hemophagocytic lymphohistiocytosis

Hemophagocytic lymphohistiocytosis (HLH), also known as haemophagocytic lymphohistiocytosis (British spelling), and hemophagocytic or haemophagocytic syndrome, is an uncommon hematologic disorder seen more often in children than in adults. It is a life-threatening disease of severe hyperinflammation caused by uncontrolled proliferation of activated lymphocytes and macrophages, characterised by proliferation of morphologically benign lymphocytes and macrophages that secrete high amounts of inflammatory cytokines. It is classified as one of the cytokine storm syndromes. There are inherited and non-inherited (acquired) causes of hemophagocytic lymphohistiocytosis.

Appendix 12.5. Macrophage activation syndrome

From Wikipedia (https://en.wikipedia.org/wiki/Macrophage_activation_syndrome)

Macrophage activation syndrome is a severe, potentially life-threatening, complication of several chronic rheumatic diseases of childhood. It occurs most commonly with systemic-onset juvenile idiopathic arthritis (SoJIA). In addition, MAS has been described in association with systemic lupus erythematosus (SLE), Kawasaki disease, and adult-onset Still's disease. It is thought to be closely related and pathophysiologically very similar to reactive (secondary) hemophagocytic lymphohistiocytosis (HLH). The incidence of MAS is unknown as there is a wide spectrum of clinical manifestations, and episodes may remain unrecognized.

The hallmark clinical and laboratory features include high fever, hepatosplenomegaly, lymphadenopathy, pancytopenia, liver dysfunction, disseminated intravascular coagulation, hypofibrinogenemia, hyperferritinemia, and hypertriglyceridemia. Despite marked systemic inflammation, the erythrocyte sedimentation rate (ESR) is paradoxically depressed, caused by low fibrinogen levels. The low ESR helps to distinguish the disorder from a flare of the underlying rheumatic disorder, in which case the ESR is usually elevated. A bone marrow biopsy or aspirate usually shows hemophagocytosis.

In many cases a trigger is identified, often a viral infection, or a medication. There is uncontrolled activation and proliferation of macrophages, and T lymphocytes, with a marked increase in circulating cytokines, such as IFN-gamma, and GM-CSF. The underlying causative event is unclear, and is the subject of ongoing research. In many cases of MAS, a decreased natural killer cell (NK-cell) function is found.

A febrile patient with known or suspected sJia must be considered for macrophage activation if:

Ferritin >684 ng/ml

and any 2 of the following:

Hemoglobin <90g/L (in infants <4 weeks: <100g/L)

Platelets <100 x 109/L

Neutrophils <1.0 x 109/L

Fasting triglycerides ≥3.0 mmol/L (i.e., ≥ 265 mg/dl)

Fibrinogen ≤1.5 g/L[3]

In addition, other specific markers of macrophage activation (e.g. soluble CD163), and lymphocyte activation (e.g. soluble IL-2 receptor) can be helpful. NK cell function analysis may show depressed NK function, or, flow cytometry may show a depressed NK cell population.

The best treatment for MAS has not been firmly established. Most commonly used treatments include high-dose glucocorticsteroids, and cyclosporine. In refractory cases treatment regimens are used similar to that in HLH.

Anakinra may also be effective.

Appendix 12.6. Abdominal compartment syndrome

This syndrome occurs when tissue fluid within the peritoneal and retroperitoneal space (either edema, retroperitoneal blood or free fluid in the abdomen) accumulates in such large volumes that the abdominal wall compliance threshold is crossed and the abdomen can no longer stretch. Once the abdominal wall can no longer expand, any further fluid leaking into the tissue results in fairly rapid rises in the pressure within the closed space. Initially this increase in pressure does not cause organ failure but does prevent organs from working properly – this is called intra-abdominal hypertension and is defined as a pressure over 12 mmHg in adults. ACS is defined by a sustained IAP (intra-abdominal pressure) above 20 mmHg with new-onset or progressive organ failure. Severe organ dysfunction syndrome: These pressure measurements are relative. Small children get into trouble and develop compartment syndromes at much lower pressures while young previously healthy athletic individuals may tolerate an abdominal pressure of 20 mmHg very well. The underlying cause of the disease process is capillary permeability caused by the systemic inflammatory response syndrome (SIRS) that occurs in every critically ill patient. SIRS leads to leakage of fluid out of the capillary beds into the interstitial space in the entire body with a profound amount of this fluid leaking into the gut wall, mesentery and retroperitoneal tissue.

Appendix 12.7. Capillary leak syndrome

Capillary leak syndrome is characterized by the escape of blood plasma through capillary walls, from the blood circulatory system to surrounding tissues, muscle compartments, organs or body cavities. It is a phenomenon most commonly witnessed in sepsis, and less frequently in autoimmune diseases, **differentiation syndrome**, **engraftment syndrome**, hemophagocytic lymphohistiocytosis [see above], the **ovarian hyperstimulation syndrome**, viral hemorrhagic fevers, and snakebite and ricin poisoning. Pharmaceuticals, including the chemotherapy medications gemcitabine and tagraxofusp, as well as certain interleukins and monoclonal antibodies, can also cause capillary leaks. These conditions and factors are sources of secondary capillary leak syndrome.

Appendix 12.8. Ovarian hyperstimulation syndrome

Ovarian hyperstimulation syndrome (OHSS) is a medical condition that can occur in some women who take fertility medication to stimulate egg growth, and in other women in very rare cases. Most cases are mild, but rarely the condition is severe and can lead to serious illness or death. Symptoms can be mild, moderate, or severe. Mild symptoms include abdominal bloating and feeling of fullness, nausea, diarrhea, and slight weight gain. Moderate symptoms include excessive weight gain (weight gain of greater than 2 pounds per day), increased abdominal girth, vomiting, diarrhea, darker urine, decreased urine output, excessive thirst, and skin and/or hair feeling dry (in addition to mild symptoms). Severe symptoms are fullness/bloating above the waist, shortness of breath, pleural effusion, urination significantly darker or has ceased, calf and chest pains, marked abdominal bloating or distention, and lower abdominal pains (in addition to mild and moderate symptoms).

The central feature of clinically significant OHSS is the development of vascular hyperpermeability and the resulting shift of fluids into the third space. As hCG causes the ovary to undergo extensive luteinization, large amounts of estrogens, progesterone, and local cytokines are released. It is almost certain that vascular endothelial growth factor (VEGF) is a key substance that induces vascular hyperpermeability, making local capillaries "leaky", leading to a shift of fluids from the intravascular system to the abdominal and pleural cavity. Supraphysiologic production of VEGF from many follicles under the prolonged effect of hCG appears to be the specific key process underlying OHSS. Thus, while the woman accumulates fluid in the third space, primarily in the form of ascites, she actually becomes hypovolemic and is at risk for respiratory, circulatory (such as arterial thromboembolism since blood is now thicker), and renal problems. Women who are pregnant sustain the ovarian luteinization process through the production of hCG.

Appendix 12.9. Engraftment syndrome

Engraftment syndrome (ES) is an early complication of hematopoietic stem cell transplantation (HSCT) that occurs around neutrophil engraftment time and is attributed to the sudden cytokine discharge associated with robust engraftment of transplanted cells. The secreted cytokines cause a clinical picture suggestive of an exaggerated inflammatory response. This complication has been described both in autologous and allogeneic transplantation.

The diagnostic clinical features include the presence of two or more of the following symptoms usually 96 hours before neutrophil engraftment time: 1. fever of unknown origin (38.0-38.5 °C) with no detectable infectious agent or other cause, 2. erythematous skin rash not related to drug reactions or viral infection (usually covering >25% of the body surface), 3. weight gain of 2.5-5% (above baseline of admission) and albumin drop to 90% of pretransplant levels, and 4. pulmonary symptoms with dyspnea, hypoxia and pulmonary infiltrates on a chest X-ray (excluding infection, thromboembolism, pulmonary hemorrhage, fluid overload, or cardiac causes). Though hepatic dysfunction, renal insufficiency and transient encephalopathy have been described in adults, they have not been reported as common findings in pediatric practice.

Risk Factors include;1. High cell doses infused on day 0, 2. Prompt increase in white blood cell (WBC) counts, 3. Autologous peripheral blood as stem cell source, and 4. Autoimmune disease as an underlying condition.

Differential diagnosis and early recognition are particularly important since corticosteroids have a critical role in the reversal of symptoms and management of the condition.

The prognosis is usually good with early corticosteroid use, and complete resolution is seen in 1-5 days in >80% of cases. Otherwise, this complication occasionally may lead to increased morbidity and mortality if not managed appropriately and timely. ES is associated with increased length of hospitalization. It may be problematic since it can resemble cutaneous acute graft-versus-host disease (aGvHD) or be complicated by capillary leak syndrome and noncardiogenic pulmonary edema. Rarely, ES can mimic aGvHD by affecting the liver and gastrointestinal tract. It has been shown that patients who develop ES receive empirical antifungal therapy more frequently than patients who do not, most likely due to persistent fever. Patients undergoing autologous HSCT for multiple sclerosis who develop ES may experience transient worsening of neurological symptoms. In pediatric patients, ES is also associated with increased transfusion requirements, need for parenteral nutrition and

increased risk of critical care requirement
Corticosteroids also have a role in the prevention of ES.

Appendix 12.10. Differentiation syndrome

Differentiation syndrome, formerly known as Retinoic acid syndrome (RAS), is a potentially life-threatening complication observed in people with acute promyelocytic leukemia (APML) and first thought to be specifically associated with all-trans retinoic acid (ATRA) (also known as tretinoin) treatment. Subsequently, so-called RAS was recognized in APML patients who had been treated with another highly efficacious drug, arsenic trioxide, and yet did not appear in patients treated with tretinoin for other disorders. These facts and others support the notion that RAS depends on the presence of the malignant promyelocytes. This has led to the growing deprecation of the term 'retinoic acid syndrome' and to an increasing use of the term differentiation syndrome to signify this APML treatment complication.

Appendix 12.11. Multiple organ dysfunction syndrome

Multiple dysfunction syndrome is the presence of altered organ function in acutely ill patients such that homeostasis cannot be maintained without intervention. It usually involves two or more organ systems. It calls for an immediate intervention. Although Irwin and Rippe cautioned in 2005 that the use of "multiple organ failure" or "multisystem organ failure" should be avoided, both Harrison's (2015) and Cecil's (2012) medical textbooks still use the terms "multi-organ failure" and "multiple organ failure" in several chapters and do not use "multiple organ dysfunction syndrome" at all.

The condition results
from infection, injury (accident, surgery), hypoperfusion and hypermetabolism. The primary cause triggers an uncontrolled inflammatory response.

Sepsis is the most common cause of multiple organ dysfunction syndrome and may result in septic shock. In the absence of infection, a sepsis-like disorder is termed systemic inflammatory response syndrome (SIRS). Both SIRS and sepsis could ultimately progress to multiple organ dysfunction syndrome. However, in one-third of the patients no primary focus can be found. Multiple organ dysfunction syndrome is well established as the final stage of a continuum: SIRS + infection → sepsis → severe sepsis → Multiple organ dysfunction syndrome.

At present, there is no drug or device that can reverse organ failure that has been judged by the health care team to be medically and/or surgically irreversible (organ function can recover, at least to a degree, in patients whose organs are very dysfunctional, where the patient has not died, and some organs, like the liver or the skin, can regenerate better than others),- with the possible exception of single or multiple organ transplants or the use of artificial organs or organ parts, in certain candidates in specific situations. Therapy, therefore, is usually mostly limited to supportive care, i.e. safeguarding hemodynamics, and respiration. Maintaining adequate tissue oxygenation is a principal target. Starting enteral nutrition within 36 hours of admission to an intensive care unit has reduced infectious complications.

Mortality, though it has lessened to a limited degree, at least in high income countries with timely access to initial and tertiary care, varies where the chance of survival is diminished as the number of organs involved increases. Mortality in MODS from septic shock (which itself has a mortality of 25-50%), and from multiple traumas, especially if not rapidly treated, appear to be especially severe. If more than one organ system is affected, the mortality rate is higher, and this is especially the case when five or more systems or organs are affected. Old age is a risk factor in and of itself, and immunocompromised patients, such as with cancer or HIV/AIDS or recipients of organ transplants, are at risk. Earlier and aggressive treatment, the use of experimental treatments, or at least modern tools such as ventilators, ECMO, dialysis, bypass, and transplantation, especially at a trauma center, may improve outcomes in certain cases, but this depends in part on speedy and affordable access to high-quality care. Measurements of lactate, cytokines, albumin and other proteins, urea, blood oxygen and carbon dioxide levels, insulin, and blood sugar, adequate hydration, constant monitoring of vital signs, good communication within and between facilities and staff, and adequate staffing, training, and charting are important in MODS.

Appendix 12.12. Graft-versus-host disease

Graft-versus-host disease (GvHD) is a syndrome, characterized by inflammation in different organs, most commonly associated with hematopoietic stem cell transplants. T cells of the donor's immune system which remain within the donated tissue (the graft) recognize the recipient (the host) as foreign (non-self). The T cells present within the transplanted tissue then attack the recipient's body's cells, which leads to GvHD. This should not be confused with a transplant rejection, which occurs when the immune system of the transplant recipient rejects the transplanted tissue. GvHD occurs when the donor's immune system's T cells reject the recipient. GvHD can also occur after a blood transfusion if the blood products used have not been irradiated or treated with an approved pathogen reduction system).

Appendix 12.13. Immune reconstitution inflammatory syndrome (IRIS)

From Wikipedia
(https://en.wikipedia.org/wiki/Immune_reconstitution_inflammatory_syndrome)

Immune reconstitution inflammatory syndrome (IRIS) is a condition seen in some cases of AIDS or immunosuppression, in which the immune system begins to recover, but then responds to a previously acquired opportunistic infection with an overwhelming inflammatory response that paradoxically makes the symptoms of infection worse.

HIV infection and immunosuppression

The suppression of CD4 T cells by HIV (or by immunosuppressive drugs) causes a decrease in the body's normal response to certain infections. Not only does this make it more difficult to fight the infection, it may mean that a level of infection that would normally produce symptoms is instead undetected (subclinical infection). If the CD4 count rapidly increases (due to effective treatment of HIV, or removal of other causes of immunosuppression), a sudden increase in the inflammatory response produces nonspecific symptoms such as fever, and in some cases a worsening of damage to the infected tissue.

There are two common IRIS scenarios. The first is the “unmasking” of an occult opportunistic infection. The second is the “paradoxical” symptomatic relapse of a prior infection despite microbiologic treatment success. Often in paradoxical IRIS, microbiologic cultures are sterile. In either scenario, there is hypothesized reconstitution of antigen-specific T cell-mediated immunity with activation of the immune system following HIV therapy against persisting antigen, whether present as intact organisms, dead organisms, or debris.

Though these symptoms can be dangerous, they also indicate that the body may now have a better chance to defeat the infection. The best treatment for this condition is unknown. In paradoxical IRIS reactions, the events will usually spontaneously get better with time without any additional therapy. In unmasking IRIS, the most common treatment is to administer antibiotic or antiviral drugs against the infectious organism. In some severe cases, anti-inflammatory medications, such as corticosteroids are needed to suppress inflammation until the infection has been eliminated.

Infections most commonly associated with IRIS include *Mycobacterium tuberculosis* and cryptococcal meningitis. Persons living with AIDS are more at risk for IRIS if they are starting HAART for the first time, or if they have recently been treated for an opportunistic infection (OI). It is generally advised that when patients have a low initial CD4 T cell count and opportunistic infection at the time of their HIV diagnosis, they receive treatment to control the opportunistic infections before HAART is initiated approximately two weeks later. This is true for most OIs, except for OIs involving the central nervous system.

In cryptococcal meningitis

IRIS is particularly problematic in cryptococcal meningitis as IRIS is fairly common and can be fatal.

IRIS has been described in immunocompetent hosts who have meningitis caused by *Cryptococcus gattii* and *Cryptococcus neoformans var. grubii,* environmental fungi which often affect immunocompetent hosts. Several weeks or even months into appropriate treatment, there is a sudden onset deterioration with worsening meningitis symptoms and progression or development of new neurological symptoms.

Magnetic resonance imaging shows increase in the size of brain lesions, and CSF abnormalities (white cell count, protein, glucose) increase. CSF culture is typically sterile, and there is no increase in CSF cryptococcal antigen titer.

The increasing inflammation can cause brain injury or be fatal.

The general mechanism behind IRIS is increased inflammation as the recovering immune system recognizes the antigens of the fungus as immunosuppression is reversed. Cryptococcal IRIS has three phases:

- before HAART, with a paucity of cerebrospinal fluid (CSF) inflammation and defects in antigen clearance;
- during initial HAART immune recovery, with pro-inflammatory signaling by antigen-presenting cells without an effector response; and
- at IRIS, a cytokine storm with a predominant type-1 helper T cell interferon-gamma response.

Three clinical predictors of cryptococcal-related paradoxical IRIS risk include:

- lack of initial CSF pleocytosis (i.e. low CSF white blood cell count);
- elevated C-reactive protein;
- failure to sterilize the CSF before immune recovery.

IRIS may be the cause of paradoxically worse outcomes for cryptococcal meningitis in immunocompetent compared with immunocompromised hosts, in whom *Cryptococcus neoformans* is the usual pathogen. Treatment with systemic corticosteroids during IRIS may be beneficial in preventing death or progressive neurological deterioration. Corticosteroids given to persons with anti-fungal treatment failure / cryptococcal relapse (in whom CSF cultures are not sterile) can be a fatal iatrogenic error.

11. GLOSSARY

Abbreviations used (other than those explained in Table1, Table 2 and in the FDA-derived text). This list includes abbreviations used in other books in the series Medicine 2020 and the series Modern Medicine 2021.

AC, adriamycin and cyclophosphamide (combination chemotherapy)

ACE, angiotensin-converting-enzyme

ADC, antibody-drug conjugate

ADCC, antibody-dependent cellular cytotoxicity

ADCC, antibody directed enzyme prodrug therapy

AGEP, acute generalized exanthematous pustulosis

AI, aromatase inhibitor

ALK, anaplastic lymphoma kinase

ALL, acute lymphoblastic leukemia

ALT, alanine aminotransferase

AML, acute myeloid leukemia

aPTT, activated partial thromboplastin time

ARR, administration-related reaction

AS, adverse reaction

AS, ankylosing spondylitis

ASCT, autologous stem cell transplant

AST, aspartate aminotransferase

ATA, anti-therapeutic antibody

ATM, ataxia telangiectasia mutated (gene)

AUC, Area Under the Concentration – time curve

AUC (0-inf): AUC curve to infinite time. As we cannot get the assays to go to infinity, we have to extrapolate to infinity. This can be calculated from the AUC(0-t) by the addition of a constant (Clast/λz), where Clast is the last observed quantifiable concentration and λz is the terminal phase rate constant.

BCG, Bacille Calmain-Guerin

BCMA, B cell maturation antigen

BCR-ABL, breakpoint cluster region/Abelson

BCRP, breast cancer resistance protein

b DMARD, biologic disease-modifying anti-rheumatic drug

BRACA1, breast cancer susceptibility gene 1

BTK, Bruton's tyrosine kinase

CAT, cyclophosphamide, adriamycin and taxane (combination chemotherapy)

CDC, complement-dependent cytotoxicity

CDK, cyclin-dependent kinase

C-G, Cockoft-Gault (formula)

cHL, classical Hodgkin Lymphoma

CINV, chemotherapy-induced nausea and vomiting

CIS, carcinoma in situ

CLL, chronic lymphocytic leukemia

Clcr, creatinine clearance rate

CMF, cyclophosphamide, methotrexate, and fluorouracil (combination chemotherapy

CML, chronic myelogenous leukemia (also known as chronic myeloid leukemia)

CPS, combine positive score

CR, complete remission

CRC, colorectal carcinoma

CRS, cytokine release syndrome

CS, cytokine storm

csDMARD, synthetic disease-modifying anti-rheumatic drug

CSF1R, colony-stimulating factor receptor 1

CT, computed tomography

CTCAE, Common Terminology Criteria for Adverse Events

CVVHD, continuous veno-venous hemodialysis

DBCL, diffuse B cell lymphoma

DCIS, ductal carcinoma in situ

DFS, disease-free survival

dMMR, deficient mismatch repair

DLBCL, diffuse large B cell lymphoma

DMSO, dimethyl sulfoxide

DPP4, dipeptidyl peptidase-4

DRESS, drug reaction with eosinophilia and systemic symptoms. DRESS syndrome is classified as one form of severe cutaneous adverse reactions (SCARs). In addition to DRESS, SCARs includes four other drug-induced skin reactions, the Stevens–Johnson syndrome (SJS); Toxic epidermal necrolysis (TEN), Stevens–Johnson/toxic epidermal necrolysis overlap syndrome (SJS/TEN)

EBC, early breast cancer

ECG or EKG, electrocardiogram

EFS, event-free durvival

EGF, epidermal growth factor

EGFR, epidermal growth factor receptor

EN, erythema nodosum

ER, estrogen receptor

ET, endocrine therapy

ErbB, derived from erythroblastic leukemia viral oncogene

FBG, fasting blood glucose

FEC, fluorouracil, epirubicin and cyclophosphamide (combination chemotherapy)

FGF, fibroblast growth factor

FGFR, fibroblast growth factor receptor

FISH, fluorescence in situ hybridization

FKBP12/mTOR, FK Binding Protein-12/mammalian target of rapamycin

Flt3, fms like tyrosine kinase 3

FPG, fasting plams glucose

FSH, follicle-stimulating hormone

FU, fluouracil

gBRCAm, BRCA mutated

GBS, Guillain-Barré Syndrome

G-CSF, granulocyte colony-stimulating factor

GD, gestational day

GI, gastro-intestinal

GIST, gastrointestinal stromal tumor

GFR, glomerular filtration rate

GMR, geometric mean ratio

GVHD, graft-versus-host disease

HBV, hepatitis B

HCC, hepatocellular carcinoma

HCV, hepatitis C

HER, human epidermal receptor

HER2, human epidermal growth factor receptor 2

HIV, human immune deficiency virus

HNSCC, head and neck squamous carcinoma

HR, hormone receptor

HRR, homologous recombination repair

HSCT, hematopoietic stem cell transplant

JAK, Janus kinase

KLIFS-3, kinase-ligand interaction fingerprint and structure residue-3

IAP, intra-abdominal pressure

IBC, inflammatory breast cancer

IC, immune cell

ICANS, immune effector cell–associated neurotoxicity syndrome

IFN, interferon

IL, interleukin

ILD, interstitial lung disease

ILN, interstitial lung disease

iNHL, indolent non-Hodgkin lymphoma

IRIS, immune reconstitution inflammatory syndrome

IRR, infusion-related reaction

ITAM, immunoreceptor tyrosine-based activation motif

ITP, idiopathic thrombocytopenic purpura

LBCL, large B cell lymphoma

LCIS, lobular carcinoma in situ

LFT, liver function test

LH, luteinizing hormone

LLN, lower limit of normal

LVEF, left ventricular ejection fraction

Mab, monoclonal antibody

MATE, multi-antimicrobial extrusion protein

MBC, metastatic breast cancer

MCC, Merkel cell carcinoma

mCRPC, metastatic castrate resistant prostate cancer

MEK, mitogen-activated protein kinase

MRI, magnetic resonance imaging

MSI-H, microsatellite instability – high

MUGA, multigated acquisition

NCI-CTC, National Cancer Institute – Clinical Toxicity Criteria

Nib, small i**n**h**ib**itory molecule

NMIBC, non-muscle invasive bladder cancer

NRH, nodular regenerative hyperplasia (of the liver)

NSCLC, non-small cell lung cancer

OHSS, ovarian hyperstimulation syndrome

OS, overall survival

PARP, poly(ADP-ribose) polymerase

PDGF, platelet-derived growth factor

PDGFR, platelet-derived growth factor receptor

PFS, progression-free survival

Ph+, Philadelphia chromosome positive

PI3K, phosphatidylinositol 3-kinase

PI3KA, phosphatidylinositol-4,5-bisphosphate 3-kinase catalytic subunit alpha

PJIA, polyarticular juvenile idiopathic arthritis in patients aged 2 years or older

PJP, *Pneumocystis jiroveci* pneumonia

PK, pharmacokinetic analysis

PKA, protein kinase A

PMBCL, primary mediastinal B cell lymphoma

PML, progressive multifocal leukoencephalopathy

PNET, progressive neuroendocrine tumor (of the pancreas)

PR, progesterone receptor

pRb, retinoblastoma protein

PsA, psoriatic arthritis

PsO, plaque psoriasis

RA, rheumatoid arthritis

RAF, rapidly accelerated fibrosarcoma

RCC, renal cell carcinoma

REMS, Risk Evaluation and Mitigation Strategy

RET, "rearranged during transfection"

ROCK, Rho-associated protein kinase

ROS, 'orphan' receptor tyrosine kinase

rb, retinoblastoma (gene or protein)

r/r, relapsed/refractory

scFv, single-chain Fv fragment

SCARS, severe cutaneous adverse reactions

SCLC, small cell lung cancer

SERD, selective estrogen receptor degrader

SEGA, subependymal giant cell astrocytoma

SIRS, systemic inflammatory response syndrome

SLAM, signalling lymphocytic activation molecule family (CD319)

SJS, Stevens–Johnson syndrome

SLL, small lymphocytic lymphoma

SYK, spleen tyrosine kinase

SWFI, sterile water for injection

TBC.tuberose sclerosid complex

TCH, docetaxel, carboplatin, and trastuzumab (combination chemotherapy)

TCR, T cell receptor

TEN, toxic epidermal necrolysis

TNBC, triple negative breast cancer

TMB- high, tunor mutational burden - high

TNF, tumor necrosis factor

TRK, tropomyosin receptor kinase

ts DMARD, targeted synthetic disease-modifying anti-rheumatic drug

Tyk, tyrosine-protein kinase

UGT1A1, uridine diphosphate-glucuronosyl transferase 1A1

ULN, upper limit of normal

VEGF, vascular endothelial growth factor

VEGFR, vascular endothelial growth factor receptor

Made in the USA
Las Vegas, NV
03 November 2026

57423534R00181